# Status of Vascular Surgery in Europe

# Status of Vascular Surgery in Europe

An ESVS/EDBVS Collaboration for the XVIII Annual Meeting of the European Society for Vascular Surgery held in Innsbruck, Austria between 17 and 19 September 2004


*Editors:*

**Christos D. Liapis**
Vascular Surgery Clinic
Athens University Medical School
Athens
GREECE

and

**William P. Paaske**
Department of Cardiothoracic and
Vascular Surgery
Aarhus University Hospital, Skejby Sygehus
DENMARK

*Co-editors:*

**Fabrizio Benedetti-Valentini**
2a Cattedra di Chirurgia Vascolare
School of Medicine
La Sapienza University
Rome
ITALY

**John Wolfe**
Regional Vascular Unit
St. Mary's Hospital
London
UK

**Michael Horrocks**
Department of Surgery
Royal United Hospital
Bath
UK

**Mauri Lepäntalo**
Department of Vascular Surgery
Helsinki University Central Hospital
Helsinki
FINLAND



ELSEVIER

**2004**

**ELSEVIER B.V.**
**Sara Burgerhartstraat 25**
**P.O. Box 211, 1000 AE**
**Amsterdam**
**The Netherlands**

ELSEVIER Inc.
525 B Street, Suite 1900
San Diego, CA 92101-4495
USA

ELSEVIER Ltd
The Boulevard, Langford Lane
Kidlington, Oxford OX5 1GB
UK

ELSEVIER Ltd
84 Theobalds Road
London WC1X 8RR
UK



First edition 2004

Library of Congress Cataloging in Publication Data
A catalog record is available from the Library of Congress.

British Library Cataloguing in Publication Data
A catalogue record is available from the British Library.

International Congress Series No. 1272
ISBN: 0-444-51762-6
ISSN: 0531-5131

∞ The paper used in this publication meets the requirements of ANSI/NISO Z39.48-1992 (Permanence of Paper).
Printed in The Netherlands.

**Acknowledgements**

Collecting data on conditions that prevail in Vascular Surgery across the European Continent is not a task that could have been achieved without the dedicated support and cooperation of the membership and "outside" collaborators, who were kind enough to put pen to paper and share their knowledge and experience for the good of all concerned.

The spectrum of participation on this compilation is wide; it comprises chapters by eminent colleagues either associated with the founding of the UEMS Division and Board of Vascular Surgery in the early 90s or other respected individuals associated, through their expertise, with issues concerning this specific area of interest. *No less important* are the country-specific reports kindly provided by the UEMS national representatives on the Division and Board of Vascular Surgery from Austria, Belgium, Czech Republic, Croatia, Cyprus, Denmark, Finland, France, Germany, Greece, Hungary, Ireland, Italy, Luxembourg, Netherlands, Norway, Portugal, Slovakia, Spain, Sweden, Switzerland, and UK. The valuable input of *all* members during council meeting discussions since early 2003, was instrumental in the realization of this project.

The endeavours and time taken off demanding surgical schedules, by all who so munificently contributed to the enhancement of this valuable reference book, are enormously appreciated. The efforts of the Administrator at the Athens Secretariat Mrs Vivienne Rose, in getting this project off the ground, are greatly valued.

We are also deeply grateful for the generous support of the ESVS Executive, past and present Presidents, the Secretary and all the Council Members, which resulted in the gracious decision to partially finance this project.

(On behalf of the UEMS Division and Board of Vascular Surgery)

Fabrizio Benedetti-Valentini, President of the Division
John H. N. Wolfe, President of the Board
Klaus Balzer, Vice President of the Board
Christos D. Liapis, Secretary General of the Division and Board

## COUNCIL OF THE DIVISION AND BOARD OF VASCULAR SURGERY 2003 AND 2004

### EXECUTIVE BOARD

Fabrizio Benedetti-Valentini (Italy)
**President, Division of Vascular Surgery**

John H.N. Wolfe (UK)
**President, European Board of Vascular Surgery**

Klaus Balzer (Germany)
**Vice President, European Board of Vascular Surgery**

Christos D. Liapis (Greece)
**Secretary/Treasurer, Division and European Board of Vascular Surgery**

## NATIONAL REPRESENTATIVES, ASSOCIATE MEMBERS AND SOCIETIES
(BY ORDER OF COUNTRY OR ASSOCIATION)

| | |
|---|---|
| AUSTRIA | Johann Strassegger<br>Reinold Perkmann<br>Josef Klocker |
| BELGIUM | J.O. Defraigne<br>Robert Verhelst<br>André Nevelsteen |
| CROATIA | Tomislav Šoša |
| CYPRUS | Nicos Angelides |
| CZECH REPUBLIC | Pavel Sebesta<br>Milos Adamec |
| DENMARK | Henrik Sillesen<br>Jes Sandermann<br>Franz von Jessen |
| FINLAND | Juha Salenius<br>Mikael Railo |
| FRANCE | Olivier Goëau-Brissonnière<br>Jean-Baptiste Ricco |
| GERMANY | H.H. Eckstein |
| GREECE | Elias Bastounis<br>Panagiotis Panoussis |
| HUNGARY | Csaba Dzsinich |
| IRELAND | Dermot Moore<br>Cathal Kelly |
| ITALY | Domenico Palombo<br>Piergiorgio Settembrini |
| LUXEMBOURG | Patrick Berg<br>Fernand Marxen |
| NETHERLANDS | Peter Kitslaar<br>J. Hajo van Bockel<br>Jan D. Blankensteijn |
| NORWAY | Hans O. Myhre<br>Anne Karin Lindahl<br>Tor Florenes |
| PORTUGAL | José Fernandes e Fernandes<br>José Daniel Menezes<br>Armando Mansilha |
| SLOVAKIA | Vladimir Sefranek |
| SPAIN | Marc Cairols<br>Jordi Maeso Lebrún |
| SWEDEN | Lars Norgren<br>David Bergqvist<br>Hakan Parsson<br>Eric Wahlberg |
| SWITZERLAND | Amadee Genton<br>Jon Largiadèr |
| TURKEY | A. Alaçayir |
| UK | Peter Lamont<br>Julian Scott |
| EAVST | Jean-Noel Albertini<br>Thomas Nyheim |
| EBS | Roger Greenhalgh<br>Patrick Rutten |
| ESVS | Michael Horrocks |
| ESCVS | Jean-Claude Schoevaerdts |
| IUA | Jill Belch |
| UEMS | Bernard Maillet |

## COUNCIL OF THE EUROPEAN SOCIETY FOR VASCULAR SURGERY 2004

| | | |
|---|---|---|
| Mauri Lepäntalo | President | Finland |
| Michael Horrocks | Secretary | UK |
| Jean Baptiste Ricco | Treasurer | France |
| Michael Jacobs | Chairman Editorial Board | The Netherlands |
| Christos Liapis | President Elect | Greece |
| Tomislav Šoša | Past President | Croatia |
| Henrik Sillesen | Secretary Elect | Denmark |
| Andreia Andreev | Councillor | Bulgaria |
| Steinar Aune | Councillor | Norway |
| Selcuk Baktiroglu | Councillor | Turkey |
| Jan Brunkwall | Councillor | Germany |
| Piergiorgio Cao | Councillor | Italy |
| Albert Flamme | Councillor | Belgium |
| Asterios Katsamouris | Councillor | Greece |
| Alexandre Kirienko | Councillor | Russia |
| Heinrich Magometschnigg | Councillor | Austria |
| Lajos Matyas | Councillor | Hungary |
| Luis Mendes Pedro | Councillor | Portugal |
| Manuel Miralles Hernandez | Councillor | Spain |
| Kevin O'Malley | Councillor | Ireland |
| Jan Rauwerda | Councillor | The Netherlands |
| Jes Sandermann | Councillor | Denmark |
| Torben Schroeder | Councillor | Editor, EJVES |
| Walerian Staszlewicz | Councillor | Poland |
| Alexi Svetlikov | Councillor | Junior Members Representative |
| Jesper Swedenborg | Councillor | Sweden |
| Jan Tomká | Councillor | Slovakia |
| Vladislav Treska | Councillor | Czech Republic |
| Pius Wigger | Councillor | Switzerland |

OUTGOING COUNCIL MEMBERS IN 2003

| | | |
|---|---|---|
| André Nevelsteen | Past President | Belgium |
| Gustav Fraedrich | Councillor | Austria |
| José Gonzalez Fajardo | Councillor | Spain |
| Mehmet Kurtoglu | Councillor | Turkey |
| Jan Marusiak | Councillor | Czech Republic |
| Dr Axel Marx | Councillor | Switzerland |

International Congress Series 1272 (2004) ix–xi

ELSEVIER

www.ics-elsevier.com

Preface

# VASCULAR SURGERY AND ITS RELATIONSHIP TO OTHER SURGICAL SPECIALTIES

The Management Council of the UEMS is inclined to consider the creation of a new Section wherever that specialty is recognised in greater than one-third of the member states of the European Union. The specialty must also fulfil three conditions as laid down by the Management Council in 1979:

a) Competent specialists must effectively carry on the specialty as such, essentially in exclusive practice.
b) The number of these specialties must be sufficient to establish from among their members, panels of examiners or recognition committees in that discipline.
c) The specialty must be practiced in institutions with sufficient training facilities available for them to be designated as training centres. Specialists of such seniority and experience as to be acknowledged as directors of training must control these institutions.

In addition, the Management Council considers a new specialist Section only if the parent Section agrees to the creation.

A request to establish proper status for vascular surgery began in my case in approximately 1980 when a group of us, who by 1982 became the Association of International Vascular Surgeons, commenced a ski group together. The AIVS continues to meet as a group of friends on an annual basis. During mountain discussions amongst vascular surgeons in the 1980s, the concept and need for a European Society for Vascular Surgery was visualised and created in the minds of several of us. It fell to me to convene the first European Society for Vascular Surgery at Charing Cross in May 1987 and I also had the pleasure of writing the first constitution. I became the Chairman of the Editorial Board because I regarded the Society's publication to be crucial in the development of the specialty.

In the early 1990s an important initiative occurred in the Val d'Aosta. While there, a group of surgeons called for a "European Council of Vascular Surgery." The problem was that this "Council" had no official status. Colleagues from the European Society for Vascular Surgery dispatched me to Brussels to investigate the official links. I was a little disappointed, but the only official organisation I could find was the European Union of Medical Specialties, the UEMS.


doi:10.1016/S0531-5131(04)01285-3

I was shocked to find that the UEMS had no vascular surgery; indeed, I believe it had not really heard of vascular surgery at the time! I was elected to the Section of Surgery and had a most welcoming reception at a meeting in Leuven in 1993. I was received from the pouring rain with Professor Hero van Urk, Secretary of the ESVS and my Austrian wife, Karin. We were made most welcome and this led to election on behalf of the United Kingdom as a member of the Section of Surgery on the retirement of my friend Georges Jantet. I was to serve as President of the Section from 1998-2002.

The restructuring of surgery commenced almost at once and I have to be blamed for the concept of the so-called "grapefruit structure" in which I saw the Section of Surgery as an envelope, which would be divided into Divisions such that each Division could have its own full European Board without asking the permission of the Management Council. We were encouraged to do this by the Management Council, and in 1996 with their full knowledge, the Division of Vascular Surgery was created as an "Associate Section." From that moment, the Division of Vascular Surgery has been invited to Management Council in May of each year, along with the Section of Surgery. The European Board of Vascular Surgery has been most effective and, indeed, has shown the way for other surgical specialties. It has been like a shining light.

Initially, vascular surgeons were delighted with the creation of the full Board and worked in a fairly autonomous way, meeting at the same time each year for the European Society for Vascular Surgery where they had a successful time. The Vascular Board has been an important part of the European Board of Surgery and shares the EBSQ office in London. This has been a cost-effective way of running the exam and assessing eligibility.

In 1998, following vascular surgery, coloproctology launched its European Board followed by trauma in 1999, general surgery in 2000, and endocrine surgery and surgical oncology more recently.

In 2003, an exciting link with the Section of Cardiothoracic Surgery has been achieved in that cardiothoracic surgeons have accepted that vascular surgery is established with its own Board, and thoracic surgeons can be trained either in association with cardiac surgeons or in association with more general surgeons. Accordingly, a single European Board of Thoracic Surgery is recommended with input from the 2 Sections, Cardiothoracic Surgery and Surgery. This has led to the concept of a more formal linkage with other sections of surgery, such as ophthalmology, neurosurgery, oro-maxillo-facial, orthopaedic, otorhino-laryngology, paediatric surgery, plastic surgery, urology and, possibly, gynaecology.

There is somewhat of a conflict of interest between the specialties who wish to be separate and somewhat autonomous and the European Union lobbying potential of the UEMS, which is much better achieved in larger groups. Thus, an aggregation of the surgical Sections in some sort of "federal" structure would be admirable from the point of view of lobbying politicians in the European Union. One of the shortcomings in Europe is the paucity of representation in health. The lobbying needs to be much more effective for each branch of surgery.

What of the Section of Surgery? Vascular, coloproctology, trauma, endocrine, general, and surgical oncology have already established their Boards, but perhaps vascular is the only one that would satisfy the UEMS requirements for the creation of a new Section. Accordingly, the Section of Surgery must examine this issue with a view to recommending the creation of a stand alone Section of Vascular Surgery, taking the European Board of Vascular Surgery with it. We envisage that coloproctology, trauma, endocrine, general and surgical oncology will come along behind in the future, but perhaps these subjects do not satisfy the Management Council criteria at the present time, whereas it is likely that vascular does.

Therefore, we come to the view that the Management Council could be confronted with a gradual increase in the number of surgical Sections. That may not be pleasing to the Management Council, but the payoff would be an aggregation of the existing, separate Sections with surgery and vascular surgery to form much more of a "federal" structure, a united grouping. There is considerable enthusiasm for this endpoint provided that it is a new structure with voluntary membership. Each of the Sections, and indeed the Divisions within the Section of Surgery, will have their own full specialist European Board of Surgery and so the present *European Board of Surgery* will no longer have a significant role to play. It could become the "federation" mentioned above. The benefit of this solution would be that, for example, the President and Secretary of each separate Section could voluntarily form a linkage with other surgical Sections within this newly created "*European Board of Surgery.*" The new European Board of Surgery would assemble these surgical groups and it would request that the Secretary-General of the Management Council would attend such a grouping, which could be highly influential in political lobbying. For this to occur it could produce a sensible new structure within the UEMS; in all probability, medicine, pathology and other aggregations could follow.

Once again then, vascular surgery is in the vanguard fighting the way. Vascular surgery has come a long way and is ready to stand alone, but does not wish to turn its back on the rest of surgery but remain part of the grand plan. If there is enthusiasm for this endpoint, it will be important that in my remaining time as President of the European Board of Surgery, I work on behalf of the Sections to create the linkages described for potential benefit.

Roger M. Greenhalgh
President, European Board of Surgery 2002–2006

# Contents

International Congress Series 1272 (2004) 1–3

www.ics-elsevier.com

# Introduction

William P. Paaske[a,*], Christos D. Liapis[b,1]

[a] *Department of Cardiothoracic and Vascular Surgery T, Aarhus University Hospital, Skejby Sygehus, DK-8200 Aarhus N, Denmark*

[b] *2nd Department of Propedeutic Surgery, "Laiko" General Hospital Vascular Laboratory, 16 Sevastoupoleos Street, 115 26 Athens, Greece*

*Keywords:* Vascular surgery; Speciality; Vascular surgeon

*Vascular surgery is the clinical and scientific discipline concerned with the diagnosis, treatment and prevention of diseases affecting arteries, veins, and lymphatics.*

This precise definition of our speciality is deceptively simple; it was formulated after long discussions between the national representatives of the scientific societies for vascular surgery in Europe coming together in the Aosta valley in 1990 [1] with the purpose of setting up a formal system for collaboration between vascular surgeons, and their professional organizations, within the European Economic Community, the forerunner of the present European Union (EU). At the time it became very clear, how many interests were at play to influence the future of vascular surgery—and how diverse they were [2]!

The definition includes the adjectives "clinical" and "scientific"—not a fortuitous conjunction when considered in the light of the spectacular advances for the basic vascular sciences, the diagnostics, and the treatment options within only a couple of generations. Vascular surgery has intense interactions with a long list of basic sciences as well as the other clinical specialities, but only the vascular surgeons enjoy the privilege of treating diseases in the vessels of the whole body—with the exception of those of the heart and those inside the brain, the domains of cardiac surgeons and neurosurgeons, respectively.

One of the difficulties in creating a coherent organizational system in Europe was that vascular surgery was not a distinct, officially recognised speciality in some countries. In this, as in so many other cases, the advancement of medicine is not reflected in the administrative and political support structures. However, professionals should never allow this factor to play a decisive role since the principles of the Hippocratic Oath must,

* Corresponding author. Tel.: +45-89-49-69-85; fax: +45-89-49-69-79.

*E-mail addresses:* william@paaske.org (W.P. Paaske), liapivas@panafonet.gr, liapis@hol.gr (C.D. Liapis).

*URLs:* http://www.paaske.org, http://www.uems-vasc.org.

[1] Tel.: +30-210-7456128; fax: +30-210-7456130.


doi:10.1016/j.ics.2004.05.024

at any time and under any circumstances, override immature or fossilized bureaucratic systems.

Vascular surgery has now acquired a well-established identity throughout the EU in spite of many difficulties [3]. Proper diagnosis and treatment are, of course, dependent on proper training of dedicated surgeons, and since vascular surgery is a speciality highly dependent on maximum aptitude, it is becoming clear to the public that it is totally unacceptable to practice vascular surgery without first class, well-structured training.

The local traditions for training, authorisation, practice, etc. vary greatly throughout Europe [4]; local needs have defined the structures and traditions that have developed over the course of time, so one of the truly amazing facts about vascular surgery on this continent has been that it was at all possible to create the framework for collaboration in such a relatively short time. After the initial formation of the Council of Vascular Surgeons in Aosta, it became possible for vascular surgery to become part of the European Union of Medical Specialists, UEMS. In practical terms, the Council was transformed into the Division of Vascular Surgery, and a European Board of Vascular Surgery was created [5]. Much work has gone into the creation of the European Board of Surgery Qualification in Vascular Surgery, a—so far—optional opportunity to document proficiency to practice independently as a vascular surgeon in the EU [6,7]. Further, national training centres have been identified throughout Europe and a simple system for recognition, on a European scale, of events for continuing medical education and continuing professional development has been developed; it is now in operation and is gaining widespread, even transatlantic, acceptance [8,9]. A system for collaboration between national and international vascular registries has been created [10,11], and it would be natural, in due course, to consider a format for the profession's input into the device (grafts, stents, etc.) evaluation and recognition systems.

The close collaboration between these organizations and the main scientific society, the European Society for Vascular Surgery, ESVS [12], has been excellent throughout the last decade, and it has been a priority to involve the young vascular surgeons in training in as many processes as possible; indeed, the European Association of Vascular Surgeons in training was created with heavy support by the ESVS as well as the European Board.

One of the great challenges of vascular surgery is to format the training of the vascular surgeon of the future [13,14]; whether we shall see a hybrid interventional radiologist/vascular surgeon/surgical engineer in the years to come is as yet unclear, but for the moment, the pressing point is to incorporate proper and sufficient training in endovascular procedures in the national curricula [15,16].

It is the purpose of the present book to present as a series of review contributions prepared by eminent colleagues, all of whom have been intimately involved with developing the system and contents for European collaboration within vascular surgery. The aims are not only to give historical accounts of the background for the present situation but also to describe possible future scenarios. The texts are not hyperdetailed descriptions of intra-organizational political intricacies of interest to a few politicos; on the contrary, we wish to present a clear and easily readable overview of European topics that influence the daily practice of our speciality and, indeed, the way we perceive ourselves as European professionals.

## References

[1] D. Palombo, P. Brustia (Eds.), La Chirurgia Vascolare nella Comunità Economica Europea, Consiglio Chirurghi Vascolari nella Comunità Economica Europea, Public Health Department of the Valle d'Aosta Regional Government, Aosta, 1992, pp. 1–59.
[2] P. Harris, Vascular surgery: the European perspective, Ann. R. Coll. 81 (1999) 241–244.
[3] W.P. Paaske, Training, continuing medical education and recertification in vascular and endovascular surgery in Europe, in: E.A. Bastounis (Ed.), Proceedings of the 13th Congress of the European Chapter of the International Union of Angiology. Milan: Monduzzi, 1999, pp. 91–97.
[4] J.H. Wolfe, Training-vive la difference, Eur. J. Vasc. Endovasc. Surg. 18 (1999) 1–3.
[5] J. Buth, et al., Harmonization of vascular surgical training in Europe. A task for the European Board of Vascular Surgery, Cardiovasc. Surg. 8 (2000) 98–103.
[6] C.D. Liapis, B. Nachbur, EBSQ-Vasc examinations—which way to the future? Eur. J. Vasc. Endovasc. Surg. 21 (2001) 473–474.
[7] D. Bergqvist, C. Liapis, J.N. Wolfe, The developing European Board Vascular Examination, Eur. J. Vasc. Endovasc. Surg. 27 (2003) 339–340.
[8] J.H. Wolfe, European CME, Eur. J. Vasc. Endovasc. Surg. 18 (1999) 277–279.
[9] W.P. Paaske, Continuing medical education in Europe—the impact of endovascular therapy, in: M. Cairols (Ed.), Syllabus de las III Monografías Vasculares. Cirugía Endovascular de los AAA, Ciutat Sanitària i Universitària de Bellvitge, Barcelona, 2000, pp. 21–24.
[10] W.P. Paaske, Vascular and endovascular surgical activity in Denmark, Finland, Norway, Sweden and Northern Ireland, Eur. J. Vasc. Endovasc. Surg. 17 (1999) 537–538.
[11] W.P. Paaske, EUROVASC Report 1998: vascular and endovascular surgical activity in Denmark, New Zealand, Northern Ireland, Slovakia, Sweden and St. Petersburg region, Russia, Eur. J. Vasc. Endovasc. Surg. 20 (2000) 233–234.
[12] S.G. Darke, The European Society for Vascular Surgery and Journal origins and early days, Eur. J. Vasc. Endovasc. Surg. 27 (2004) 349–356.
[13] G.M. Biasi, The way to a new endovascular specialist—a university-certified educational program: the master in endovascular techniques (MET), J. Endovasc. Ther. 10 (2003) 168–170.
[14] W.P. Paaske, The status of vascular surgery as an independent speciality in Europe: are the relationships with general and cardiothoracic surgery a problem, Vascular 12 (2004) 7–14.
[15] C.D. Liapis, W.P. Paaske, Training in vascular surgery in Europe—the impact of endovascular therapy, Eur. J. Vasc. Endovasc. Surg. 23 (2002) 1–2.
[16] W.P. Paaske, Vascular Surgery in Europe, in: P. Gloviczki (Ed.), Perspectives in Vascular Surgery and Endovascular Therapy, Vol. 15, 2002, pp. 1-11.

International Congress Series 1272 (2004) 4–14

www.ics-elsevier.com

# The UEMS—short history

Bernard Maillet*

*Union Européenne des médecins spécialistes, 20 Av. de la Couronne, B-1050 Brussels, Belgium*

*Keywords:* Vascular surgery

## 1. The UEMS—short history

On 20 July 1958, 1 year after the treaty of Rome was signed, the representatives delegated by the professional organisations of medical specialists of the six member countries of the European Community (EEC), created 1 year earlier, met in Brussels and founded the European Union of Medical Specialists (UEMS).

Thanks to the perceptiveness of its founders and through the impetus given by its first President, French gynaecologist Jacques Courtois, and the Belgian otolaryngologist Oscar Godin, Secretary General, the UEMS soon established contacts with authorities concerning the EEC (notably with J.P. de Crayencour), and defined the basic principles in the field of training of European medical specialists.

The UEMS immediately tackled the problem of quality, in an effort to obtain from the European Commission and the Member States a comparably high level of training for future medical specialists of the six Common Market countries.

This vision of the future resulted in the elaboration of common general criteria, applicable to all specialists wishing to move from one member country to another.

To realise this ambitious objective, in 1962 the UEMS created Specialist Sections for each of the main disciplines practised in the Member States.

This groups of experts, composed of representatives of the national associations of the specialty concerned, carried out a considerable amount of work with the idea of coordinating, then harmonising the specialist training and criteria for the recognition of medical specialists.

The UEMS and its Sections developed their actions in constant cooperation with the Standing Committee of European Doctors (CP), created in 1959 to bring together the whole of the organised medical profession of the Member States.

The first European directives concerning doctors, published only in 1975, were quite largely inspired by the proposals and the surveys presented by the UEMS and its Specialist Sections.

* Tel.: +32-2-649-5164; fax: +32-2-640-3730.
*E-mail address:* uems@skynet.be (B. Maillet).


doi:10.1016/j.ics.2004.04.080

In the meantime, the European Community was enlarged, first by the addition of the United Kingdom, Denmark and Ireland, which resulted in the need to make some improvements to the proposals of the doctors' directives that were ready to be published, then progressively by the six other countries presently also belonging to the European Union, as well as Norway and Switzerland.

These successive enlargements led to important changes in the different organs of the UEMS, its statutes and the composition of its various Specialist Sections, of which the number gradually increased to 38.

The enforcement of the doctors' directives was followed by the creation by the European Commission of an Advisory Committee on Medical Training (ACMT), a community institution ensuring the link between the European professional medical organisations, the universities and the national governments on the one hand, and the Commission on the other.

The UEMS immediately established close relations with this new body, which successively auditioned all the Specialist Sections of the UEMS from 1980 to 1981. Each Section had submitted a report explaining its conceptions and proposals regarding the evolution of the specialty.

This vast consultation, organised on the initiative of Dr. Pierre Pouyaud (F), who presided over the UEMS and the Advisory Committee at the time, and of Dr. Guy Des Marez (B), Secretary General of the UEMS, led to the publication of the second and third reports and recommendations of this committee concerning the training of medical specialists.

In the 1990s, the new managing team, composed of L.P. Harvey (GB), A. Kuttner (D), J.-C.I. Schaack (L), P. Fédi (F), C.C. Leibbrandt (NL) with R. Peiffer (B) as Secretary General, gave the UEMS a real lease of vitality by creating European "Boards," working groups of the Specialist Sections in order to guarantee optimal care in the field of the specialty concerned by bringing the training of medical specialists to the highest level possible. It elaborated European charters on the training of medical specialists and on the assurance of quality in specialist medicine, a key document on the autonomy of practice of medical specialists, highlighted the role and determining action of the Specialist Sections, basic cells of the UEMS, and progressively opened the UEMS to the countries of central and eastern Europe.

During the presidency of L.P. Harvey, the UEMS was involved in the framing of the fourth report of the ACMT in 1996, which still has to be implemented. In this period, more and more emphasis in the policy of the UEMS was placed on reaching consensus between the national member organisations and the direct advising of national professional regulatory bodies on quality issues. The Charters played a prominent role in this process.

A main focus of attention became Continuing Medical Education. The importance of harmonising policy of the many national and European associations working in this field was recognised. Under its new President, C. Twomey (IRE), this led to the institution of the European Accreditation Council for CME (EACCME) in January 2000.

This institution acts as a clearinghouse for accreditation in Europe. It tries to harmonize the CME and promotes the exchange of credits between the different Member States of the European Union and of the European Economic Area and also between the different Specialities. The EACCME, as integrated body of the UEMS, has an agreement with the American Medical Association for a mutual recognition of credits.

Dr. Bernard Maillet, Secretary General, adapted for C. Paul, UEMS Managing Director 1958–1996, November 2003.

### *1.1. European Union of Medical Specialists—UEMS*

The European Union of Medical Specialists (UEMS), with a current membership of 30 countries, is the representative organization of the National Associations of Medical Specialists in the European Union and its associated countries.

Its structure consists of a Management Council responsible for and working through 38 Specialist Sections, each with its own European Board, addressing training in the specialty and incorporating representatives from academia (Societies, Colleges and Universities).

An Executive Committee comprising the President, the Secretary General, the Liaison Officer, and the Treasurer, is responsible for the routine functioning of the organization. UEMS is representative of over 1 million specialists in all the different specialties. It also has strong links and relations with the other independent European medical organizations (e.g. CPME, PWG, UEMO) and the European medical and scientific societies.

The objective of UEMS is:

- To promote the highest level of patient care in the European Union;
- To defend the title of the "medical specialist" for the doctor who practices the highest quality of medical care in his/her specialist field of expertise;
- To uphold his/her professional and ethical status;
- To promote the harmonization of high quality training programs within the various specialties throughout the EU; and
- To endorse, encourage and facilitate CME/CPD.

Debates among the representatives of the National Medical Association meeting in plenary session of the UEMS Management Council, held on a 6-monthly basis, contribute to the development of policy positions. By its agreed documents, UEMS sets standards for high quality healthcare practice that are transmitted to the authorities and institutions of the EU and the national medical associations and encourages them to implement its recommendations.

UEMS has issued Charters and Position papers on:

- Postgraduate training for all specialties,
- Continuing Medical Education/Continuous Professional Development,
- Basel Declaration on Continuing Professional Development/quality improvement,
- Quality assurance and improvement,
- Visitation of training centers,
- Autonomy of specialist medical practice.

The UEMS has established the European Accreditation Council for CME (EACCME), which will facilitate the exchange of CME credits within the European Union, its associated countries and the United States. The latter is achieved by virtue of a common memorandum of agreement on mutual recognition reached between UEMS and the American Medical Association.

## 2. The policy of UEMS: introduction

UEMS proposals classification and training durations of the specialties registered in the Doctors Directive, 1996.

## 3. The definition of specialist medicine

The specialist doctor has chosen to confine his or her practice essentially to one field of medicine. This implies that he or she shall be, and must remain, at a high level of competence in the chosen specialty by mastering advances and innovations both in data and technique.

For some specialties, the expansion of knowledge threatens to lead to super-specialties concentrating on particular techniques or a narrowly defined field of pathology. National authorities often grant official recognition to these competencies, which should however remain within the broad framework of the main specialty. These developments should not lead to the proliferation of new specialties, as the number of specialties must be kept under control. The development of techniques should not prevent awareness that specialised medicine is a clinical discipline, which must remain focussed upon the patient.

Clearly, the practice of the general practitioner and the medical specialist are complementary. Their precise roles and arrangements for access to specialist treatment vary from country to country. Patients should be able to exercise freedom of choice and should have prompt access to the treatment that they need, within the framework of the healthcare system of the country in which they live. Good practice in both disciplines depends on effective cooperation and exchange of information.

## 4. Medical specialist training

### *4.1. The competent body*

At the national level, a national authority, which may be a combination of competent professional or university bodies, a national board or a national governmental authority receiving advice from professional organisations regulates the training of medical specialists. It sets standards in accordance with national rules and EU legislation, as well as considering UEMS recommendations for recognition of training programmes, of trainers and training centres, the quality assurance of training, and the qualifications of the medical specialist and manpower planning.

### *4.2. Guarantee of the quality of training*

Basic medical training should be authenticated before the course of specialist training is started. The specialist training must be comprehensive and should omit no important field.

In the training centres, adequate numbers of teaching staff and appropriate training facilities must be available and in balance with the number of trainees in order to guarantee high quality training.

Other methods of ensuring the quality of training could include, for example, the audit, logbook, the possibility of part of the training period being spent abroad, and a national examination at the end of the postgraduate training.

### 4.3. Particular aspects of specialist training

The content and practice of the specialty inevitably determine the training that is required. A system of centralised classification, which takes into account the real content of each specialty and its historical development, shows that training in medical and surgical specialties follows different pathways. However, apart from these main groupings, there exist organ-related disciplines, which include both medical and surgical elements.

This type of classification allows one to define a specialist training programme based on a common trunk, which broadens out to include the divisions and subdivisions of both medical and surgical specialties.

A regrouping of specialties, such as was proposed in 1983 by the Advisory Committee on Medical Training (ACMT), should be adopted in place of the classification in Articles 26 and 27 of the existing Medical Directives, which take no account of the relationship of the specialties to one another (see the annex in the UEMS Web site).

As regards the content of training and the relation of the Common Trunk to specialist training, the work of the UEMS Sections and European Boards has resulted in the publication, in October 1995, of a more accurate definition. At the same time, a precise definition of the content of training should not be taken to imply that specialist practice is a system of watertight compartments. Because disciplines frequently overlap, there must be scope for flexibility, although quite clearly no specialist should carry out a procedure for which he or she is not appropriately trained.

## 5. Continuing Medical Education (CME)

Continuing Medical Education is both a necessity and an obligation, which applies as much to the medical profession as to any other. The process of education lasts throughout the doctor's entire career, beginning with basic undergraduate training, carrying on through specialist training and extending for the remainder of professional life as Continuing Medical Education.

As it is a professional, ethical and moral obligation, CME must be managed and supervised independently by the profession.

Basically, it should be a voluntary responsibility for the individual specialist. The representative national, professional organisation is free to decide in a democratic manner to impose a formal obligation to fulfil CME requirements. However, someone who does not fulfil these requirements cannot lose his/her status as a doctor or specialist, but must understand that he/she may be disadvantaged in other ways.

The content of CME must take into account the specific situation of the specialist and, in consequence, is of an individual nature. Systems of assessment, which award credit points, are preferable to those that involve re-evaluation or recertification of the specialist's knowledge. Control of such systems must remain in the hands of organisations, which represent the medical community. These systems could also include models of self-assessment.

## 6. The organisation of specialist medicine

The activity of the specialist doctor may be practised not only in a hospital or private office, but also in health centres, companies, schools and other places where the specialist's presence is required. In all cases, the specialist doctor shall be free to treat his/her patient without external constraint.

The medical specialist must have adequate medical equipment at his/her disposal. The quality of care should remain independent from the system of remuneration, and compliance with professional quality standards should be assured by peer review assessment.

Contracts with and the remuneration of specialists, whether salaried or in private practice, must provide for the expenses involved for the doctor in meeting his/her CME obligations.

Independence from outside pressure in the choice of management and treatment of the individual patient remains the cornerstone of medical care. The physician and the patient must remain free to exercise a responsible choice.

## 7. Conclusions

The UEMS, through its 38 Specialist Sections, is in a position to know the conditions that each specialty needs to meet in order to reach harmonisation, both as regards the duration and the content of training and the practice of the various disciplines registered in the Medical Directives. It can inform each EU member state of these conditions, in all countries and all specialties.

Thanks to the European Boards, which are the working groups of the Specialist Sections and include delegates appointed by scientific and academic bodies as well as representatives of the Sections, the UEMS is in a position to define for each discipline the conditions that will ensure high quality training and the necessary criteria for a training centre. It can put forward suggestions regarding methods of assessment to which individuals can submit if they so desire.

The specified recommendations are available on the UEMS Web site: http://www.uems.net.

Dr. Bernard Maillet, Secretary General, November 2003, adapted from Dr. R. Peiffer past Secretary General (1990–1999).

## 8. European Accreditation Council for Continuing Medical Education (EACCME®)

### *8.1. History and political background*

Continuing Medical Education has been a major concern of the UEMS since 1993 when the Charter on Continuing Medical Education was published. Voluntary CME is enshrined in UEMS policy, but in several European countries steps are being taken on a national level towards mandatory CME, coupled with legal or professional recertification or re-licensing, financial incentives or coupled with contracts with insurance companies and hospitals.

This will lead towards an increasing need for a European exchange of CME credits, obtained by individual doctors outside their own country.

In 1999, the Management Council decided to establish the EACCME. The EACCME will facilitate access to quality CME for European doctors, contribute to the quality of CME in Europe and make exchange of CME credits in Europe possible.

Quality control of CME activities is a key element in this process. It was decided to effect this in a decentralized manner, using the expertise of existing European and national professional bodies active in this field. This is effected by the EACCME in everyday practice with one important addition. This is the political necessity to conform to the political authority of national, professional, regulatory bodies in the field of CME. These bodies are in charge of registration of doctors' CME/CPD in their country and, therefore, insist on being in charge of accreditation of CME and the awarding of credits. In some countries this is, or may be in the near future, linked to recertification.

### *8.2. Structure of the EACCME*

The UEMS is the political representative umbrella organisation for specialists in the European Union and associated countries. Its governing body is the Management Council, in which the national associations in each member country have voting rights.

The Management Council elects an executive committee consisting of the President, the Secretary General, the Treasurer and the Liaison Officer. The Executive Committee reports to the Management Council.

The Management Council decided in 1999 to establish the EACCME, with the EACCME becoming operational in January 2000.

### *8.3. The EACCME is governed by the management council of the UEMS*

A second body of the EACCME is the UEMS Advisory Council on CME, in which the national CME regulatory bodies are directly represented. For many countries, this representation is identical to the representation in the Management Council, but there are important exceptions such as Belgium, France, Germany, Ireland and the UK. For this reason, the Advisory Council is a key element in the EACCME. In the Advisory Council, the EACCME can also accommodate relevant, professional bodies.

## 9. The daily proceedings of the EACCME are managed by the Executive Committee of the UEMS and its Brussels secretariat

Right from the start of the EACCME, it was clear that the national, professional, regulatory bodies could approve a structure making CME credits in Europe exchangeable, but only with the condition that they will remain firmly in charge of events in their own country and that they would have a decisive vote in the governing body of the EACCME. This is a political reality. In some countries, it is based upon the expectation that within a few years mandatory recertification will occur and that CME credits will play an important role in this recertification.

The EACCME received its mandate from the national regulatory bodies, but with several distinct conditions:

- National authority should be maintained. The EACCME should not become a supranational body, but a link and clearinghouse among the national regulatory bodies.
- The final word concerning accreditation of each activity should thus rest with the national regulatory body in the country where the activity takes place.
- The Brussels administration should be as lean as possible.
- Quality assurance and determination of number of credits of separate CME activities should be decentralized. Here the EACCME should rely upon the expertise of

professional bodies in each specialty, such as the UEMS Sections/Boards and national/European professional societies, thus avoiding duplication of quality assurance proceedings.
- There should be no accreditation of commercially biased activities, Internet activities and, for the time being, each activity should be judged separately. This is in order that providers are not accredited for series of activities stretching over years.
- Administrative expenses of the EACCME should be borne by the providers of activities applying for European accreditation. The expenses should be limited, avoiding duplication in Brussels of work done already in the professional bodies.

Only within the framework of these conditions do the national regulatory bodies guarantee recognition of EACCME credits obtained by doctors in their country.

The EACCME has been working strictly within this mandate. This means that the procedure is as follows:

- The provider of a CME activity requests European accreditation of that event with the EACCME at its Brussels office. Full details concerning the activity should be provided together with the application. This will be judged against the UEMS quality criteria.
- The EACCME requests professional advice from a professional body, which may not be the provider itself. The professional body, such as the UEMS Sections/Boards and national/European professional societies, has the final say in the determination of the number of credits based upon the "credit-hour." Often the provider has already obtained such accreditation, which can be forwarded to the EACCME together with the formal application.
- The EACCME requests approval from the national regulatory body of the country where the activity takes place. When this is obtained, the EACCME grants European accreditation.

This procedure meets the political requirements of the national regulatory bodies. The added value of the EACCME is the link between the professional societies and others, who are the providers of CME and the national regulatory bodies. Any change to this procedure would need the consensus of the national regulatory bodies. Any deviation from this consensus would defeat the purpose of the EACCME and it would also mean loss of the agreement with the American Medical Association concerning mutual recognition of EACCME and AMA credits.

The added value for providers is that they will attract more participants from abroad and also from the USA. The long-term benefit is the link with the national regulatory bodies. These bodies are very keen to preserve their national authority in the awarding of credits to the doctors in their own countries. The EACCME offers an institution in which they participate and have authority. In this way, the profession facilitates exchange of CME credits in Europe in a similar way to postgraduate diplomas, which are mutually recognized on the basis of European law.

At present, in 2001, the exchange of CME credits is not urgent as systems of mandatory CME are not yet operational in Europe. At the moment, providers look at European accreditation mostly as an additional mark of quality and they are willing to reimburse the administrative expenses for this reason. The EACCME started with a charge of 100 euro, but in the future there will be a sliding scale depending upon the size and duration of the actual activity. One thousand euro will be the upper limit for activities with thousands of participants and a budget of many millions.

In the Management Council, there was a debate as to the right time to start operation of the EACCME. It was judged to be better to start in a period before possible mandatory European accreditation. This provided the opportunity to gain experience and commence on a smaller scale, to develop gradually without much extra infrastructure.

The ultimate goal is to develop a system that makes life easier for our colleagues and to provide them with recognised, quality CME with the guarantee that they can use the CME credits they obtain to meet their national requirements.

The system should be decentralized, using expertise in quality assessment available in the existing professional structures, and should be governed by the responsible, national professional bodies participating in the UEMS and the EACCME structure.

### 9.1. Purpose

The purpose of the EACCME® is the harmonization and improvement of the quality of specialist medical care in Europe. In the field of Continuing Medical Education, the EACCME® will serve this purpose by improving quality of CME and accessibility to CME for medical specialists in Europe.

The practical instrument to improve the quality of CME in Europe will be the facilitation of transfer of CME credits obtained by individual specialists in CME activities that meet common quality requirements:

- Between European countries
- Between different specialties
- In case of migration of a specialist within Europe
- Between the European credit system and comparable systems outside Europe.

In order to make exchange of credits possible, the "hour of CME" equating to one credit will be used for the international awarding of CME credits. National systems should also use this unit or establish a fixed exchange rate with this unit.

The EACCME® will not provide accreditation of CME activities directly, but it will connect the existing and emerging accreditation systems in Europe and act as a clearinghouse for accreditation of CME and credits in Europe. As such, it does not supersede the national authority on accreditation of CME, nor does it create another layer of bureaucracy.

The UEMS Advisory Council on CME will link the accrediting bodies participating in the EACCME®. Partners in the EACCME® will be the UEMS Specialist Sections/Boards. As institutions of the UEMS, they will provide the EACCME® with expert knowledge in their fields. The other partners in the Advisory Council will be the institutions, national and European, active in the field of CME.

The UEMS will be committed to further evolvement of the procedures of the EACCME® in cooperation with its partners, the national professional CME authorities and professional specialist organizations and societies in Europe.

### 9.2. Procedure

#### 9.2.1. Application for European accreditation

The provider of a CME activity requests European accreditation of that event with the EACCME® at its Brussels office. Full details concerning the activity should be provided together with the application. This will be judged against the UEMS quality criteria. If available, the provider submits proof of already obtained accreditation by national or European institutions.

The provider submits the intended number of hours and the language(s) of the CME activity, and by applying for European accreditation the provider commits itself to adhere to the quality requirements as stated by the EACCME® (document D 9908).

#### 9.2.2. Quality assurance of the CME activity

The EACCME® requests professional advice from a professional body, which may not be the provider itself. The professional body, such as the UEMS Sections/Boards and national/European professional societies, judges the number of credits based upon the "credit-hour". Often the provider has already obtained such accreditation, which can be forwarded to the EACCME® together with the formal application. The number of hours of credit should be included in this statement.

#### 9.2.3. National approval

The EACCME® requests approval from the national regulatory body of the country where the activity takes place. When this is obtained, the EACCME® grants European accreditation.

Where national accreditation institutions are not in a position to do so, specialty based accreditation institutions should be mediators between the CME provider and the EACCME®.

#### 9.2.4. Continuous accreditation of providers or accreditation of single activities

Initially, European accreditation is granted for single CME activities. Presently, the mandate of the EACCME® does not extend to continuous accreditation. Providers who offer CME activities on a regular basis have to apply for accreditation on a case-by-case basis.

#### 9.2.5. Confirmation of European accreditation

The EACCME® will confirm the European accreditation to the provider and authorize the CME provider to publish the accreditation by the EACCME® with the approved number of hours of credit in brochures, advertisements and in the programme of the CME activity. For this purpose, the standard EACCME® statement must be used in printed material concerning CME activities, adapted to continuous accreditation or accreditation for single CME activities:

> The ⟨name of institution⟩ (or) ⟨title of the CME activity⟩ is accredited by the European Accreditation Council for Continuing Medical Education (EACCME) to provide the following CME activity for medical specialists. The EACCME is an institution of the

European Union of Medical Specialists (UEMS), http://www.uems.net.

The ⟨title of the CME activity⟩ is designated for a maximum of (or "for up to") ⟨number of hours⟩ hours of European external CME credits. Each medical specialist should claim only those hours of credit that he/she actually spent in the educational activity.

EACCME credits are recognized by the American Medical Association toward the Physician's Recognition Award (PRA). To convert EACCME credit to AMA PRA category 1 credit, contact the AMA.

*9.2.6. Proof of attendance*

The upper statement together with the number of granted "hours of CME credit" should be printed in the proof of attendance or diploma that the CME provider distributes to the participating medical specialists. They are themselves responsible for handling and preserving these documents and should utilise these documents when requested by local recognition authorities.

*9.2.7. Quality requirements for European accreditation*

For European accreditation, the CME provider must comply with the requirements of the national CME authority in its home country.

By application for accreditation by the EACCME®, the CME provider certifies that it complies with the basic criteria for the quality of CME as defined by the EACCME® (document D 9908).

*9.2.8. Administrative expenses for EACCME®*

The administrative expenses of the EACCME® will be met by contributions by the CME providers obtaining European accreditation. As the EACCME® will utilise the accreditation by its partners and will not supersede existing systems, the administrative expenses have to remain modest. The contribution fees for the administrative expenses of the EACCME® are determined by a sliding scale based on the number of participants to the event.

*9.2.9. Registration by the EACCME®*

The EACCME® will keep a register of these CME activities with EACCME® accreditation and will supply the relevant information to CME authorities when requested.

Dr. Bernard Maillet, Secretary General, adapted from Dr. Cees Leibbrandt, past Secretary General (1999–2002) update November 2003. http://www.uems.net.

International Congress Series 1272 (2004) 15–20

ELSEVIER

www.ics-elsevier.com

# The beginning: the Aosta initiative—the Council of Vascular Surgeons in the EEC/EU

Domenico Palombo*
With the collaboration of Dr. Simone Mambrini

*Vascular Surgery Unit, Department of Cardiothoracic and Vascular Surgery, S. Martino University Hospital, Largo Rosanna Benzi, 10 Genova, Italy*

**Abstract.** The nineties began in an atmosphere of ardent socio-economic, political and cultural innovations. The incoming waves of admittance in the Economic European Community (EEC), subsequently renamed European Union (EU), and the recent fall of the Berlin Wall (9 November 1989), generated a feeling of European unification and breakdown of the national barriers. This widespread sensation would become true with the Maastricht Treaty, which was signed in the Netherlands on 7 February 1992 and entered into force on 1 November 1993. It sanctioned the birth of the EU to promote a balanced and sustainable economic and social progress, in particular through the creation of an area without internal frontiers. 

*Keywords:* Vascular surgery

The possibility of free movement of for citizens of the EU, sensed from the beginning of the nineties and made concrete by the Maastricht Treaty, was to have important repercussions in the medical world, too. Was, with the free movement of specialist doctors within the EU, the differences in organisation, in the structure as well as in the scientific background in the various countries would need to confront each other.

The first step to empower the visionary dream of some sort of common organisation to unite vascular surgeons throughout Europe and try to harmonise rules, specialist training and to have a common "policy" had obviously to be the creation of a working group that could analyse a picture of the situation in various countries. To organise that working group, a meeting entitled "Vascular Surgery in the EEC" was arranged in St. Vincent (Aosta-Italy) by Dr. Domenico Palombo (presently Director of the Department of Vascular Surgery at San Martino University Hospital of Genoa). This meeting lasted from 11 to 14 March 1991 and gathered for the first time the representative delegates of the national societies of vascular surgery of 12 European countries: Italy, Germany,

* Tel.: +39-10555-2424; fax: +39-1055-56653.
*E-mail address:* domenico.palombo@hsanmartino.it (D. Palombo).

0531-5131/ 
doi:10.1016/j.ics.2004.05.119

France, Belgium and the Netherlands, among the six that formed the EEC in 1950, Denmark and United Kingdom, entered into EEC in 1973, Greece, entered in 1981, Portugal and Spain, entered in 1986. In addition, the representatives of the national vascular surgery societies of four East European countries took part in the meeting, too. Every official representative reported on the current situation of vascular surgery in his country replying to preordained questions [1,2]: "How many sections, services, official and autonomous units of vascular surgery are there in your country?"; "Is there a specialisation or a vascular surgery diploma recognised within the EEC?"; "Is vascular surgery autonomous or run together with cardiac surgery or with other surgical branches?"; "Is vascular surgery thought of as a degree course or as a post-graduate course?"; "How many specialists are trained every year?"; "Is the number fixed or related to demand?"; "Is it possible to estimate the number of patients and consequently the number of specialists needed?"; "What is the ratio between the number of vascular surgery centres and the population or the estimated patients per year?"; "Is the specialist training carried out following EEC regulations or others?". The picture that appeared was not homogeneous. In the majority of European countries vascular surgery was not independent of general surgery or cardio-thoracic surgery. Indeed, in most cases, vascular surgery was carried out by a general surgeon with an interest in this matter. In various states, there was not a diploma in vascular surgery. In some cases, all general or cardio-thoracic surgeons could practise vascular surgery without more training, in some cases, it was the result of a postgraduate course after the surgery diploma without recognition within EEC. In other words, vascular surgery was not recognised both as an autonomous branch of surgery and as an autonomous speciality in numerous European countries. Moreover, the number of vascular surgeons and general or cardio-thoracic surgeons performing vascular surgery was usually superior to real requirement. Among these, most had only a minor interest in this field and performed just a small number of operations per year. Hence the need to concentrate vascular surgery into fewer centres, which were better equipped and staffed by surgeons with an exclusive interest in vascular disease. Lastly, there often was no clearly defined training programmes for vascular surgery.

From this meeting, various suggestions for the future of vascular surgery transpired. Among these the principal objectives were: (1) vascular surgery had to be defined with precision and recognised as an independent surgical specialisation within the EEC; (2) this speciality had to be carried out exclusively by competent specialists; (3) the number of specialists in vascular surgery had to be established according to the real local demand in each European country; (4) vascular surgery must only be practised in institutions with appropriate equipment; (5) a prearranged and harmonised training programme in vascular surgery had to be defined to guarantee an improvement of the quality of medical practice provided to patients with vascular disease; (6) the mobility of vascular surgeons within the EEC should be brought to be carried into effect; (7) an official authority had to be created to supervise the training in vascular surgery within the EEC with the aim of a European Diploma of Vascular Surgery.

As a consequence of this meeting, the Council of Vascular Surgeons of the EEC was created to carry out these ambitious objectives. The Council, later named "Aosta group" or "Aosta initiative", was composed of one representative from each national vascular surgery society of EEC countries and was the first attempt to formalize a supranational organization in vascular surgery for a pan-European approach to the upgrading of surgical practice, training and certification.

Despite difficulties due to concern in some of the national vascular societies which feared limitations in their autonomy, it was the right time for the birth of the Council which had a permanent site (St. Vincent-Aosta) and a permanent organising secretary (Domenico Palombo).

It promptly worked and rapidly developed, overcoming many "political" obstacles, a clear-cut definition of vascular surgery, training programmes and various general policy papers, aiming at the unification of vascular surgery speciality [3,4].

Results were disseminated with the return of the national representatives to their respective national vascular societies, collecting also at that level opinions and proposals of vascular surgeons.

As a first step, a statute attested by a notary was drawn up defining of vascular surgery and objectives of the Council of Vascular Surgeons in the EC. The following text was subscribed and signed by:

- Prof. M. D'Addato (Italy)
- Prof. P.C. Maurer (Germany)
- Prof. H.G. Nicaise (France)
- Prof. R. Vanmaele (Belgium)
- Prof. J. Barbosa (Portugal)
- Prof. J. Buth (Netherlands)
- Prof. P.L. Harris (Great Britain and Ireland)
- Prof. M.A. Cairols (Spain)
- Prof. P. Balas (Greece)
- Prof. W.P. Paaske (Denmark).

The Council of Vascular Surgeons in the EC is formed of official representatives of the specialist vascular surgical societies of all the member states of the European Community.

## 1. Definition of vascular surgery

Vascular surgery is the clinical and scientific discipline concerned with the diagnosis, treatment and prevention of diseases affecting blood vessels and lymphatic system.

Vascular disease is the most common cause of death and disability in European countries. Its surgical management has become a clearly defined, highly specialised and progressively expanding discipline with specific training requirements.

## 2. Objectives of the Council of Vascular Surgeons in the EC

The objectives of the Council are to ensure optimal care of patients with vascular diseases in the EC by:

(1) promoting adequate provision of facilities and qualified personnel relative to the prevalence of vascular diseases in our countries;

(2) setting high educational standards in vascular surgery and defining the requirements for training institutions and trainers;
(3) encouraging effective audit of clinical vascular surgical practice;
(4) promoting programmes of research into vascular diseases, their treatment and prevention; and
(5) reducing the prevalence of vascular diseases in the Community by promoting initiatives to eliminate or reduce risk factors (e.g., cigarette smoking).

Our ultimate aim is to optimise patient care in vascular surgery. This is achieved most effectively in specialist units by people who are engaged in vascular surgery full time or nearly full time.

It is our intention to realise our objectives by exerting an influence over government and community agencies with responsibilities for professional accreditation and resource allocation for medical services.

In a more precise document, definition of vascular surgery was developed in the following sections:

- detailed specifications of vascular surgery;
- application of basic knowledge;
- relevant pathologies;
- clinical diagnosis;
- special investigation techniques;
- non-invasive vascular laboratory;
- X-ray angiography;
- intra-operative investigations;
- prevention of vascular disease;
- treatment of vascular diseases;
- endovascular surgery;
- general management;
- research, audit and education.

After approximately 2 years of activity, the Council of Vascular Surgeons approached the UEMS, in order to be more effective in Europe and to eventually give the necessary autonomy to vascular surgery in the bosom of UEMS, which, created by the national trade unions for specialist medical doctors, was actively present in Brussels.

Although the European Union of Medical Specialists (Union Européenne des Médecins Spécialistes-UEMS) formed, from 1962, a Specialist Section for each of the main disciplines practised in the member States, vascular surgery was not represented. For this reason, in that new cultural climate, we observed the necessity of towards the UEMS.

The UEMS [5] was created in Brussels on 6 December 1954, less than 1 year after the Treaty of Rome, by the representative delegates of the professional organisations of medical specialists from the six member countries (Belgium, Germany, France, Italy, Luxembourg and the Netherlands) relevant. This non-profit organisation, which is not an official agency of the EU, established contacts with the authorities of the EEC, working in principle as a lobby group and defined the basic principles in the field of training of European medical specialists. The organisation straightaway tackled the problem of quality and tried to obtain from the EEC a level of training comparably high for the future medical specialists. The statutory purpose of the UEMS and its sections is the harmonisation and improvement of the quality of medical specialist practice, first in the EEC, then in the EU. The aim was the following objectives: first, the study and promotion of the highest level of training of the medical specialists, medical practice and health care within the EU; second, the study and promotion of free movement of specialist doctors within the EU; third, the establishment of a bureaucratic network among the medical specialist profession in the Member States of the EU, and the EU authorities, for the achievement of the aforementioned objectives.

After a phase of negotiation, the Council instituted a Subsection of Vascular Surgery in the UEMS.

At that time, it was estimated that the Council had to dissolve into the Subsection of Vascular Surgery born in the bosom of the UEMS's Monosection of Surgery. The same members of the Council had to be nominated into the Subsection.

This decision was made despite the advice of many members who were in favour of the prosecution of the activities of the Council "highly useful to prepare reports and decisions that subsequently could be formulated in the possibly more political atmosphere in Brussels...." "the Council is more suitable for strategic planning and decision making".

However, the subsection quickly became the Division of Vascular Surgery of the UEMS and the activity of the Council was stopped. The division started the European Board of Vascular Surgery.

These events developed in Edinburgh in 1993. In this way, the European era of vascular surgery was started.

## References

[1] D. Palombo, Vascular surgery across the European Community, Critical Ischaemia 1 (4) (1991 Nov.) 3–5.
[2] D. Palombo, P Brustia (Eds.), La Chirurgia Vascolare nella Comunità Economica Europea, Consiglio Chirurghi Vascolari nella Comunità Economica Europea, Public Health Department of the Valle d'Aosta Regional Government, Aosta, 1992.
[3] D. Palombo, Editorial—Council of Vascular Surgeons in the European Community, Cardiovascular Surgery 1 (3) (1993 June) 203–206.
[4] D. Palombo, H. Nicaise, J. Barbosa, W.P. Paaske (Eds.), Training for Vascular Surgeons in the European Union, Public Health Department of the Valle d'Aosta Regional Government, Aosta, 1995.
[5] P.L. Harris, Union Européenne des Médecins Spécialistes (UEMS) Section of Surgery Division of Vascular Surgery. European Board of Vascular Surgery annual report 1995, European Journal of Vascular and Endovascular Surgery 12 (1996) 383–385.

## Further reading

[1] P.C. Maurer, Vascular surgery in the European Union: current state, developments and prospects for the future, Int. Angiol. 14 (1995) 335–338.
[2] W.P. Paaske, The European Society for vascular surgery on the Internet, Endocr. Cardiovasc. Multimedia Mag. 2 (1998) 92–98.

[3] J. Buth, P.L. Harris, P.C. Maurer, B. Nachbur, H. Van Urk, Harmonization of vascular surgical training in Europe. A task for the European board of vascular surgery, Cardiovasc. Surg. 8 (2000) 98–103.
[4] C.D. Liapis, B. Nachbur, EBSQ-Vasc—which way to the future? Eur. J. Vasc. Endovasc. Surg. 21 (2001) 473–474.
[5] W.P. Paaske, Continuing professional development for vascular surgeons in Europe, in: P. Balas, X. Panoussis (Eds.), Syllabus of the 8th Pan Hellenic Conference on Angiology and Vascular Surgery. Athens. (2002) 83–93.
[6] D. Palombo, C.D. Liapis, E.A. Tzortzis, J.H.N. Wolfe, D. Bergqvist, The value of a logbook for young vascular surgeons in training: the UEMS experience. International Angiology. in press.

ELSEVIER

International Congress Series 1272 (2004) 21–31

www.ics-elsevier.com

# European origins of the vascular speciality and foundation of the European Board of Vascular Surgery (EBVS)

Peter Harris*

*Royal Liverpool University Hospital, 88 Rodney Street, Liverpool L1 9AR , UK*

*Keywords:* Vascular surgery

## 1. Introduction

While contributions of physicians and scientists from other continents merit recognition, Europe can justifiably claim to have been the cradle of vascular surgery. Fundamental principles were established throughout the twentieth century, by the end of which vascular practice had evolved into a clearly defined speciality with its own extensive knowledge base and specific diagnostic and therapeutic techniques. Today, advances in the management of vascular disease continue to progress at an accelerating pace. The modern vascular specialist must have at his command a wide range of skills bridging traditional divides between the conventional surgical, medical, and radiological specialities. The need to respond to these changes and ensure that vascular patients in European countries continues to have access to the highest possible standards of care, gave impetus to the foundation—and remains the raison d'être—of the European Board of Vascular Surgery (EBVS).

This chapter traces the origins of vascular speciality in Europe. It also describes the events that led to the inauguration of the EBVS and summarises its aims.

## 2. European firsts in vascular surgery

### *2.1. First sutured vascular anastomosis*

Before and after the turn of the century, experiments were carried out all over the world on vascular suturing and the replacement of arteries. The French school had the greatest success in this research, and it was in Lyon where Alexis Carrel and Rene Leriche first evolved modern techniques of vascular anastomosis. These two luminaries worked together under the direction of Mathieu Jaboulay. History awarded credit for eventual success to

* Tel.: +41-151-709-0669; fax: +41-151-706-5827.
*E-mail address:* findplh@hotmail.com (P. Harris).

0531-5131/ © 2004 Published by Elsevier B.V.
doi:10.1016/j.ics.2004.05.030

Carrel [1]. He met a fate shared by a number of outstanding European physicians and scientists; he could not find satisfactory working conditions at home and therefore emigrated. First, he went to Canada and then to Chicago where he teamed up with Guthrie. In 1912, he was awarded the Nobel Prize for medicine for his work on vascular suturing and anastomosis. But the original ideas and experimental work took place in Europe!

The first to apply Carrel's techniques clinically, with success, was a Spaniard, Goyanes [2], in 1906.

### 2.2. First angiograms

Angiography was developed in Portugal. Moniz [3] performed the first cerebral angiogram in Lisbon in 1927, and Reynaldo Cid dos Santos performed the first aortogram in the same city in 1929 [4].

### 2.3. First application of heparin

Heparin was actually discovered in America by William Howell and Jay McLean between 1916 and 1925. But, it was first manufactured in crystalline form by Fischer and Schmitzin Copenhagen in 1933, and it was first used clinically to treat patients with deep vein thrombosis by Crafoord [5] in Stockholm in 1937.

### 2.4. First endarterectomy

The first endarterectomy on the superficial femoral artery was carried out in Lisbon in 1946 by Jean Cid dos Santos, son of Reynaldo [6]. This was a semiclosed endarterectomy which he carried out under local anaesthesia.

### 2.5. First bypass using autologous vein graft

Jean Kunlin (Fig. 1) performed the first femoropopliteal bypass using a reversed saphenous vein graft in Paris in 1948 [7]. His boss was Rene Leriche (Fig. 2) who was apparently highly sceptical about the idea because he believed that arterial pressure would rupture the vein. Faced with this opposition from his superior, Kunlin waited until Leriche was out of town before operating upon his first patient who had critical limb ischaemia with

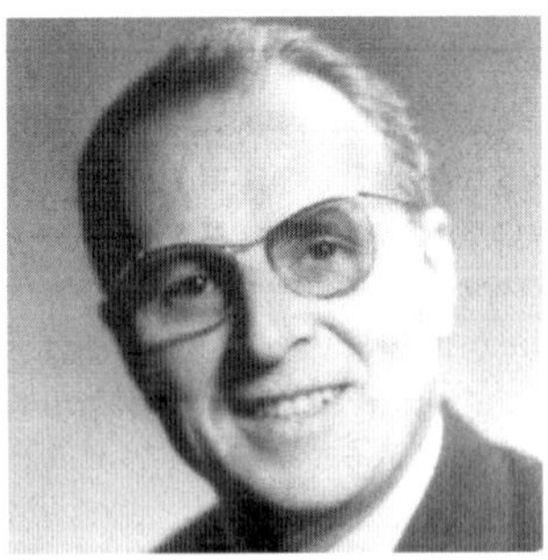

Fig. 1. Jean Kunlin.

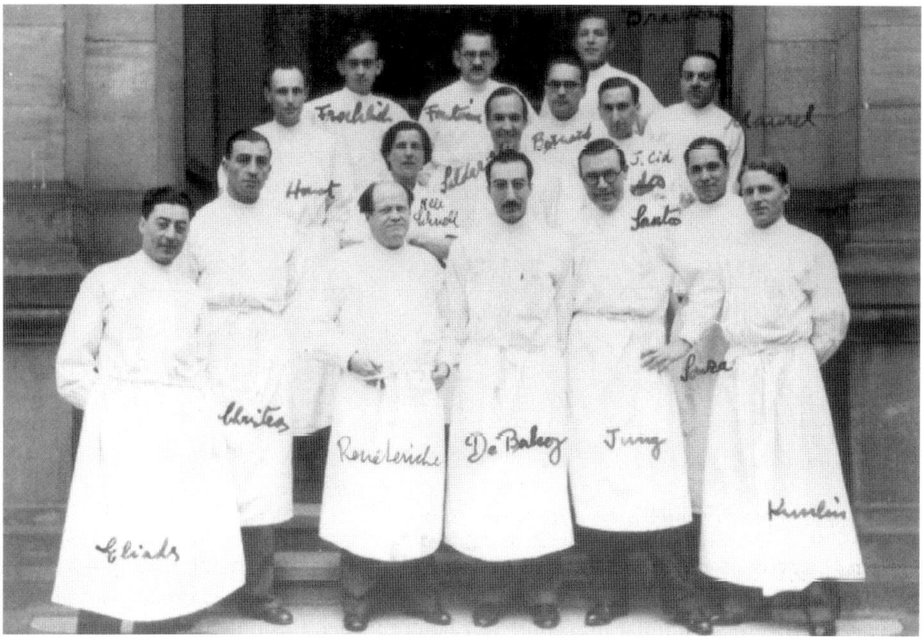


Fig. 2. Members of the 'Service of Rene Leriche', Strasbourg, 1936. Michael DeBakey is standing to the left of Leriche.

a necrotic foot. Fortunately for the patient, Jean Kunlin, and the rest of the world, it worked. Despite the outstanding success of this first ever femoropopliteal vein graft, Leriche and other leading European surgeons remained unconvinced, and it was the Americans, most notably, Linton, who took up the idea and exploited it fully.

### *2.6. First aortic bifurcation reconstruction*

The first operation to replace an occluded bifurcation of the aorta was carried out in 1950, again in France, by Jacques Oudot (Fig. 3) [8]. He used an aortic allograft from a young victim of an accident. Oudot was an interesting man with a highly developed sense of adventure. Some months prior to undertaking the first aortic graft, he participated in another notable 'first'—the ascent of Annapurna. During the course of this expedition, he experimented with intra-arterial injections of vasodilators for the treatment of frostbite. In 1953, he crashed his high-powered sports car, sustaining fatal injuries. He was just 40 years old.

### *2.7. First repair of an abdominal aortic aneurysm*

Yet another Frenchman, Charles Dubost (Fig. 4), was responsible for the first operation to repair an abdominal aortic aneurysm [9]. This was in 1952. A 14-cm length of preserved thoracic aorta from a young accident victim was used to replace an aneurysmal abdominal aorta. The patient lived for another 8 years before dying from myocardial infarction.

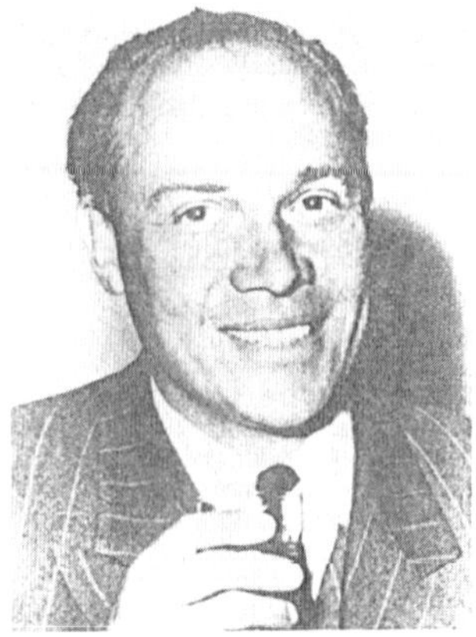

Fig. 3. Jacques Oudot.

### 2.8. First reported carotid artery reconstruction

Felix Eastcott is credited with the first carotid reconstruction for recurrent cerebral transient ischaemic attacks in London in 1954 [10]. It has been claimed that Michael DeBakey carried out a similar procedure just before Eastcott. But he was slower in getting his report into print.

### 2.9. First balloon angioplasty

As we move into the era of endovascular surgery, we again find Europeans leading the way. Charles Dotter had been working in the States dilating arteries with solid catheters, but it was the invention of a really effective balloon for arterial dilatation by Andreas Gruntzig (Fig. 5) that really opened the floodgates for endovascular interventions [11]. He carried out the first femoral and iliac angioplasties with a balloon catheter in 1972 and the first coronary PTA in 1977, both in Zurich. Andreas Gruntzig also carried out the first renal PTA with Felix Mahler in Bern in 1977.

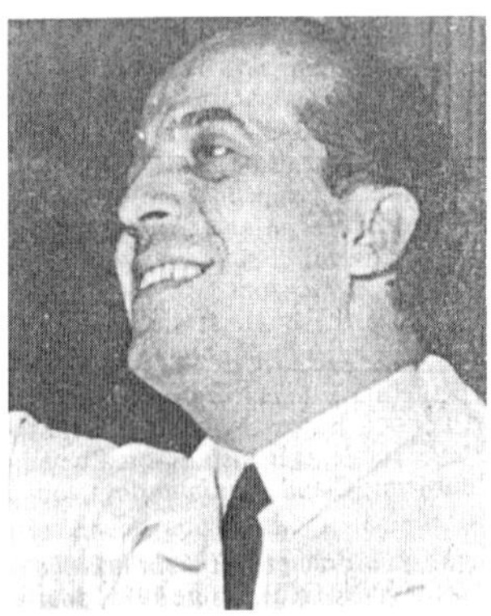

Fig. 4. Charles Dubost.

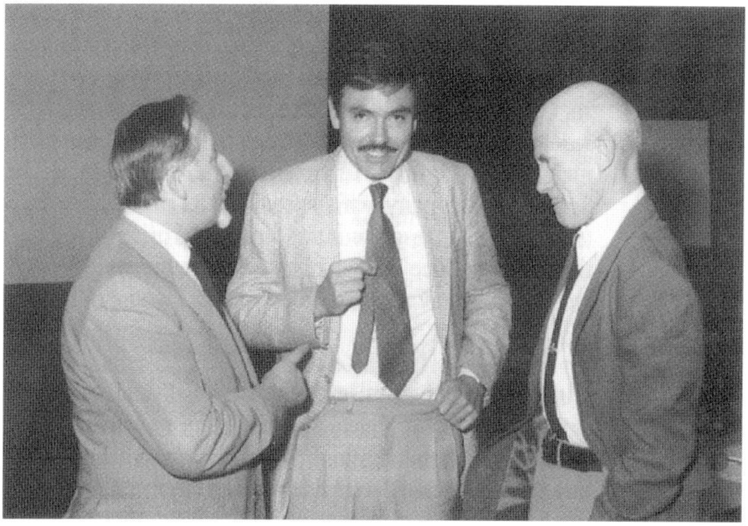

Fig. 5. Andreas Grunzig with Charles Dotter to his left and Felix Zeitler to his right.

## *2.10. First endovascular aneurysm repair with a modular stent/graft*

Juan Parodi attempted endovascular repair of an abdominal aortic aneurysm in Buenos Aires in 1990 using a tube graft stented at the proximal end only [12]. But, Claude Mialhe (Fig. 6) was the first to use a modular intraaortic stent/graft which was the forerunner of the bifurcated modular devices in use today [13].

And so, it can be seen that it has been in Europe where most of the major advances in modern vascular surgery have occurred. Despite this incredible record of innovation, vascular surgeons in many parts of the continent have been slow to organise themselves into a vascular speciality. Exceptions are Austria, France, Spain, Portugal, Italy, and

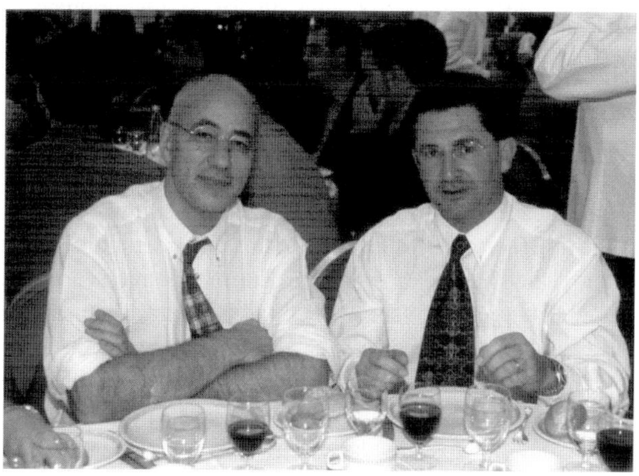

Fig. 6. Claude Mialhe (left) with Jean-Pierre Becquemin.

Denmark. It took an inordinately long time also for vascular specialists in the different member states of the European Union to join together to work for the recognition of the speciality within the medico-political institutions of Europe, an essential prerequisite for appropriate levels of funding. Europe harbours a wide diversity of cultures, there are marked differences in the structure and organisation of basic medical and specialist training, and above all, in language. But, we have much more in common than that which divides us, and the last decade has seen major changes on a Europe-wide scale in many facets of life. The first signs of a recognisable vascular surgical identity in Europe became apparent through evolution of the scientific societies for vascular surgery.

### *2.11. European scientific societies for vascular surgery*

Until the late 80s, the European Chapter of the International Society of Cardiovascular Surgery was the only scientific society for vascular surgeons in Europe. In the meantime, in America, the Society for Vascular Surgery had become well established, and in Europe itself, the cardiac surgeons had split off to form their own society. There was clearly a need for change. In 1987, the inaugural meeting of the European Society for Vascular Surgery took place in London.

It is now a matter of record that the birth of this new society, like that of the International Society for Cardiovascular Surgery before it, was not achieved without some angst. Initially, a majority of vascular surgeons in some European countries, most notably, France, declined involvement in the ESVS. However, there has been a gradual 'meeting of minds', and in 1999, the annual meeting of the European Society took place in Paris with a French surgeon being elected as president. The ESVS was highly influential in securing a place for vascular surgery within the Union Européene des Médecins Spécialistes (UEMS).

### *2.12. Union Européene des Médecins Spécialistes*

It is part of the 'European ideal' that medical specialists should be able to travel freely and work throughout the European Union. This ideal was originally enshrined in two medical directives that were adopted as laws in 1976. One relates to basic medical qualifications and the other to specialist qualifications. The principles were restated in revisions of these directives in1996. Refusal of the General Medical Council in the UK to recognise the specialist qualifications of two doctors from the continent led to the successful prosecution of the British government in European courts and a radical revision of specialist training in Britain.

For a specialist qualification awarded in one European country to be recognised by all other European countries, there has to be agreement on acceptable standards of training. The UEMS is the body that has been set up in Europe to oversee the harmonisation of specialist training in the EU member states. There are similar organisations for generalists, i.e., GPs, and for the trainees themselves. These bodies report to a central committee of doctors, the *comite permanent*, which in turn reports to the European Healthcare Committee of politicians. Finally, this committee impacts upon the European Parliament in Strasbourg and the Council of Ministers in Brussels.

In order to secure a foothold in this system, the type of practice in which one works must first be recognised as a speciality by the UEMS. Prior to 1995, a speciality had to be recognised in at least two thirds of EU countries in order to be accepted by the UEMS. In 1995, the rule was changed so that recognition in one third of the countries was sufficient to justify a place in this committee. Prior to 1995, vascular surgery could be represented on the UEMS only through the Section of General Surgery because it was recognised as an independent speciality in six EU countries only (of a total of 15). After 1995, vascular surgery had a right to independent representation.

### *2.13. The European Society for Vascular Surgery and the Council of Vascular Surgeons in the EU*

The founding in 1987 of the European Society for Vascular Surgery stimulated considerable interest in vascular surgery as a speciality in Europe. In 1991, as a result of an initiative of an Italian vascular surgeon, Domenico Palombo, a group called the Council of Vascular Surgeons in the EU was established. This group was also known as the Aosta group because the meetings were held in Aosta valley. Its objective was to discuss standards of vascular training in Europe, directed towards the achievement of a consensus. As a result of pressure from the Aosta group and especially from the ESVS, a Division of Vascular Surgery was established within the UEMS in 1992 (Fig. 7). Being prior to 1995, this division was, in effect, a subsection of the Section of General Surgery.

### *2.14. A vascular surgical subsection of the Section of General Surgery of the UEMS*

The remit of the Division or Subsection of Vascular Surgery was to agree and encourage implementation of common standards of training in vascular surgery in Europe.

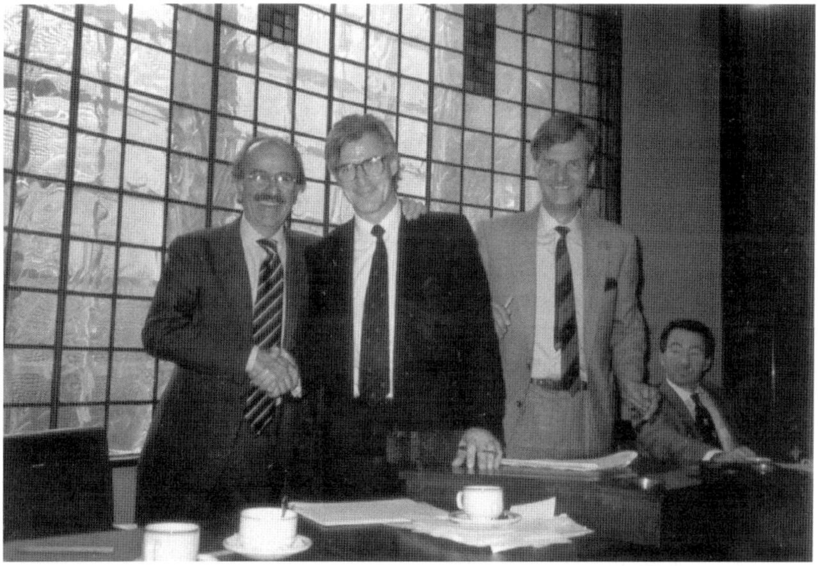

Fig. 7. L to R: Massimo D'Addato, Peter Harris, Jaap Buth, and Joe O'Donnell after formation of the UEMS Division (Subsection) of vascular surgery, Edinburgh, 1992.

This was essential in order to make possible the reciprocal recognition of vascular surgical qualifications in Europe, which EU law demanded. The fact that specialist vascular surgical qualifications did not and still do not exist at all in a majority of countries in the EU posed considerable problems to the committee in achieving these aims. Inconsistent recognition of speciality status of vascular surgery in different EU member states has been a source of considerable difficulty within the UEMS.

In some countries, the establishment of a European committee for vascular surgery, with official recognition by the EU bureaucracy in Brussels, was perceived to be a threat to long-established national institutions.

It would not be an exaggeration to say that the impact of the Subsection of Vascular Surgery of the UEMS on standards of training in Europe was negligible. The pronouncements and recommendations made by it were simply ignored by the national bodies responsible for setting and evaluating training in the individual countries. Subsequently, two developments occurred that impacted significantly upon the situation. First, and most importantly, the division was permitted by the Council of the UEMS to form a Board of Vascular Surgery empowered not only to set standards of training but also to assess candidates against those standards and to issue certificates of quality in training. This provided an opportunity to appeal directly to the trainees themselves. Secondly, the two-thirds rule was changed to a one-third rule and vascular surgery was entitled to representation in the UEMS independently of the Section of General Surgery.

### *2.15. The European Board of Vascular Surgery*

Opposition to the formation of a European board of vascular surgery was considerable. First, opposition came from the UEMS Section of General Surgery, which saw this as an unacceptable step towards the disintegration of the speciality of general surgery in Europe. Second, there was fierce opposition from the national licensing authorities of some countries. It might be surmised that those who felt most threatened objected the most.

The change in the rules governing the acceptance of a speciality, from recognition in two thirds of EU countries to recognition in one third, effectively rendered the Section of General Surgery impotent in its opposition to a board of vascular surgery. In 1996, a vote was held on the question whether ‘vascular surgery should be represented by an independent section on the UEMS’. The result was overwhelmingly favourable; only Britain and the Netherlands voted against it on the instruction of their national vascular surgical societies. However, a compromise was engineered whereby not only vascular but also other surgical specialities were allowed to form their own speciality boards. It was intended that these boards would relate with each other within a confederate structure or ‘common envelope’ represented by what was previously the Board of General Surgery.

### *2.16. European Board of Surgery certification of quality of training in vascular surgery*

The European Board certification, in all specialities, is an entirely voluntary qualification. National specialist qualifications only have a legal status in the EU. It was reasoned that in countries where the currency of the national qualification in vascular surgery was considered by the trainees to be of low value, they would opt for European Board certification as an added qualification. However, this strategy would be successful only if the EBSQvasc was considered to be of a higher standard. It was reasoned that a successful EBSQvasc would impact, in turn, upon national institutions and would cause them to respond by adjusting their own standards of training. Equally important, this initiative would make available a specialist qualification in vascular surgery to trainees whose country of origin did not provide one.

The concept of the EBSQvasc assessment is that it should be competency-based. The award of the qualification is evidence of training in vascular surgery to a standard set by the European Board of Vascular Surgery. It was never intended to be an academic examination and it is definitely not to be regarded as another academic accolade. In order to achieve its aims, the standard was set at a relatively high level.

Competency is assessed by a review of the training log books that have been validated by the principal trainer and backed up by a viva voce examination. To ensure consistent standards of adjudication, both the questions and the answers are carefully defined. The examination is being revised constantly to reflect changing vascular practice, strengthen its validity as a reliable assessment of competence, and improve the standard further. A recent interesting additional innovation is a test of dexterity skills, which is undergoing a process of validation within the setting of the EBSQvasc.

European Board certification is open only to citizens of EU member states who have already gained a national CCST in the relevant speciality.

The first EBSQvasc assessments took place in 1996 in Venice (Fig. 8) and subsequently each year in different European cities in conjunction with the annual meeting of the ESVS.

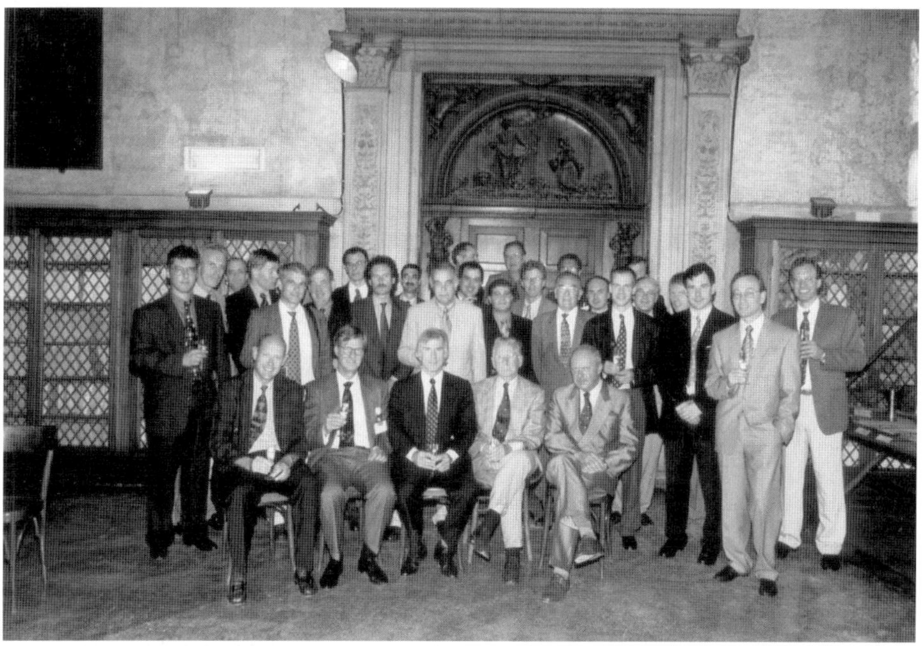

Fig. 8. First EBSQvasc Assessments, Venice, 1996. Examiners and successful candidates.

## 2.17. The future

There are indications that the European Board of Vascular Surgery and EBSQvasc certification may about to play more prominent roles in setting and regulating the standard of training for the vascular specialities in Europe than has been the case so far. There are two reasons for this. First, throughout Europe, vascular training is undergoing radical revision to incorporate the new vascular technologies. At the same time, training is becoming much more focussed to achieve the desired aims in the face of shorter training programmes demanded by most national governments and the severe restriction on the hours available for training resulting from full implementation of the European Working Time Directive (EWTD). In response to these pressures, the vascular speciality is moving progressively further away from its general surgical roots towards multidisciplinary training and competency-based exit assessments. The EBVS is well placed to respond to these developments with the added advantage of setting a marker for the standard of training throughout Europe. There is a good chance that some member states may adopt the EBSQvasc as their exit qualification in the vascular specialities.

Second, those formerly east-block countries that are about to accede to the EU are likely to look at EU institutions to set new standards in vascular speciality training as in many other areas of professional, commercial, and scientific life.

Given the preeminent history of achievement in the vascular specialities in Europe, the European Board of Vascular Surgery is built upon very solid foundations. But in a rapidly changing world, it also needs to be flexible and adaptable. To be accepted as the pivotal organisation for speciality in Europe, it will be essential for it to promulgate the principles of multidisciplinary practice and develop a framework for training that encompasses all of the many and varied skills that will be expected of vascular specialists in the future.

## References

[1] A. Carrel, Les anastomoses vasculaires et leurs technique operatoire, Union Med. Can. (1904) 33–97.
[2] D.J. Goyanes, Nuevos trabajos d:e cirugia vascular. Substitution plastica dc las arterias por las venas o arterioplastica veoosa, aplicada, como nuevo metodo, al triatamiento de los aneurismas, Siglo Med. 53 (1906) 5–16.
[3] E. Moniz, L 'encephalographic arterielle, son importance dans la localization des tumeurs cerebrales, Rev. Neurol. (Paris) 2 (1927) 72.
[4] R. dos Santos, A. Lamas, J. Caldas, L'arteriographic des membres, de l'aorte et ses branches abdominales, Bull. Mem. Soc. Natl. Chir. (Paris) 55 (1929) 87.
[5] C. Crafoord, Preliminary report on post-operative treatment with heparin as a preventive of thrombosis, Acta Chir. Scand. 79 (1937) 407.
[6] J.C. Dos Santos, Sur la desobstruction des thromboses arterielles ancieenes, Mem. Acad. Chir. 73 (1947) 409.
[7] I. Kunlin, Le traitment de l'arterite obliterante par la greffe veineuse longue, Arch. Mal. Coeur. 42 (1949) 371.
[8] I. Oudot, Un deuxieme cas de greffe de la bifurcation aortique pour thrombose de la fourche aortique, Mem. Acad. Chir. 77 (1951) 644.
[9] C. Dubost, M. Allary, N. Oeconomos, Resection of aneurysm of abdominal aorta; re-establishment of continuity by a preserved human arterial graft, with result after 5 months, Arch. Surg. 64 (1952) 405.
[10] H.H.G. Eastcott, G.W. Pickering, C. Rob, Reconstruction of internal carotid artery in a patient with intermittent attacks of hemiplegia, Lancet ii (1954) 994.

[11] A. Grunzig, H. Hopp, Perkutane rekanalisation chronischer arterieller Verschlusse mit einem neuen Dilatationskatheter; Modifikation der Dottcr Technik, Deutsch. Med. Wochenschr. 99 (1974) 2502.
[12] J.C. Parodi, J.C. Palmaz, H.D. Barone, Transfemoral intraluminal graft implantation for abdominal aortic aneurysms, Ann. Vasc. Surg. 5 (1991) 491–499.
[13] C. Mialhe, C. Amicabile, Taitement endovasculaire des aneurysmes de l'aorte sous-renale par endoprothese Stentor, Serie preliminaire, J. Mal. Vasc. 20 (1995) 290–295.

International Congress Series 1272 (2004) 32–37

www.ics-elsevier.com

# The division of vascular surgery of the UEMS

Fabrizio Benedetti-Valentini*

*Division of Vascular Surgery of the UEMS, School of Medicine, La Sapienza University, Via Cassiodoro 6, Rome 00193, Italy*

**Abstract.** The "vascular surgery" (VS) specialty in Europe, as elsewhere, was created as a side branch of General Surgery. At the time, only a few reconstructive procedures were possible and extensively applied, but many "firsts" were performed in Europe, from carotid endarterectomy to graft repair of an abdominal aortic aneurysm. Some of our old Masters were proud to practice vascular procedures so effectively for bowel, kidney or thoracic surgery. Technology with its progressive achievements in materials, instruments and methodologies, as well as medical applications of several principles of physics and clinical use of biological discoveries and pharmacological research with the introduction of new drugs, led to rapid and incredible developments in VS. Hence, in the late 1960s in the universities it began to be recognized as a well-defined discipline and a specific specialty. 

*Keywords:* Vascular surgery

A parallel pathway was formed in 1950 by the European Economic Community (EEC), followed by the European Union (EU) in 1992. Fifteen "Western" European Countries are at present Member States of the EU, which is scheduled to expand in 2004 with the accession of 10 new Member States, mostly "Eastern" European Countries, as well as Turkey and Cyprus. The Union Européenne de Médecins Spécialistes (UEMS) was founded in Brussels in 1958 in this political, economic and social framework, 1 year after the signing of the Treaty of Rome. A specific paper in this same book is devoted to UEMS and its organization, aims and achievements. For the purpose of this contribution it is enough to recall that from 1962 Specialist Sections were created within the UEMS according to the main disciplines present in the EU. Some Sections are divided into Divisions or have associated Divisions. The Division of Vascular Surgery (DVS), associated with the Section of Surgery, was created in Edinburgh in 1993 after a preliminary loose aggregation of the representatives of most vascular surgical societies of the EEC in 1991, named the Council of Vascular Surgeons in the EEC. Art. 1 of the statute [1] states that "The Division of Vascular Surgery within the UEMS is an associate

* Tel.: +39-6-490255; fax: +39-6-49970230.
*E-mail address:* chvs.rm@flashnet.it (F. Benedetti-Valentini).


doi:10.1016/j.ics.2004.04.078

section of the UEMS Section of Surgery, which was formed in 1993 to prepare specific advice on issues relating to training and professional practice in vascular surgery within the countries of the European Union for the benefit of the EU political administration."

The Division consists of one Representative from each EU Member State (who must be a vascular surgeon), appointed by the national medical union which is part of the UEMS. The European Board of Vascular Surgery, as a function of the Division (UEMS Statute—IV Specialist Section—. 21—it. IV "Each specialist section may create its own European Board as a working Group ..."), was subsequently created and consists of the national Representatives in the Division (1st Representative), plus one additional member from each country appointed by the national vascular surgical society (2nd Representative). The delegated Member States are *voting members* and each Member State (comprised of representatives) has one vote. The Council (both Division and Board) works mainly by consensus, as it is politically sound and decisions are reached unanimously; however, a majority decision cannot be ruled out like in every true democracy. Associate Members participate in the Council without voting rights, but their contribution is most valued particularly on major issues. There are also Associate Member delegations of some non-EU Member states, such as Hungary, Switzerland, Czech Republic, Slovenia, etc., on the Division and Board of VS, as well as the Secretaries of the European Society of Vascular Surgery (ESVS) and of the European Chapter of the International Union of Angiology (IUA), the President of the European Board of Surgery, the Secretary of the UEMS and some other Representatives of professional or scientific institutions involved in vascular surgery (VS). Voting members are 15 at present, but will be many more once the EU becomes enlarged.

The definition of Vascular Surgery, as stated by the DVS, is "the clinical and scientific discipline concerned with the diagnosis, treatment and prevention of diseases affecting arteries, veins and lymphatics". It should be noted that there is no emphasis on the "surgical" perspective, but conversely a strong one on the "vascular" perspective. The field was left wide open. On the one side is the concept of a vascular surgeon who is "a specialist in vascular sciences equipped to take responsibility for the complete management of patients with vascular diseases," as clearly defined by Liapis and Paaske [2] in agreement with Sillesen's vision: "thus, the future vascular surgeon will be a vascular specialist capable of treating the whole patient with PAD" [3]. On the other side is the view of an intensive and close cooperation of all "vascular specialists," mainly the Angiologist, the Interventional Radiologist and the Vascular Surgeon (but also the Physiologist, the Pharmacologist, the Psychiatrist and so forth) to provide the best care for the whole spectrum of vascular diseases. These two conceptions are not necessarily contradictory since any vascular specialist, through appropriate training and subsequent updating (continuing professional development—CPD) can broaden his/her knowledge and professional skills in various fields of vascular science, but no vascular specialist can succeed in mastering all facets of vascular care and research. Better, more articulated and multidisciplinary training for each "vascular" speciality, intertwined with close cooperation of all vascular specialists, is the ideal recipe.

Up to the first few months of 2002, both the DVS and the Board were managed by the same executives with full success. Yet, the growing and in-depth involvement of both the Division and Board in the many issues and problems of VS in Europe indicated a need for the workload to be segmented and different members of the Council to be involved in specific areas of responsibility and management. Therefore, after appropriate discussion and agreement by the Executives and Council members, it was decided to distinguish, not divide, the activities of the Division from those of the Board and to create Committees and Working Groups devoted to specific issues. The new "internal" organization in the UEMS-Division and Board of Vascular Surgery was launched in London, on 7 April 2002, as stipulated by Christos Liapis [4], Secretary-General, and reported in Fig. 1. It should also be stated "The separation of labour between Division and Board has been defined for the purpose of enhancing progress and not to separate the entities, and to make use of the valuable expertise of more council members. Nominations for the new committees listed above are based on membership categories as stated in the statutes" [4].

As is evident, the main function of the Division is a political one, the first top priority being management and enlargement of membership. This issue is under constant evolvement by the admission of Associate Members, such as Croatia, Hungary, the Czech Republic, and Slovakia, and is expected to become more intensive with the forthcoming expansion of the EU. Many more countries will be involved with differences in organization of VS and relations with other specialties, mainly General Surgery, Cardiac Surgery and Angiology. This has led to the subsequent creation of a Committee for

Item 10

**STATUTORY ELECTIVE PROCESS**

**CHANGE OF STRUCTURE IN THE DIVISION AND BOARD**

REPORT CHRISTOS LIAPIS

**EXECUTIVE MEMBERS OF THE UEMS DIVISION AND BOARD OF VASCULAR SURGERY**
(as at the last elections in London on 7 April 2002)

**DIVISION**

| | |
|---|---|
| President | Fabrizio Benedetti-Valentini (Italy) |

**BOARD**

| | |
|---|---|
| President | John H N Wolfe (UK) |
| Vice President | Klaus Balzer (Germany) |

**DIVISION AND BOARD**

| | |
|---|---|
| Secretary/Treasurer | Christos D Liapis (Greece) |

**COMMITTEES - AREAS OF RESPONSIBILITY**

**DIVISION**
1. Membership
2. Relations with other specialties and UEMS
3. Registry
4. New Products and CE
5. Quality Assurance
6. Relations with health systems of EU countries

**BOARD**
1. CME/CPD
2. Vascular Training/Examinations
3. Logbook
4. Visitation
5. Regulations for Vascular Surgery Specialist Training in EU countries

Fig. 1.

"Territorial expansion and implementation of vascular events"; it is already at work delineating the actual situation of VS in most Eastern European countries and looking at ways to accommodate them into the frame of an enlarging EU.

The issue of relations with other specialities and UEMS focused particularly on cooperation with our medical and radiological "counterparts." Angiology, or Vascular Medicine as some like to call it, is not yet a fully established and recognized specialty in most countries of the present EU, nor in the incoming ones. However, there are some angiological units, albeit a few of them, in many European countries and indeed there are many colleagues interested in the medical problems of the vascular patient [5]. There are also national and international scientific societies of Angiology and some of them are comprised of vascular surgeons, interventional radiologists and cardiologists.

This DVS decided to open up to other vascular specialists, particularly the Angiologists, and get them engaged in a common organizational effort. Therefore, the International Union of Angiology (IUA) was invited to join us as an Associate member in 2003, formally on the same status as ESVS, and to take part in all our activities and functions. The IUA was a strong foundation as the leading angiological society, is highly reliable and very representative of its profession throughout Europe and the world. The second step was to form a Working Group on Vascular Centres with the purpose of studying the possibility of starting the formation of "vascular centres" in Europe, where vascular patients receive coordinated multidisciplinary, specialized care. The Secretary of the European Chapter of the IUA is directly involved in this group, as well as a leading representative of the Interventional Radiologists. The Working Group is expected in 2004 to set the guidelines for the organization of a vascular centre, specialists working in it and their coordination, equipment, management, rules of procedures, location, etc. It should also be able to estimate the number of Vascular Centres needed in the European countries and suggest their ideal locations. This kind of work is in line with politics in Europe since the perception of "vascular centres," although still smoky, is now common among the public health authorities of the majority of the EU Countries and those of the near future.

The *Registry* is a multivaried and thorny issue. Ideally, we should keep count of a large series of factors such as vascular surgeons in the EU and in every single Member State, number of vascular patients and surgical procedures, vascular units, training centres and so forth. Number, location, organization and management of training centres in VS were the first part of the problem that had to be faced by the Division with a large measure of patience, effort and goodwill. All the training centres of each country had to be identified and recorded, as well as all the different legislation and regulations; all the Representatives in the Council were involved in this process. Subsequently, each centre would be registered with all its features: number of trainees, facilities, equipment, trainers, management, etc. This is indeed the most difficult part of the task since many directors of the training centres seem to be wary of this kind of investigation and are slow to cooperate. We should be aware that for years, and in part even today, Brussels and the European institutions have been feared as prone to curtail identity and independence of the national institutions and the academic world is always very defensive of its positions. Nevertheless, we should try to convince them that getting their training centre into a complete European Registry will not only contribute to a better knowledge of the general setting of VS in Europe, but will also be in their interest, providing international recognition, easier access to CME for their educational events, easier access to European examinations for people who were trained with them, and possibly easier recognition by the EU in the future.

Obviously the issue of a uniform and high standard of training in Europe will be more and more important with the progressive integration of the European countries and will affect the movement of patients and surgeons within the EU, thus the private and public insurance systems and, in turn, the educational and occupational process. So, we are in the field of the relations with health systems of EU countries and of the present and foreseeable European regulations. The main involvement in such problems came for the Division when the European Commission, through its Internal Market Directorate on 7 March 2002, presented a proposal for a new Directive on "Recognition of professional qualifications"—Directive (COM 2002) 119, which became known as the new Doctors' Directive for its partial dealing with the medical profession (Chap. III: Sect 1, Art 20–21; Sect 2, Art 22–23 (training of medical specialist)—24 plus Annex V point 5.1.4—25–26–27–28). If passed in its present form, it will be a terrible blow to the entire medical profession and in particular to VS and some other specialities. In short, it divides the 52 Medical Specialities, recognized at present in the EU, into two groups: the first 17 specialities, present as a monospecialty in all the EU countries, maintain the current sectoral system, whereas the second 35 specialities not present in all the EU Countries, are moved to the general system.

The *sectoral system*, successfully applied till now [6], is based on two levels: first, coordinating directive, standardizing training courses; second, automatic recognition once it has been established that the training course corresponds to the directive. The *general system* is based on the principle of mutual recognition on a case-by-case consideration. In other words, the sectoral system sets European level and standard and everything else follows accordingly; the general system throws back the entire matter to national and, sometimes even, regional level. The new Doctors' Directive is heavily discriminating against VS, which is downscaled into the general system. VS is an independent specialty in 9 member states of the EU and in all the other ones it is precisely recognizable and specific, since there are surgeons with special training in this discipline devoting their professional life to it. In those countries there are also units named after "Vascular Surgery" and meant for vascular care, as in the UK, Germany, Norway and so forth. We felt that such discrimination was completely unacceptable as it was purely formal and void of scientific and professional substance. A specialty should not be relegated to the corner of neglect only because it is not "recognized" (translate "not a monospeciality") in some member states, but, conversely, perhaps the national academic and health authorities of those countries should be encouraged to recognize it in a European perspective! Therefore, since the summer of 2002, this DVS started a strong opposition, with continuous action since that time, and is still pressing hard against the Directive (COM 2002) 119. This opposition is in cooperation with the Management Council of the UEMS, with the UEMO (European Union of General Practitioners) and the CPME (Standing Committee of European Doctors) and with many other professional organizations. We also received the support of the Referee for the Committee on Legal Affairs and the Internal Market of the European Parliament who was highly critical of the entire proposal. Among other statements, he wrote "In view of the complexity and specific nature of the individual professions and the individual national rules governing them, it will be futile to endeavour to force them into a single mould and the European Parliament does not wish to do so" and "... leaving the organizations representing the professions ... the freedom to decide in consultation between the general and sectoral system" [7].

All the Executives of our Division and Board of VS and many Members of the Council participated in the lobbying effort. Even now, at the time of this manuscript, the battle continues in the European Parliament. Let's hope that common sense and legitimate positions will prevail.

Quality Assurance (QA) is a very complicated matter, but it should be faced, analysed, looked at under every possible angle and, possibly, fixed along the lines of reasonable suggestions, advice and regulations. That is as true for VS as for any other field in the medical profession. It is a difficult task, but we have in our council many people with adequate expertise and we can take advantage of the excellent preliminary work done within the UEMS, Management Council [8]. First, it should be stipulated that QA is "the regular review against defined standards of clinical practice" and that it is different from Quality Control, which is limited to regulations, and Quality Improvement, which has much to do with Continuing Professional Development. Then, it should be taken into account that as vascular surgeons (and the medical profession in general) are only one of the stakeholders in the process of QA, the others being of course the patient, but also the entire society and the health service employers, as well as the providers of funding and the regulatory authorities. It is a six-partner system. Since in a correct QA process all stakeholders must take their responsibility, we should care for our CPD and prove our adequacy at the highest possible standards. However, of course, every other stakeholder should concur and cooperate for its part, such as providing resources, setting fair regulations, smoothing daily operations and so forth. Our main contribution as a UEMS Division will be to set European standards for performance of vascular surgeons, but also suggesting what should be provided for them to be effective and how they should be regulated.

No doubt the DVS has a lot of work to do, but it is very challenging and we are keen to do it.

## References

[1] Internet website: http//www.uems-vasc.org.

[2] C.D. Liapis, W.P. Paaske, Training in vascular surgery in Europe—the impact of endovascular therapy, Eur. J. Vasc. Endovasc. Surg. 23 (2002) 1.

[3] H. Sillesen, Who should treat patients with peripheral arterial disease—the vascular specialist? Eur. J. Vasc. Endovasc. Surg. 24 (2002) 1.

[4] C.D. Liapis, Change of structure in the Division and Board Report of the Secretary General to the Council of the UEMS-Division and Board of Vascular Surgery, Minutes of the Meeting, Istanbul, Sept. 25th 2002.

[5] J. Ostergren, B. Fagrell, Is there a need for the medical angiologist? Eur. J. Vasc. Endovasc. Surg. 24 (2002) 4.

[6] Directives 93/16/CEE, 97/50/CE, 98/21/CE, 98/63/CE and 99/46/CE.

[7] S. Zappalà, On the proposal for a directive of the European Parliament and of the Council on the recognition of professional qualifications. Working Document—Committee on Legal Affairs and the Internal Market-PE 324.175 (2002).

[8] E. Borman, Quality assurance of clinical practice, UEMS Policy Paper, Draft 6—Meeting of the Sections with the Management Council—Brussels May 7th 2003.

International Congress Series 1272 (2004) 38–40

ELSEVIER

www.ics-elsevier.com

# Introduction to the European Board of Vascular Surgery

John H.N. Wolfe*

*Consultant Vascular Surgeon, St Mary's Hospital, Praed Street, London, W2 1NY, UK*

Within the UEMS, we have opted to divide the responsibilities for vascular surgery between the Division and the Board. Broadly speaking, the President of the Division, with the support of the Council, looks outward towards cooperation with other specialists (most recently, in particular, with the angiologists) and the relationship with central committees that affect the delivery of vascular services around Europe. Note, for example, our successful lobbying regarding Directive COM (2002) 119. Alterations to the text allow vascular specialists to be recognised among different European countries. The Division also looks towards the Section of Surgery and our relationship with other surgical specialties. We strongly believe that this should be on an equal footing and that all surgical specialties should form a federation, but that each surgical specialty should have a section of its own.

Conversely, the Board looks inwards to the orchestration and delivery of vascular education within our specialty. It is most important in the complex relationship between national societies, European societies, the European Board of Vascular Surgery and other European boards that we all recognise our own particular roles and fulfil these obligations whilst not attempting to embark upon commitments that are beyond our remit.

European organisations have a clear responsibility to provide a service for the European Community and cannot, and should not, attempt to impose upon national organisations within each country. These activities are focussed on their own vascular surgeons and provided for by national societies. European bodies have no role in these activities, but should a national group wish to encourage the involvement of other Europeans it can call upon the support of the European Board.

The European vascular societies have the responsibility for encouraging and providing education in the form of annual meetings, symposia and workshops. This is clearly not the remit of the European Board of Surgery, whose role is to judge and encourage these activities through its role as an accreditor of CME. Societies and organisers provide CME, the European Board accredits CME. As the Board, we have recognised this responsibility and have transparent and clear principles relating to CME activity so that our methods of

* Tel.: +44-207-886-6666; fax: +44-207-631-5341.
*E-mail address:* John.Wolfe@st-marys.nhs.uk (J.H.N. Wolfe).


doi:10.1016/j.ics.2004.04.077

accreditation are accepted and respected [1]. Johan van Bockel, as the current Chairman of the CME Committee, deals with this in more detail in chapter X, but suffice it to say that that we now have clear and transparent guidelines on CME accreditation for meetings and symposia, workshops and, most recently, on the important relationship with industry [2]. We hope that this CME activity provides a template for all European societies and universities within which to provide educational opportunities that are recognised throughout Europe.

The European Board is also proud of the progress it has made with the European Vascular Exam (EBSQ-Vasc); now those who pass it are Fellows of the European Board of Vascular Surgery (FEBVS). This exam is reported in greater detail by David Bergqvist, Chairman of the Examiners, in chapter Y. The exam was started in 1996 and is now developing into an exam that will be of value to most Europeans. It is the first modern exam to introduce a technical skills exercise into a surgical exam [3]. With the cooperation of the various nation states of Europe, this could be a unifying process that provides a standard of vascular training to which all countries can aspire. The strength of Europe is its cultural diversity and variations in approach to surgery. This rich variety of inspiration and abilities need not be homogenised into a grey mass, and I hope that variations in training, surgical approach and priorities will continue to be a source of amicable discussion between the various countries. This diversity of talent enriches us all. Nevertheless, the provision of an exam available to all vascular surgeons who are European citizens allows equal opportunity and a qualification that will, we hope, be respected throughout Europe. The provision of CCST and admission to the Surgical Specialist Register as a vascular surgeon remains the responsibility of each nation. I stress that a European qualification cannot, and does not, wish to bypass national accreditation but, as a respected qualification, may be used by the countries as part of the accreditation process. As a service to the medical associations of these countries, we hope that we can provide a fair and respected qualification, which is available to all.

In order to sit this exam, the trainee must perform a minimum number of vascular operations and meet other criteria. In order to facilitate the documentation of these operations, the European Board has also suggested a logbook that allows easy documentation of experience for the trainee (this is discussed in more detail by Domenico Palombo in chapter Z). We also hope that by documenting experience the trainee will be empowered to discuss his/her training needs with his/her trainers. It is quite clear that the level of experience obtained in different programmes in Europe is almost infinitely variable.

We have also started the documentation of vascular centres in various countries and educational facilities and clinical experience available in these vascular centres. In Germany, this process is well developed and their experience is useful to us all. In the future, these vascular centres may be accredited for the vascular training they provide, but we are currently at a very early stage of this process. All activities of the Board should be seen to encourage education and training and also to support innovative initiatives. To designate units as vascular centres without careful consideration of the consequences could become divisive and counterproductive, but in due course, when carefully considered criteria have been developed, this system should allow the free flow of both trainees and mature surgeons between different European units and thus further enrich our specialty.

## 1. Conclusion

The European Board is a young and vital body that has already developed a transparent and effective CME process that is utilised by European vascular meetings. The Exam has also proved a success and we hope that this will be used as a benchmark by young surgeons throughout Europe. These initiatives must not ossify, but grow and develop with an exciting and fast changing specialty.

## References

[1] J.H.N. Wolfe, European CME (editorial), Eur. J. Vasc. Endovasc. Surg. 18 (1999) 277–279.
[2] J.H. van Bockel, et al., Guidelines for CME Activities Accredited by the EBVS, Eur. J. Vasc. Endovasc. Surg. (2004) (in press).
[3] V.A. Pandey, et al., on Behalf of the European Board of Vascular Surgery, Validity of an exam assessment in surgical skill: EBSQ-VASC pilot study (ESVS 2003 Winning Article), Eur. J. Vasc. Endovasc. Surg. 27 (4) (2004) 341–348.

International Congress Series 1272 (2004) 41–45

www.ics-elsevier.com

# The role of the European society for vascular surgery

Michael Horrocks*

*European Society for Vascular Surgery, Royal United Hospital, University of Bath, 6th Floor, Norwood House, Bath BA2 7AY, UK*

*Keywords:* European Society of Vascular Surgery; Scientific and clinical research; New treatments and technology

The European Society of Vascular Surgery was first proposed at a meeting to take place in London in July 1986 with representatives of the European Chapter of the ISCVS and the Vascular Surgical Society of Great Britain and Ireland.

The proposal was as follows:

> It is proposed to discuss the formation of a European Society of Vascular Surgery to meet annually for the presentation and discussion of papers on vascular topics. It is intended that membership should be open to Vascular Members of the European Society for Cardiovascular Surgeons and members of National Societies and other of similar standing.

Those interested were invited to meet in the Clarence Room of the Metropole Hotel on Friday 4th July.

In any event, the meeting did not take place, probably because of a conflict of interest with the European Chapter of the ISCVS, but the proposal did not go away and was then discussed again at the following meeting of the Vascular Surgical Society of Great Britain and Ireland. In the meantime, the European Journal of Vascular Surgery was launched and publishers Grune and Stratton were selected. The Society managed to retain ownership of the title of the Journal in what has proven to be an extremely wise move and the European Society of Vascular Surgery Company Limited was set up in order to retain ownership of the title and management of the Journal.

From this modest beginning has grown a large and vibrant Society with its Journal, which has also proven to be a great success. The inaugural meeting of the ESVS was held on the 7th and 8th May 1987, and this took place at Charing Cross Hospital in London. Dr. Michael DeBakey gave the invited lecture on "Significant Vascular European Advances". The first President was Professor Hans Mhyre from Trondheim and the first Honorary

* Tel.: +44-1225-383770; fax: +44-1225-383669.
*E-mail address:* S.Needham@bath.ac.uk (M. Horrocks).

0531-5131/
doi:10.1016/j.ics.2004.06.012

Secretary was Hero Van Urk. Simon Darke was appointed as the first Honorary Treasurer. The first meeting turned out to be a great success with Presidents of most of the European Vascular Societies present and an excellent cross section of prominent Vascular Surgeons from throughout Europe.

The following year, the meeting was in Rotterdam, and this proved to be even more of a success with an excellent Scientific Programme and an enjoyable social calendar. Presentations at the Society were converted into original articles for the European Journal of Vascular Surgery and the whole enterprise became increasingly successful. In the early days, membership was in the order of 200 people but has steadily increased, and last year, in Dublin, there were 1750 registrants for a packed 2-day Programme. This was comprised of a mixture of scientific papers and symposia on current topics. In addition, there were specific educational and training initiatives and opportunities to review new technologies presented in the large trade exhibition. At the same time, many collaborative research projects were being reviewed and discussed at satellite meetings.

The role of the Society can now be divided into a number of separate interactive activities. The Society is run on a day-to-day basis by the Secretariat, which moves from country to country with the appointment of each successive Secretary General. Full details of the constitution and workings of the Society can be found on the website www.esvs.org.

The Society is organised by the Council, and each country with 10 or more Society members is entitled to a Council Member. As the Society has grown in size and new member countries have come on board, the Council has gradually increased in size. The members of the ESVS in each country vote for their Council representative who sits on Council for 3 years. Council meets at least twice a year, usually once in London at the Charing Cross Meeting and then again before the Annual General Meeting (wherever that might be). The Annual Meeting moves from country to country providing a wonderful opportunity for members to visit the many capital cities of Europe and to experience the local culture and slant put on to the meeting by the Local Organising Committee.

As the Society has grown in size and influence, its roles have become more extensive and are outlined in the following.

## 1. Presentation of scientific and clinical research

This has been the most important role of the Annual Meeting of the Society and remains the primary reason for the Society's existence. We try to attract the principal research output from all major Vascular Units throughout Europe to be presented at the plenary session of the Annual General Meeting. The Scientific Sessions are greatly competed for and approximately 10 papers are submitted for each one accepted. A condition of acceptance is that an original article must be written and presented to the Editor of the European Journal of Vascular Surgery (now the European Journal of Vascular and Endovascular Surgery), prior to presentation. A large panel of Reviewers are used to score papers submitted according to their category and may be scored by up to 10 Reviewers in order that the Society obtains the very best papers presented. The whole exercise has become so successful now that the Reviewing Panel has to be increased year by year in order to accommodate the increasing number of submissions. More than 90% of papers presented are subsequently published providing a permanent reference to this work. Papers are only published after they have been critically reviewed by the Editorial Panel of the Journal.

The Annual General Meeting is now themed so that each session has a central topic, which is relevant to all the papers, allowing comparisons and more fruitful discussion. Approximately 15 min is allowed for each paper, half for the formal presentation and half for discussion and it is often the discussion which creates the most interest, allowing free and unrehearsed comments and questions from the floor. A major feature of the Society has been the brisk and incisive questioning at the discussion, a feature not found in many other Societies. It is widely regarded as a great honour to be chosen to present at these plenary Scientific Sessions and a large attentive audience always ensures careful preparation and high quality presentations. The best Scientific Paper and the best Clinical Paper are rewarded with Society prizes.

## 2. New treatments and technology

A very important part of the Society's function has been to allow presentation of new treatments and technologies to the membership. This has been done in the form either of an original paper or as part of a Society Symposium. The constant interchange of ideas, treatment regimes and new technologies between the members of different countries has proven to be a fertile area for mutual education for Vascular Surgeons. The gradual breakdown of language barriers and the increased travel between countries has enabled a much broader spread of treatment regimes across the European continent. The ability to present large series of patients with a particular management regime has led to changes in practice with consequent improvement in patient care.

The presence of so many influential Vascular Surgeons in one site has encouraged industry to invest in the Society and in the Annual Meeting with sponsorship of many activities within the Society, notably the Symposia with schedules agreed between the Society and the Companies so that the best speakers are brought to air the important topics. These symposia have proven to be extremely popular and are an established integral part of the Annual General Meeting.

## 3. Training courses

We have been fortunate to have members who have been enthusiastic teachers and who have set up a series of training courses not only for surgeons in training but also for established surgeons who wish to learn new vascular or endovascular techniques. The growing use of models and simulators have complimented the increasing difficulty of training surgeons within restricted timetables. This has led to more emphasis on the use of training courses for honing skills and learning new techniques.

For the past few years, the Society has run skills courses in open and endovascular surgery which, although relatively costly in time and equipment, have proven to be extremely valuable and popular for those who have attended. In the future, the Society intends to build on these courses and to have additional training opportunities in partnership with industry. Across Europe, there are many excellent training facilities for endovascular and open surgery, and there are some animal laboratories in which it is possible to learn new techniques and to become competent to treat vascular disease without putting patients at risk. With the growing sense of shared responsibility from industry with regard to the introduction of new and potentially dangerous techniques, there has been an ever increasing sense of responsibility to ensure that training is complete before new techniques are employed. The European Society for Vascular Surgery has entered into a partnership allowing trainees to gain technical expertise without putting patients at risk. These new ventures are undoubtedly going to expand and will become an increasingly important part of the role of the ESVS.

## 4. Clinical research

With a move to large Multi-Centre Trials, necessary to answer important clinical questions, and with increasing collaboration with industry, the ESVS has hosted large research groups trying to answer some of these difficult clinical questions. The ability to attract large numbers of like-minded surgeons keen to participate in such research has resulted in many fruitful research projects with positive outcome. Fortunately, Vascular Surgery has already proven to be one of the most well-researched and evidence-based branches of surgery with an in-built culture of demanding good evidence for new treatments. The value of the Society in facilitating and promoting these research projects remains fundamental.

## 5. Interface with industry

The relationship between ESVS and industry has changed notably in the past few years from uneasy collaborators to one of a clear partnership. The ESVS could not have existed without support from industry, nor could industry survive without the input and experience of vascular surgeons. At the present time, we have an excellent relationship between the leaders of interested companies and the ESVS Council, leading to more collaborative education and training opportunities for the benefit of all. In the future, it is likely that there will be fewer and fewer larger companies with much more critical financial control of how they spend their money. The development of more education and training courses with increasing collaboration over research projects and the increased engagement of vascular surgeons in advising industry should further cement this relationship.

The presence of strong support of companies at the Annual General Meeting, particularly within the large trade exhibition, allows members of the Society to review all of the currently available products and to have an opportunity to see new products being developed for the market. This is also an important forum for industry allowing access to a large number of influential vascular surgeons ensuring future products will be relevant to the treatment of vascular disease.

## 6. Certification and examination

The ESVS has worked closely with UEMS to develop the European Board of Surgery Qualification in Vascular Surgery (EBSQ-VASC), and to provide Examiners for this important Examination. This has grown in stature and importance over the past few years, and the Society is proud of its contribution towards this development with Examiners being largely appointed from within the membership of the Society. There seems little doubt that a European Qualification in Vascular Surgery will be increasingly important, particularly as it seems likely that vascular surgery will become a recognised mono-specialty across Europe. It may be that the EBSQ-VASC will become the recognised Qualification for Vascular surgery across Europe in the future.

## 7. Personal benefits

Perhaps one of the most important aspects of the European Society is that of friendship and camaraderie. Year on year, like-minded surgeons meet at the Annual General Meeting to exchange views on the art and science of Vascular Surgery, in the process forming firm friendships which have proven to be enduring and fruitful. Out of these friendships have spawned many important collaborative research projects, clinic trials, and exchange of trainees, all of which have been to the benefit of vascular surgery. Equally important, members have had the opportunity to travel all over Europe visiting quite distinct destinations with their own customs and culture. Each local organiser has stamped their personal mark on the Annual Meeting, with colourful social events, which have proven to be both enjoyable and educational. The continuing increase in membership, particularly amongst the young vascular surgeons, with the Society's ability to sponsor new members from poorer countries, has been an important feature of the ESVS and one which consecutive Councils have been keen to promote.

## 8. Conclusion

The ESVS has proven to be an enduring and steadily improving focus for the practice and development of vascular surgery throughout Europe. Its success was founded on a clear vision for the development of vascular surgery as a mono-specialty coupled to a Journal which has been successfully promoted so as to attract the best original scientific vascular work from within Europe. Increasing time restraints in training and rapid advances in the methods of treating vascular disease have both required a central organisation to facilitate education and teaching. The ESVS has been successful in achieving this aim, but the engagement of future generations of vascular surgeons will remain crucial in ensuring the Society's continued success in the future.

International Congress Series 1272 (2004) 46–51

www.ics-elsevier.com

# The European Board of Surgery Qualification in Vascular Surgery

David Bergqvist*

*Department of Surgery, University Hospital, Uppsala SE-751 85, Sweden*

*Keywords:* Vascular surgery

Vascular surgery has different status among the surgical specialities in Europe. Right now, there are three models: a specialty on its own, a specialty after a variable period of the so-called common trunk surgery or a profile domain within the specialty of general surgery. It would be rather naïve to insist upon just one way to look at the organization and training of vascular surgery within Europe, and perhaps it is even better with some variations and possibilities to focus on differences, which sometimes may lead forward to a fruitful synthesis and thereby, a strength [1]. With the new opportunities for increased manpower mobility between EU countries, it seems, however, important to have a common level of knowledge and an agreed basic standard among vascular surgeons, despite the country they come from. The motivation for an examination in vascular surgery, therefore, would be

- to harmonize knowledge and skills
- to indicate that the candidate has passed a structured training programme
- to guarantee a minimal level of competence, which would seem important for the patient, the hospitals and also the candidates sitting the examination, i.e., the future vascular surgeons.

The harmonization of required knowledge and skills throughout Europe would have the potential to also harmonize vascular surgical education and training between the countries [2]. This would then facilitate the free movement of vascular surgeons among the EU countries, which actually has been adopted in an EC directive from 1975.

Throughout the history of the Division and Board of Vascular Surgery, there has been discussion on a formalized examination that was stimulated and decided upon under the presidency of Peter Harris. The development and structuring of the format

* Tel.: +46-18-611-4633; fax: +46-18-611-4632.
*E-mail addresses:* david.bergqvist@surgsci.uu.se, david.bergqvist@kirurgi.uu.se (D. Bergqvist).


doi:10.1016/j.ics.2004.04.076

was very much the dedicated work of Bernhard Nachbur from Switzerland, with valuable and professional support from the two Secretaries-General, first Jaap Buth from the Netherlands and then Christos Liapis from Greece [3,4]. The examinations have taken place in direct connection with the annual meeting of the European Society for Vascular Surgery (ESVS), the first examination being held in Venice in 1996 and yearly thereafter.

## 1. The structure of the examination

In the first part of the examination, the candidates' credentials are checked to see whether they fulfil the requirements based on the CCST (Certificate of Completion of Specialist Training) and the operation logbook listing to reflect surgical experience, and thus are eligible for the second part of the examination. The administrative and screening part is provided in cooperation with the EBSQ Eligibility Office, previously in Guernsey and now in London, U.K. This is all based on the applicant's written information, which must be signed by his or her supervisor. The training in vascular surgery must have taken place in one of the 15 EU countries, a UEMS country (Cyprus, Iceland, Norway, Switzerland) or an associated UEMS country (Croatia, Hungary, Malta, Poland, Slovakia, Slovenia, Czech Republic, Turkey, Estonia, Romania, or Azerbaijan). The required numbers of operations are listed in Table 1. The assessment committee, under the chairmanship of the EBSQ-VASC chairman, makes the final decision in the selection process for eligibility to participate in the second part of the examination. Supplementary information may be considered necessary and will be provided by the national representatives. Having passed this first part of the examination, the candidates are admitted to the second part, the viva voce assessment.

Table 1
Number of surgical procedures needed to be allowed to take part in the second viva voce part of the EBSQ-VASC examination (these figures are currently being amended to reflect the 2 years of surgical practice before the examination)

| | A | B | C |
|---|---|---|---|
| Femoropopliteal bypass | 15 | 15 | 10 |
| Femorodistal bypass | 15 | 10 | 10 |
| Aortic aneurysm—elective | 10 | 10 | 10 |
| Aortic aneurysm—rupture | 10 | 5 | 5 |
| Aortofemoral bypass | 10 | 10 | 10 |
| Carotid | 15 | 10 | 5 |
| PTA and stenting | 15 | 15 | – |
| Varicose veins | 10 | 10 | 10 |
| Others, complex procedure[a] | 25 | – | – |
| | | | |
| Credit point/procedure | 1 | 4 | 2 |
| Credit points per category | 125 | 340 | 120 |
| Total for vascular surgery | 585 | | |

A: First assistant; B: principal surgeon assisted by trainer; C: principal surgeon not assisted by trainer.

[a] Includes thoracoabdominal aneurysm, carotid body tumour, deep vein reconstruction, vascular malformation, vertebral artery reconstruction, pediatric vascular surgery.

Here, the candidates meet six to nine assessors. The examination consists of three parts:

1. Case analysis. For one hour, the candidates analyse and discuss three patients, randomly selected by numbers within three main groups of clinical problems (one aneurysm case, one case with limb ischaemia and one belonging to a miscellaneous group). With the majority of cases, relevant illustrations are included, such as clinical pictures, X-ray films, details from operations, etc. During the examination in Dublin in 2003, the 34 cases were on CD-ROMs, whereas previously there were 24 cases in books. The questions are accompanied with expected answers to try to have as little subjectivity and bias as possible when the assessors give points to the candidates' answers. In Table 2, one case presentation with the first question is exemplified.
2. Scientific article. During the first years, this part was more of an examination in statistics and trial methodology, but it has been changed to deal with the candidates' ability to read, analyse and assess the quality of a scientific paper. Although the majority of vascular surgeons sitting the examination are not scientists, it is important that a scientific paper can be read critically, leading to the right conclusions, not necessarily the same as those drawn by the authors. The candidates are requested to read for 30 minutes one paper relevant to vascular surgery. In the paper, the abstract, the conclusions and the discussion are deleted and the candidate has to answer specific and relevant questions regarding the paper.
3. Overall assessment. In this part, the candidates' logbooks are scrutinized and discussed. This is a way of assessing that the candidates have the surgical knowledge, which is in keeping with their given numbers of operations. There are also questions on how patients are followed up, which quality control they receive postoperatively, which kind of continuous medical education (CME) or continuous professional development

Table 2
An example of a case from the Case Analysis part of the examination (no longer included, but used here to illustrate the format)

Case number 7

G.M., 84 years of age, female

The patient is sent to the vascular unit for critical ischaemia of the left leg with stage IV disease (rest pain since 4 weeks and necrosis of the large toe). Ankle systolic pressure as measured by Doppler ultrasound is 40 mm Hg at the dorsum of the foot, not measurable over the posterior tibial artery. Digital subtraction contrast angiography is performed on the basis of which a PTA procedure was tried without success.

| | |
|---|---|
| 1 Question | Four sequential figures, 25, 26, 27 and 28, show the angiography of the affected leg. Now you<br>a. read the angiograms and comment<br>b. propose a form of treatment |
| Expected answers | Ad a: detailed verbal description of the four pictures.<br>Ad b: a femorodistal bypass but foot runoff must be better visualized. |
| Notes for candidate answers: Assessment | 3 points if (a) and (b) are answered to the full satisfaction of the assessors.<br>2 points if the assessment is correct, but better angiographic runoff visualization is not asked for.<br>0 points if assessment of angiography and the therapeutic solution are not correct. |

(CPD) the candidates take part in and how they deal with morbidity and mortality conferences.

In the declaration of principles, which all candidates have to read, it is clearly stated that they must achieve a 2/3 (67%) success rate in each and every one of the three parts of the examination. The country representatives on the UEMS Division and Board of Vascular Surgery, in collaboration with their national societies, choose the assessors. The examination is held in English. There is no formal translation, but the candidates can ask for assistance in the various European languages. It is important to differentiate between lack of knowledge and linguistic difficulties. After assessment, the assessors check and discuss the results and decide on pass or fail. So far, there have been between 13 and 26 eligible candidates every year, making a total of 145 through the 8 years and the overall passing rate is 78%. (Table 3). Comparing the two 4-year periods during which there has been an examination, the failure rate has increased. The expected failure rate is not known but the present level seems to guarantee a certain level of difficulty, representing an examination, which is relevant and demanding. Thus, there is a certain risk of failure. After having passed the examination, the candidates are awarded the EBSQ-VASC diploma, in future rendering them the title, Fellow of the European Board of Vascular Surgery.

## 2. The future

One question that has been repeatedly discussed is whether the number of operations required to be able to sit the examination is unrealistically high and this is a matter for revision at the moment. Whatever the numbers will be in the future, it is important to keep them on a level that guarantees that the vascular trainees reach a certain technical skill and competence reflected in morbidity and mortality rates not differing from normative values. With a dedicated and supervised training programme, this EBSQ-VASC goal could be obtained as has recently been shown for carotid endarterectomy at a vascular centre in Amsterdam [5]. That supervised training in carotid surgery is safe for the patients has been reported previously [6–8]. Another question is the length and contents of the so-called common trunk, and here the solution will probably be to stick to the national requirements in the various countries. With the new European working time directive [9,10], it also seems important to evaluate the effect of training in the various countries within the EU.

Table 3
Number of candidates sitting and passing the EBSQ-VASC examination

| Year and place | Number of eligible candidates | Number of passed candidates |
|---|---|---|
| 1996 Venice | 15 | 13 |
| 1997 Lisbon | 20 | 16 |
| 1998 Paris | 16 | 13 |
| 1999 Copenhagen | 13 | 13 |
| 2000 London | 17 | 12 |
| 2001 Lucerne | 26 | 17 |
| 2002 Istanbul | 24 | 17 |
| 2003 Dublin | 14 | 12 |
| | 145 | 113 (78%) |

At the moment, the case histories are 34, but the aim is to build up a large stock of cases, covering the majority of problems that may confront a vascular surgeon. Most of the preparation of the examination obviously comes from everyday clinical experience together with reading textbooks and vascular surgical journals. Today, there is also a book that should help in preparing potential candidates for the examinations, both the EBSQ-VASC and the American Board in vascular surgery [11]. Real-life case scenarios are given with clinical relevant questions, followed by commentaries with key references and motivations for the answers. With the expansion of endovascular treatments for vascular patients, it has been considered appropriate to include specific questions on endovascular technique, and this problem is now under evaluation. PTA and stenting have already been included in the indicator procedures for a couple of years [4,12] (Table 1). Training in endovascular interventions shows, however, rather great variations among European countries.

We have tried to reduce subjectivity in assessment by using several assessors at every examination station, rotating the candidates between the assessors and having predefined correct answers for the various questions.

Another important question is how this theoretical examination reflects the practical surgical skills of the candidates. During the examination in Istanbul and Dublin, a technical skills assessment was included, in 2002 with selected candidates and in 2003 at full scale, but both years on a voluntary basis without influencing the outcome of the examination. The present President of the board, John Wolfe, has brought this experiment forward in a timely fashion. Analysing these data, one thing is clear, namely that there is no correlation between theoretical knowledge as marked in the viva voce examination and performance in practical skills exercise [13]. Every surgical teacher would perhaps have foreseen that, and the real question is how surgical skills should be assessed. This is at present a matter for discussion and evaluation. So far, the format for the pilot practical evaluation has been a three-station bench assessment evaluating dissection and ligation of the saphenofemoral junction on a bespoke model, anastomosis to the anterior tibial artery in a leg model and dexterity using a knot-tying simulator with electromagnetic motion analysis (the Imperial College Surgical Assessment Device). It is also important to have test models that are feasible and applicable throughout various countries [14]. A difficult and delicate, but important, point in this discussion is how to define criteria for a practical skills failure. Ideally, the unpractical colleagues must be identified and counselled much earlier so that he/she has the possibility to alter direction into a part of medicine where their knowledge is optimally utilized.

The number of candidates every year has varied between 13 and 26, and getting a more general acceptance for the examination will only be obtained if the successful candidates get something out of it. In the first place, they have verification that their experience and knowledge obtained during training has been satisfactory. From next year, the diploma will give the owner a title (Fellow of the European Board of Vascular Surgery, FEBVS), but for the majority of colleagues it would be a motivation to sit the examination if this quality mark would lead to a higher position in their professional career and/or a higher salary. The EBSQ-VASC examination is also considered for use as the speciality examination in countries where such an examination is not required yet. For instance, the Swedish Society for Vascular Surgery has expressed interest in having the European examination as their specialist examination. With the above in mind, my guess is that the number of candidates that will sit the EBSQ-VASC examination will increase in the future, which in turn will introduce some logistical problems and probably make it necessary to have it as a special administrative unit, not only at the ESVS meetings.

The format of the examination, with the above-mentioned possible revisions, will continue. One further problem, however, is how to weight the various parts of the examination in relation to each other and this problem is under evaluation at the moment. The case discussions are mainly clinically oriented and an open question is how much of basic science should be included in the curriculum of vascular surgery [15], and to which degree this should be part of the examination.

## References

[1] J.H. Wolfe, Training—vive la difference? Eur. J. Vasc. Endovasc. Surg. 18 (1) (1999) 1–3.

[2] J. Buth, et al., Harmonization of vascular surgical training in Europe. A task for the European Board of Vascular Surgery (EBVS), Cardiovasc. Surg. 8 (2) (2000) 98–103.

[3] J. Buth, B. Nachbur, European Board of Surgery Qualifications in Vascular Surgery (EBSQ-VASC) assessments. Three years' experience, Eur. J. Vasc. Endovasc. Surg. 18 (4) (1999) 360–363.

[4] C.D. Liapis, B. Nachbur, EBSQ-VASC examinations—which way to the future? European Board of Surgery Qualifications in Vascular Surgery, Eur. J. Vasc. Endovasc. Surg. 21 (5) (2001) 473–474.

[5] A. Rijbroek, W. Wisselink, J.A. Rauwerda, The impact of training in unselected patients on mortality and morbidity in carotid endarterectomy in a vascular training center and the recommendations of the European Board of Surgery Qualification in Vascular Surgery, Eur. J. Vasc. Endovasc. Surg. 26 (3) (2003) 256–261.

[6] A.M. Graham, G.C. Salasidis, A.M. Ferneini, Carotid endarterectomy in a vascular fellowship training program: good results with a consistent technique, Can. J. Surg. 38 (1) (1995) 39–41.

[7] A.W. Bradbury, et al., Supervised training in carotid endarterectomy is safe, Br. J. Surg. 84 (12) (1997) 1708–1710.

[8] A.R. Naylor, et al., Provision of training in carotid surgery does not compromise patient safety, Br. J. Surg. 85 (7) (1998) 939–942.

[9] T. Pickersgill, The European working time directive for doctors in training, BMJ 323 (7324) (2001) 1266.

[10] C.D. Liapis, Effects of limited work hours on surgical training, J. Am. Coll. Surg. 196 (4) (2003) 662–663.

[11] G. Geroulakos, et al., Vascular Surgery. Cases, Questions and Commentaries, Springer Verlag, London, 2003.

[12] C.D. Liapis, W.P. Paaske, Training in vascular surgery in Europe—the impact of endovascular therapy, Eur. J. Vasc. Endovasc. Surg. 23 (1) (2002) 1–2.

[13] V. Pandey, et al., Validity of an exam assessment in surgical skills: EBSQ-VASC pilot study, Eur. J. Vasc. Endovasc. Surg. 27 (2004) 341–348.

[14] S. Bann, et al., Objective assessment of technical skills of surgical trainees in Hong Kong, Br. J. Surg. 90 (10) (2003) 1294–1299.

[15] A.N. Sidawy, et al., Basic science curriculum in vascular surgery residency, J. Vasc. Surg. 33 (4) (2001) 854–860.

International Congress Series 1272 (2004) 52–55

www.ics-elsevier.com

# Training centres: differences in training[☆]

Jes Sandermann*

*Vascular Surgery Unit, Viborg Hospital, 8800 Viborg, Denmark*

**Abstract.** In order to provide optimal vascular surgical services in the future, it is essential to have good training centres, to provide good training programmes, have good trainers and basically to see that young doctors really want to become vascular surgeons. © 2004 Elsevier B.V. All rights reserved.

*Keywords:* Training centres; Vascular surgery; Training standards

The responsibility for the national training standards and the certification of specialists lies independently with the National Health Authorities. Apart from this, great work is being done within the European Union of Medical Specialists (UEMS) and especially in the EBVS (European Board for Vascular Surgery) in trying to harmonize the training standards in European countries.

The Charter on Training Medical Specialists in the European Community (1993) puts the above aspects into perspective together with overall guidelines for the training, the training institutions, the trainers and trainees. To secure this setup, UEMS has worked out a Charter on Visitation of Training Centres (1997) with guidelines for visits to training institutions to control that "all" is up to the defined high standards. Such inspections are taking place in several individual countries on a national basis. Inspection on the European level has not yet started in vascular surgery.

The way vascular surgery is organized in European countries varies a lot and owing to a rapid development towards mono-speciality status in some countries, the information soon differs from its actuality. At the moment, vascular surgery is a mono-speciality in Denmark, Finland, France, Greece, Italy, Portugal and Spain, a recognized sub-speciality in Austria, Germany, Luxemburg, Norway, (Switzerland) and the Netherlands and a surgical area of interest in Belgium, Ireland, Sweden and UK (mainly European Registry of Training Centres for Vascular Surgery data (EuReg-Vasc)). Because vascular surgery is becoming more and more delicate and thus able to justify a full-time job, it has taken

☆ EuReg-Vasc including national data, centre data and a list on specialist training centres in Europe can be found on www.uems-vasc.org under the Division for Vascular Surgery.

* Fax: +45-8927-3580.

*E-mail address:* jes.sandermann@sygehusviborg.dk (J. Sandermann).

0531-5131/ 
doi:10.1016/j.ics.2004.04.070

surgeons with a vascular interest more and more off the main surgical workload. Not dealing with general surgery for some time inevitably will bring the surgeon into pure vascular surgery and through time this will provide the foundation for the mono-speciality.

To describe this process, vascular surgery in Denmark became a recognized sub-speciality under surgery in 1983, the Danish Society for Vascular Society was founded and a pure vascular surgical training programme was set up. From 1994, all vascular operations were performed by vascular surgeons with the "old general surgeons" being retired or the last few having given up their vascular part. And today where vascular surgery is a mono-speciality, already less than 50% of the Danish vascular specialists/consultants are specialists in surgery as well as vascular surgery—this majority is doing very well as pure vascular surgeons. Of course the geographic conditions in Denmark has made our model with nine major vascular centres easy to achieve.

Today a training centre for upcoming vascular surgical specialists must deal with vascular cases 24 h a day all year round and have a sufficient case load for training. During the same hours, facilities and manpower for doing arteriograms must be available—most often performed by radiologists. Endovascular interventions must be available during daytime—optimal of course around the clock. To be responsible for vascular surgery that way it is hard to see this possibility without at least four vascular consultants to cover the on-call rota. Sharing the call for acute patients with another hospital still leaves the responsibility for the patients in your own unit with your team. A background population of at least 4–500,000 have shown to be an adequate size as the workload in the units must be sufficient to cover "the need" for both the consultants and the trainees which means around 70–100 operations per year for all.

Available EuReg-Vasc data from 1999 and 2002 are seen in Tables 1 and 2. The above-mentioned demands for a training unit seem to be satisfactorily fulfilled in many units. Italy, particularly, has a problem with too many trainees for a very small workload. The data are scarce, as many units are not registered. Only in Denmark, Sweden and the Netherlands are almost all the training units included. No register is better than the data put into it.

Based upon EuReg-Vasc data, the common trunk lasts median 4 years (range 1–8 years), where the countries with the mono-speciality lie lowest. Pure vascular training lasts median 3 years (range 2–4 years) where the countries with vascular surgery as a surgical interest lie lowest. Eight countries have a training programme and five have an examination before

Table 1
EuReg-Vasc data

| 1999 Data | Number of units | Vascular consultants | Background population | Number of operations | Number of trainees |
|---|---|---|---|---|---|
| Austria | 6 | 4 (2–6) | 1,250,000 (0.3–2.5 M) | 1649 (417–2077) | 3 (2–9) |
| France | 11 | 3 (2–9) | 850,000 (0.4–4 M) | 660 (226–1272) | 3 (1–5) |
| Italy | 11 | 7 (3–12) | 1,240,000 (0.25–5 M) | 698 (290–1255) | 9 (2–21) |
| Spain | 12 | 5 (4–10) | 600,000 (0.38–1.5 M) | 781 (365–1189) | 5 (0–8) |
| the Netherlands | 8 | 3 (2–5) | 750,000 (0.25–3 M) | 550 (342–1340) | 1 (1–2) |

The figures are given in median and range.

Table 2
EuReg-Vasc data

| 2002 Data | Number of units | Vascular consultants | Background population | Number of operations | Number of trainees |
|---|---|---|---|---|---|
| Belgium | 8 | 4 (2–6) | 275,000 (0.014–1.1 M) | 814 (606–1475) | 2 (1–4) |
| Croatia | 4 | 3 (3–6) | 425,000 (0.3–0.5 M) | 595 (226–760) | 2 (1–12) |
| Cyprus | 1 | 3 | 800,000 | 1009 | 2 |
| Denmark | 7 | 5 (3–5) | 630,000 (0.472–0.8 M) | 930 (625–1438) | 1 (1–3) |
| Finland | 3 | 4 (4–7) | 470,000 (0.25–1.4 M) | 490 (250–822) | 2 (1–6) |
| Germany | 5 | 2 (?–4) | 300,000 (0.17–1.5 M) | 1511 (624–2730) | 4 (2–5) |
| Ireland | 1 | 3 | 750,000 | 854 | 4 |
| Norway | 3 | 5 (4–7) | 550,000 (0.4–0.65 M) | 430 (340–475) | 2 (2–4) |
| Slovak Republic | 1 | 5 | 5,000,000 | 1354 | 5 |
| Sweden | 7 | 5 (2–7) | 550,000 (0.275–0.8 M) | 487 (206–1300) | 2 (0–4) |
| Switzerland | 3 | 2 (1–4) | 800,000 (0.3–1.3 M) | 582 (531–1400) | 2 (2–3) |
| UK | 1 | 3 | 400,000 | 617 | 2–5 |

Figures are given in median and range.

specialist recognition. Seven countries express a required number of operations of median 200 (range 105–820)—only three countries can specify the types included.

In general the training programmes contain less surgical skills the more purely vascular the country aims to be. With vascular surgery as an area of interest of course a full range of surgical skills must be included. Information on the training in the various countries can be obtained from the national members of the UEMS Division and Board of Vascular Surgery. The training programmes from the five Scandinavian countries were published in the EAVST Newsletter Vol. 6, Number 1, April 2002. A document on Training in Vascular Surgery in Great Britain and Ireland was published a couple of years ago by The Vascular Surgical Society of Great Britain and Ireland. The Austrian training programme was mentioned in an article in VascularNews June 2001, page 2.

Since April 1996, a vascular training programme from Spain is available in Spanish. Table 3 roughly shows the Spanish training programme. Relevant surgical and angiological competences are described.

Table 3
Spanish vascular surgical training programme (1996)

| | | | |
|---|---|---|---|
| First year | general surgery (9 months) | | thoracic surgery (2 months) |
| Second year | cardiology (2 months) | U.V.I. (3 months) | vascular surgery and angiology (6 months) |
| Third year | general surgery (3 months) | neurology (2 months) | vascular surgery and angiology (6 months, 1 month angioradiology) |
| Fourth year | cardiac surgery (4 months) | vascular surgery and angiology (7 months, 1 month angioradiology) | |
| Fifth year | vascular surgery and angiology (11 months) | | |

The technical skills to be achieved in general surgery are not very heavy and consist of explorative laparotomy through various abdominal incisions, appendectomy, groin hernia repair, biopsy from mammary gland, drainage of perianal abscess, excision of various cutaneous tumours, tracheostomy and paracenthesis.

The optimal training programme in vascular surgical specialist training must be the basis for the overall recognition of the vascular specialist all over Europe. Working in a purely vascular surgical unit the patients are very select, as the main abdominal catastrophe will be admitted to a surgical unit then transferring the ruptured aneurysms to vascular surgery. Ruptured aneurysms mistaken for a stone in the urinary tract will come from the urologists. If a patient coming to us is suspected of a ruptured aneurysm, but is suffering from something else, most often we will solve this problem by clinical examination or a CT-scan. For a vascular surgeon, having a patient with an acute abdomen, it does not matter which none-vascular disease is underlying. The patient is referred to the surgeons for further evaluation and treatment. I know that these thoughts can be difficult to handle for the surgical vascular surgeons, but at the end of the day this is the way it goes. Based upon this, just a very short introduction to surgery is necessary for the upcoming vascular surgeon. None of the surgical operations will ever be independently performed by a vascular surgeon, and then probably no surgeon will ever train the vascular surgeon to do them. Being a mono-speciality, the speciality itself will provide the trainee with the technical skills needed and the appropriate surgical attitude. The common trunk probably can be reduced to duration of less than a year where focused stays can be an option instead of being employed in some of the other surgical areas.

These days in Denmark the mentioned situation/discussion is running full steam. New specialist training programmes have been written and basically accepted by the National Health Authorities based strictly upon defined goals/objectives to be obtained, how to learn/teach them and how to evaluate them. The objectives are defined within seven areas, where the first is medical expertise (well known to us all) and the others being communication, collaboration, health advocating, management, professionalism and academic attitude. Besides the above-mentioned, there will also be economical/political aspects to discuss, and it is exciting to see whether these aspects, to some degree, will win over the objectives to be obtained as put forward. After specialisation another 2 years must be spent in one or two other vascular units to qualify as a consultant in vascular surgery.

The result of the implementation will be clear during 2004, and the new Danish training programmes hopefully will be available in English, too.

Harmonization of the European vascular surgical training should optimally end up with a uniform training programme containing the required minimum competences to become a vascular surgery specialist in Europe. Should any country, besides these requirements, want to have additional training for the qualification of consultant in vascular surgery they have to describe this. And should any country need more training in surgery to fulfil certain distant posts, they can add this training to the vascular training.

Then there just remains a language problem as the last obstacle.

International Congress Series 1272 (2004) 56–63

www.ics-elsevier.com

# European Board of Vascular Surgery: CME and CPPD activities

J.H. van Bockel*

*Department of Vascular Surgery, Leiden University Medical Center, P.O. Box 9600, 2300 RC Leiden, The Netherlands*

## 1. Introduction

Vascular surgeons, like all doctors, have been trained to provide patient care of the highest possible quality. Training includes medical school, specialist training and various additional courses. However, the medical world changes rapidly and much knowledge is usually outdated within several years. In order to keep updated, medical education should continue. Thus, medical education can be seen as a continuum. After medical school and residency training, continuing medical education (CME) is required to keep doctors up to date.

CME can be defined as "educational activities that serve to maintain, develop or increase the knowledge, skills and professional performance (and) relationships used by a physician to provide services for patients, the public or the profession [1]". It is widely agreed that continuing education is a professional responsibility for all practicing physicians and it has become increasingly important. However, the result of adequate CME should be broader than just an update of knowledge and should result in an improvement of the performance of doctors.

## 2. How effective is CME

Many feel that CME is often not successful in improving the performance of doctors. As a result, the effectiveness of CME has been studied during the last decade. The impact of various CME interventions on physician performance and health care outcomes were assessed by Davis et al. by performing a meta-analysis of randomized trials of educational programs, activities, or other interventions. They found that broadly defined CME interventions using practice-enabling or reinforcing strategies consistently improved physician performance and, in some instances, health care outcomes [2].

Davis et al. again reviewed the literature relating to the effectiveness of education strategies designed to change physician performance and health care outcomes. They

* Tel.: +31-71-5263610; fax: +31-71-5266750.
*E-mail address:* bockel@lumc.nl (J.H. van Bockel).


doi:10.1016/j.ics.2004.04.103

reviewed randomized, controlled trials of education strategies or interventions that objectively assessed physician performance and/or health care outcomes. These intervention strategies included educational materials, formal CME activities, outreach visits, such as academic detailing, opinion leaders, patient-mediated strategies, audit with feedback and reminders. They found 99 trials containing 160 interventions that met our criteria. Almost two-thirds of the interventions (101 of 160) displayed an improvement in at least one major outcome measure; 70% demonstrated a change in physician performance and 48% of interventions aimed at health care outcomes produced a positive change. Effective change strategies included reminders, patient-mediated interventions, outreach visits, opinion leaders and multifaceted activities. Audit with feedback and educational materials were less effective, and formal CME conferences or activities, without enabling or practice-reinforcing strategies, had relatively little impact. They concluded that widely used CME methods, such as conferences, have little direct impact on improving professional practice. CME providers seldom use more effective methods, such as systematic, practice-based interventions and outreach visits [3].

There is an increasing demand on doctors to ensure and improve care of their patients. A variety of approaches claim to provide solutions to the problems of health care delivery. Grol critically evaluated some of the approaches that gained popularity during the last decades: evidence-based medicine and clinical practice guidelines, professional development, assessment and accountability, patient empowerment and total quality management. He found that evidence regarding the impact and feasibility of the various approaches is mixed or simply lacking and that none of the popular models for improving clinical performance appear to be superior [4].

## 3. Efforts to make CME more effective

Classical CME approaches, providing educational materials, conferences and courses, seem to be not very effective for changing clinical performance [5–8]. Therefore, new approaches are being developed like continuous professional development, self-directed learning, problem-based learning, etc. that are based on theories of adult learning [9]. These techniques are more individualized, based on personal learning needs, require more active involvement and use educational materials, continuing medical education, interactive educational meetings, feedback on performance or combinations of these. However, it is not completely clear how effective these new approaches are since thorough evaluation has not yet been performed. A recent review suggests that these approaches are more effective than the traditional ones [7]. Several aspects of approaches aiming at better performance and improved patient care are reported by Grol (Table 1) [10].

Scientific evidence within clinical guidelines is probably an effective approach to improvement in clinical performance. However, currently too many guidelines are of questionable quality [11]. Guidelines are often not based on the best evidence available and the role of opinion leaders is not always clear [12]. Not many practice guidelines in surgery, and more specifically not in vascular surgery, are available. Only the Journal of Vascular Surgery has published some practice guidelines. This

Table 1
Aproaches to quality improvement and their assumptions on improving medical care

| Approach | Assumptions |
|---|---|
| Evidence-based medicine | Provisions of best evidence and convincing information leads to optimal decision-making and optimal care |
| Clinical practice guidelines | |
| Decisions aid | |
| Professional education and development | Bottom-up learning based on experiences in practice and individual learning needs leads to performance change |
| Self-regulation | |
| Recertification | |
| Assessment and accountability | Providing feedback on performance relative to peers, and public reporting of performance data, motivate change in practice routines |
| Feedback | |
| Accreditation | |
| Public reporting | |
| Patient-centered care | Patient autonomy and control over disease and care processes lead to better care and outcomes |
| Patient involvement | |
| Shared decision-making | |
| Total quality management and continuous quality improvement | Improving care comes from changing the systems, not from changes in individuals |
| Restructuring processes | |
| Quality systems | |
| Breakthrough projects | |

From Ref. [4].

lack is probably due to a lack of evidence of many surgical procedures and treatments.

## 4. CME and CPD

Over several years, continuing professional (physician) development (CP(P)D) has replaced CME. Currently, CME and CPD are used for the same activities. The objective of CME and CPD has become much more focused on ensuring that the learning activity contributes to an improvement of clinical practice and, thus, in better health care. The concept of CPD is much broader than CME and does not focus exclusively on lectures, symposia and participating in a course, but includes other activities as well. Examples are quality assurance systems (e.g. including output, feedback, registries of complications, etc.), looking at ways to credit the physicians for their activities in daily practice and outcome, long distance learning, "peer reviewing" for medical journals, searching and downloading articles (including answering questions) etc.

## 5. Accreditation of CME

Traditionally, CME activities are credited as 1 h of activity equals one "credit hour". Since CPD includes much more than lectures, the "credit hour" is a difficult denominator for a wide variety of learning activities. Therefore, the term "credits" has replaced the "credit hour" and can be used for "combined activities"; sometimes many hours (internet surfing) can be "packaged" for, say, 10 h. For example, setting up a complication registry takes many hours and may count for several "credits".

Since the sixties, the American Medical Association (AMA) has played an important role in stimulating CME in the USA. The AMA has given providers of CME (medical schools, etc.) clear instructions on how CME has to be organized. This is an important difference from the European system. In Europe, the events are being accredited, whereas in the USA providers are being accredited. For several years, the AMA has had reciprocity of credits with the UEMS (EACCME) [13]. A problem is that the recognition of credits from international activities by the National Authorities of the various European member states varies. These authorities have the right to accredit meetings, but they have no time and skills to do the evaluation. The specialist sections of the UEMS, like the European Board of Vascular Surgery (EBVS) [14,15], are better equipped to do this. The European Accreditation Council for Continuing Medical Education (EACCME) of the UEMS [16,17] and the Specialist Sections work closely together to accredit meetings. For example, the EBVS has been very active and accredits many European vascular meetings each year, according to simply published criteria [18]. CME activities have now been extended to technical skills workshops, again with specific and transparent criteria.

Currently, there is a voluntary system of CME in most European countries. In several countries, there is a tendency to make CME more strict and obligatory. In some member countries, there is a link to re-registration of medical specialists. It is expected that CME and CPD will become obligatory in the majority of the member states of the European Community in order to demonstrate that he or she is competent.

## 6. Summary

The emphasis of CPD is on maintaining the competence of practicing physicians. In that respect, CPD aims at bringing the research, as much evidence-based as possible, into practice by turning knowledge acquired by CME into performance of the participants. In addition, aspects such as patient safety, risk assessment, peer review of practice and quality management are all very important to achieve this goal.

## 7. The role of the European Board of Vascular Surgery in accreditation of CME and CPD activities [19]

Many CME activities are organized on a national level. For CME organized on a European level, the European Board of Vascular Surgery of the UEMS (Union Européenne des Médecins Spécialistes) has accepted a responsibility concerning the quality of these CME activities. It is important to realize that the EBVS is not a provider of CME, but must be seen as an independent authority that by its activities may assist as a clearinghouse for CME credits from a European to a national level. The EBVS has proposed accreditation for European Vascular CME activities since 1999 [20]. The CME Committee has been very active and credits many European vascular meetings each year, according to simply published criteria. Criteria for CME initially focussed on major meetings in order to ensure that our criteria were reliable. CME activities have now been extended to technical skills workshops, again with specific and transparent criteria.

In addition to accreditation, the EBVS may stimulate those activities that particularly aim at improving skills and knowledge that may be directly applied to improve clinical performance. This implies that activities in European meetings, like symposia with best evidence on a particular topic, overviews, state of the art lectures, etc. deserve special attention because these activities can be anticipated to improve the performance of vascular specialists. In the future, distant learning using internet technology may be a very useful addition to CPD as well.

Traditionally, the pharmaceutical and medical device manufacturers have generously supported CME for physicians. Without industrial support, the quality of many activities would have been less optimal and sometimes impossible. During the last decade, both physicians, editorial boards of scientific journals and authorities have increasingly scrutinised the role of industry in support of these activities [21–23]. The basis for the concern is that scientific activities may be used for promotional activities without clearly identifying these activities as such. Even in 1993, Mannick reported on the "scientific symposium", grafted onto the national meetings. For many of these, both the program and the speakers were picked and sponsored by a company. Under these circumstances, an unbiased presentation is difficult to attain [24]. It is clear that a conflict of interest may easily occur if organizers of CME activities need the support of the industry. In fact, travel funds, honoraria for nominal consultancies, free lunches, elegant dinners accompanied by product demonstrations and guest lectures with favourable views of the sponsors' products all threaten our integrity [25]. Fortunately, both CME providers and the industry have recognized this issue and both are keen to resolve the issue.

The CME Committee of the European Board of Vascular Surgery has discussed this issue at length and believes that for both CME providers and industry, as well as for the participants of CME activities, it would be helpful to provide clear and objective guidelines describing the relationship between the various parties. These guidelines are meant to stimulate a healthy and clear relationship between organizers of CME activities and the industry. The EBVS of the UEMS approved these Guidelines at the meeting of 2nd September 2003 in Dublin. The Guidelines are published on the website of the EBVS and will be given to both CME providers and the industry where appropriate. For practical purposes, the Guidelines have been subdivided into those for providers of CME activities, speakers and faculty, and industrial sponsors. The guidelines will be evaluated at regular time intervals and comments are encouraged, which will be used by the CME Committee to propose improvement of these guidelines to the European Board of Vascular Surgery in the future.

## 8. Guidelines

### *8.1. For organizers of CME activities*

Physicians involved in providing CME activities should ensure that the program is balanced.

Physicians who serve as presenters, moderators, or other faculty at CME conferences should ensure that research findings and therapeutic recommendations are based upon scientifically accurate, up-to-date information and are presented in a balanced, objective manner.

All conflicts of interest or biases, such as a financial connection to a particular commercial company or product, should be disclosed by faculty members to the audience in the programme and/or at the beginning of a presentation. Thus, faculty with specific expertise due to relations with the industry can be invited but should disclose the relationship.

A direct financial relationship between speakers and industry should be discouraged. Speakers and faculty should not accept direct subsidies from industry to pay for the costs of travel, lodging or other personal expenses. Costs should be reimbursed by the organizer/provider of the CME activities.

The scientific programme committee is responsible for moderators, presenters and other faculty and welcomes suggestions from those companies that have been generous enough to support the programme. Clearly, the final responsibility for the moderators, presenters and other faculty lies with the scientific committee.

Non-CME activities, i.e. primarily promotional seminars, should be clearly identified as such in the programme.

### *8.2. For speakers and other faculty*

Speakers and other faculty involved in providing CME activities should present a broad range of scientifically supportable viewpoints related to the topics.

Speakers and other faculty who present, chair or moderate, at CME conferences should ensure that research findings and therapeutic recommendations are based on scientifically accurate, up-to-date information and are presented in a balanced, objective manner.

All conflicts of interest should be disclosed by faculty members to the audience in the programme and/or at the beginning of a presentation.

A direct financial relationship between speakers or other faculty and industry should be discouraged. Speakers and faculty should not accept direct subsidies from industry to pay for the costs of travel, lodging or other personal expenses. Costs should be reimbursed by the organizer/provider of the CME activities.

Non-CME activities, i.e. primarily promotional seminars, should be clearly identified as such in the programme.

### *8.3. For industrial sponsors*

Financial support of CME activities is greatly appreciated by the organisers of CME activities, and it is gratefully recognized that these activities would not be viable without industrial sponsorship. The support should be provided by educational grants to the organisers of the CME activities.

A direct financial relationship between speakers or other faculty and industry should be discouraged. Speakers and faculty should not accept direct subsidies from industry to pay for the costs of travel, lodging, or other personal expenses. Costs should be reimbursed by the organizer/provider of the CME activities.

The scientific programme committee is responsible for moderators, presenters and other faculty and welcome suggestions from those companies that have been generous enough to support the programme. Clearly, the final responsibility for the moderators, presenters and other faculty lies with the scientific committee.

CME symposia, supported by a sponsor, should be fully acknowledged in the appropriate section of the programme. However, a company name in the title of the symposium unintentionally suggests a promotional relationship. For this reason, sponsor names should not be included in the title of the CME symposium.

Non-CME activities, i.e. primarily promotional seminars, should be clearly identified as such in the programme.

## References

[1] AMA PRA Information Booklet for Physicians V3.0. (http://www.ama-assn.org/ama/pub/category/2923.html).

[2] D.A. Davis, et al., Evidence for the effectiveness of CME. A review of 50 randomized controlled trials, JAMA 268 (9) (1992) 1111–1117.

[3] D. Davis, et al., Impact of formal continuing medical education: do conferences, workshops, rounds, and other traditional continuing education activities change physician behavior or health care outcomes? JAMA 282 (9) (1999) 867–874.

[4] R. Grol, Improving the quality of medical care: building bridges among professional pride, payer profit, and patient satisfaction, JAMA 286 (20) (2001) 2578–2585.

[5] A.D. Oxman, et al., No magic bullets: a systematic review of 102 trials of interventions to improve professional practice, CMAJ 153 (10) (1995) 1423–1431.

[6] D.A. Davis, et al., Changing physician performance. A systematic review of the effect of continuing medical education strategies, JAMA 274 (9) (1995) 700–705.

[7] D. Davis, et al., Impact of formal continuing medical education: do conferences, workshops, rounds, and other traditional continuing education activities change physician behavior or health care outcomes? JAMA 282 (9) (1999) 867–874.

[8] J.H. Tanne. Requiring doctors to take part in continuing medical education doesn't improve heart attack care. BMJ 328 (7441) (2004) 664.

[9] N.L. Bennett, et al., Continuing medical education: a new vision of the professional development of physicians, Acad. Med. 75 (12) (2000) 1167–1172.

[10] R. Grol, Improving the quality of medical care: building bridges among professional pride, payer profit, and patient satisfaction, JAMA 286 (20) (2001) 2578–2585.

[11] T.M. Shaneyfelt, M.F. Mayo-Smith, J. Rothwangl, Are guidelines following guidelines? The methodological quality of clinical practice guidelines in the peer-reviewed medical literature, JAMA 281 (20) (1999) 1900–1905.

[12] N.K. Choudhry, H.T. Stelfox, A.S. Detsky, Relationships between authors of clinical practice guidelines and the pharmaceutical industry, JAMA 287 (5) (2002) 612–617.

[13] http://www.uems.be/d-0234-e.htm.

[14] http://www.uemssurg.org/vascsurg.html.

[15] http://www.uems-vasc.org/.

[16] http://www.uems.be/eaccme.htm.

[17] http://www.euro-prm.org/board/cme/continuous_med_education.htm.

[18] http://www.uems.be/vasu-cme.htm.

[19] J.H. van Bockel, et al., Guidelines for CME Activities Accredited by the EBVS, Eur. J. Vasc. Endovasc. Surg. 27 (5) (2004) 534–536.

[20] J.H. Wolfe, European CME, Eur. J. Vasc. Endovasc. Surg. 18 (4) (1999) 277–279.

[21] L. Tritsmans, et al., Pharmaceutical company trials and the integrity of medical research, Lancet 347 (9015) (1996) 1628–1629.

[22] E. Wager, How to dance with porcupines: rules and guidelines on doctors' relations with drug companies, BMJ 326 (7400) (2003) 1196–1198.
[23] K. Abbasi, R. Smith, No more free lunches, BMJ 326 (7400) (2003) 1155–1156.
[24] J.A. Mannick, Vascular surgeons—are they for sale? J. Vasc. Surg. 17 (2) (1993) 245–248.
[25] J.W. Jones, L.B. McCullough, Surgeon–industry relationships: ethically responsible management of conflicts of interest, J. Vasc. Surg. 35 (4) (2002) 825–826.

International Congress Series 1272 (2004) 64–71

www.ics-elsevier.com

# Clinical governance

Roger N. Baird*

*Royal Infirmary, Bristol BS2 8HW, UK*

## 1. Introduction

Primum non nocere—first do no harm.

Human error in surgery can never be completely eliminated, but the opportunities for it to occur can be reduced. When error does happen, its impact can be minimised. As Napoleon said of his generals, the best vascular surgeon is the one who makes the fewest mistakes.

Research has shown that avoidable adverse events are much more common in vascular surgery than previously recognised. It may come as a surprise that the public and politicians feel that the medical profession has tolerated much higher levels of error and risk than would be acceptable in other sectors in which the public is being served.

Studies from the UK [1,2] have focused on claims arising from the treatment of varicose veins. In one of these studies, the authors concluded that the likely cause of most claims was failure to advise patients about potential risks and expected benefits of the treatment concerned [2].

| Cause | Number of cases | Percentage |
|---|---|---|
| Nerve damage | 76 | 31.2 |
| Incorrect or unsatisfactory surgery | 36 | 14.8 |
| Discoloration and scarring | 21 | 8.6 |
| Femoral vein damage | 16 | 6.6 |
| Infection | 15 | 6.1 |
| Femoral artery damage | 13 | 5.3 |
| Deep vein thrombosis | 11 | 4.5 |
| Tourniquet damage | 5 | 2 |
| Miscellaneous | 51 | 20.9 |
| Total | 244 | 100 |

Similar considerations apply to arterial surgery. Examples include late referrals and technical failures in diabetics who undergo major amputations and in ruptured aortic aneurysms.

* Tel.: +44-117-928-5141.

*E-mail address:* Roger.Baird@ubht.swest.nhs.uk (R.N. Baird).



doi:10.1016/j.ics.2004.05.029

Bad outcomes after surgical operations cause misery for patients and their families. The effects of a serious adverse and unexpected operative outcome go beyond the impact of the physical injury itself. Patients and their families feel let down by the surgeon. Powerful feelings are aroused, and although grief is a private matter, the injured and the bereaved can have feelings of blame, which are directed at the surgeon. Feelings of anger and bitterness persist despite explanation and an apology and can become a life-long preoccupation. The confidence of the surgical team is also shaken by unexpected serious adverse outcomes.

## 2. Professionalism

A profession is a vocation in which learning is used for the benefit of others. Medicine is a learned profession, along with divinity and the law. Surgery is a specialised skill requiring knowledge and judgment, which often involves uncertainty rather than total expertise, with the initially uncomfortable risk of being wrong. There are moral and ethical dimensions, and the capacity is required to develop and retain a fiduciary relationship in which the trust and confidence of the patients are gained. Clinical governance issues arise when the surgeon loses the trust and confidence of his patient. Self-regulation, to the greatest possible extent, is a hallmark of a profession.

### *2.1. The role of the team*

Good clinical practice depends on good professional relationships between the individual members of the clinical team. The best regulatory method for clinical performance is local, educationally based, multidisciplinary audit, including all those involved with the clinical work of the team. When clinical problems arise, any disagreements are discussed openly so that lessons are learned and changes in working practices discussed with a view to reducing the chance of similar problems recurring in the future, leading to better patient care.

If for any reason open discussion does not occur, there is the risk that someone who feels marginalized may form the view that the truth has been covered up and may criticize the surgeon outside the group to the hospital authorities and even to the patient, relatives or a journalist.

### *2.2. Internal review of serious clinical incidents*

Until reliable analytical methods exist to judge a surgeon's results against national norms, we continue to rely on the detailed investigation of individual serious clinical incidents. Examples include the following:

- late referral, with loss of the chance of cure;
- failure to diagnose a condition by proper and timely investigations;
- intra-operative injury to an adjacent vessel or nerve;
- failure of an arterial reconstruction by haemorrhage or thrombosis; and
- unexpected death during or after an operation.

The initial and best way of reviewing a serious clinical incident is from audit by the local multidisciplinary team, as mentioned above [3,4]. In this way, the incident can be analysed and lessons can be learned while the facts are fresh in the minds of the operating team. However, there are instances in which the trust of patients and relatives in the surgeon is undermined to such an extent that the facts have to be considered independently and an outside investigation is required.

## 3. Clinical governance

Governance is defined in the Oxford English dictionary as:

Promoting the happiness of society by punishment and reward.

Where substandard care has occurred, the main avenues open to patients and their relatives are the following. The most common course of action is a *complaint* to the hospital, which is dealt with locally. In more serious cases, a lawyer lodges a *claim* in the civil courts for financial compensation. Where the care has been grossly substandard, even reckless, severe sanctions are available, and the surgeon can face dismissal from his hospital appointment, withdrawal of his license to practice and even criminal prosecution. If a medical scandal has caused the confidence of the public in the healthcare service to be seriously undermined, the government may order a judicial inquiry.

### *3.1. Complaint to the hospital authorities*

Nowadays, the chief executive/managing director of a hospital is accountable for ensuring appropriate standards of care. In consequence, if a patient is dissatisfied and makes a complaint to the hospital, a manager institutes an internal investigation.

### *3.2. Local resolution*

An internal, managerially led inquiry, with the report signed by the chief executive of the hospital, often leads to local resolution, with an explanation and an apology, and achieves closure for the complainant. Procedures exist for the independent review of unresolved complaints by lay committees and the health service *ombudsman* can be approached to bulldoze any intractable administrative obstruction.

### *3.3. Independent professional review*

If a complaint raises issues about the surgeon's competence, conduct or health, the medical director may seek independent advice initially within the hospital and from outside experts.

There are several forms of independent professional review. Most involve the appointment of outside assessors, whom are nominated by national professional bodies. In Great Britain, these are the Royal College of Surgeons and the specialist surgical societies such as the Vascular Surgical Society of Great Britain and Ireland. The government has recently set up a National Clinical Assessment Authority to assist in these matters.

The results of an investigation may cause the medical director to withdraw or suspend the practice privileges of a surgeon and to institute disciplinary proceedings leading to dismissal.

In the UK in 2001/2002, no fewer than 206 consultants and doctors of all specialties were suspended from their NHS appointments for an unseemly long average time of almost a year, while allegations against them were being investigated, 40% of whom subsequently returned to work, according to a recent report from the National Audit Office (NAO) [5]. Unsurprisingly, the NAO recommends that the initial investigation be done very much more quickly, within 2 weeks.

### *3.4. Claim leading to financial compensation*

An aggrieved patient may consult a solicitor with a view to making a claim of negligence against those involved that, if successful, will result in the financial remedy of compensation. Indemnity is provided in the commercial markets for hospitals and doctors in private practice. The government indemnifies the NHS and pays the legal costs of most claimants.

The civil courts rightly demand rigorous proof that damage has been caused by substandard care. An important corollary is that not all damage is caused by substandard care. The test, which is known as causation, fails when a bad outcome was deemed inevitable from the underlying disease although the treatment might have been wrong or unacceptably delayed. Lawyers draw a distinction between damage caused by substandard care, which is negligent, and damage that would have occurred in any event, despite any substandard care, which is nonnegligent.

Medical negligence is broadly comparable with many other forms of legal action based upon fault in which someone seeks compensation for a personal injury that they have suffered. This area of civil law is called *tort* law, which imposes a duty where one person can reasonably foresee that his or her conduct may cause harm to another. No fault compensation is an alternative remedy where the need to prove negligence as a criterion for making payments is removed, although most schemes retain a test of causation.

*Tort-based* law systems are in place in the UK, the USA, Canada and Australia.

The first *no fault* compensation scheme was introduced in New Zealand in 1972 followed by the Scandinavian countries in the 1980s and by France in 2002. In these systems, there are higher levels of claims and compensation payments are lower than those awarded by courts in the UK and elsewhere.

### *3.5. Withdrawal of the state license to practice*

A patient may also lodge a complaint with the state professional regulatory body, which in the UK is known as the General Medical Council. If following an investigation the surgeon is found guilty of serious professional misconduct, then his or her license to practice may be suspended or revoked and his or her name may be struck off the specialist register.

The licensure to practice of doctors is affected by three factors: *health*, *conduct* and *performance*. It is likely that about 1 in 20 doctors will have significant problems at some stage in their careers. When a problem develops, there may be a lack of insight and a state of denial.

*Health* problems include physical and mental infirmity and excessive alcohol intake. Sickness affects surgeons just as it does their patients.

Surgeons are vulnerable to shortcomings in their *conduct* in the same way as everyone else. A surgeon can behave in an inconsiderate way to patients, their relatives, and to members of staff. If deficiencies in their personal conduct outside the hospital become widely known, their professional reputation may be undermined.

The acceptability of the clinical *performance* of surgeons varies within and between specialties. The specialty of vascular surgery includes procedures, particularly emergencies, which can be technically very challenging. Some trainees acquire surgical judgment and skills more easily than others. A few are so slow and inept that they have to withdraw from vascular surgical training and pursue less onerous careers.

New vascular procedures emerge and established operations are constantly being refined to make them more effective. Surgeons have to learn endovascular and minimal access techniques during the course of their careers. As time passes, a few lose confidence and adapt poorly.

A technically competent surgeon may fail his patient by his unavailability and by his failure to honour his commitments by his absence without adequate arrangements for cover.

### 3.6. Criminal law

A social intolerance of fatal medical mistakes has long caused them to be criminalised. Recently, a doctor was given a custodial sentence after pleading guilty to the manslaughter of his patient by gross negligence [6]. In the past, such prosecutions were rare. However, in each of the last 2 years, three doctors have been prosecuted in the UK for gross negligence manslaughter although there is a much lower medical conviction rate compared with the prosecutions of others for manslaughter.

### 3.7. Governmental inquiry

Reports in the media of unnecessary deaths after surgical procedures inevitably undermine confidence in the surgical profession, which can sometimes only be restored by an inquiry, in which lawyers expose the events surrounding the tragedy to detailed public scrutiny.

In the 1990s, the poor results of neonatal operations for the Tetralogy of Fallot by paediatric cardiac surgeons entered the public domain, and their judgment and operative techniques were called into question in a public inquiry [7].

The underlying cause was poor clinical performance, in which the outcome for arterial switch procedure in cyanotic babies in the first month of life was much worse than could reasonably have been expected. The poor surgical results had been a matter of unresolved internal debate within the hospital and some members of the clinical team felt that insufficient attention had been paid to their concerns.

A lesson was that once a serious disagreement or criticism emerged, the leader of the team needed to get to the bottom of the matter so that it became resolved and the issue became closed.

Underlying problems, such as underinvestment in the service, poor teamwork and low morale, made it much more difficult to provide clinical care of high quality.

## 4. A historical perspective

One of the earliest Kings of Babylon was an able ruler named Hammurabi (1948–1905 BC). His laws were engraved on stone and are preserved in the Louvre Museum in Paris. He regulated medical practice by a strict code including the following:

> If the doctor shall treat a gentleman and shall open an abscess with a bronze stylet and shall preserve the eye of the patient, he shall receive ten shekels of silver.

Physicians were probably of the priestly caste. A bad clinical outcome led to a drastic penalty:

> If the doctor shall open an abscess with a bronze stylet and shall kill the patient or shall destroy the sight of his eye, his hands shall be cut off.

The ancient Egyptians wrote on papyrus that no blame was incurred if the patient dies as long as the physicians adhered closely to the Hermetic books of the god Thoth. If, however, the physician departed in the least from the accredited methods of teaching and the case ended fatally, his own life was forfeited. Thus, the Egyptian code meted out even more severe punishments than those of the Babylonian code.

Hippocrates (460–355 BC) set high standards in his oath and aphorisms although with less draconian consequences for those who transgressed:

> If I carry out this oath, and break it not, may I gain for ever reputation amongst all men for my life and my art; but if I transgress it and forswear myself, may the opposite befall me.

Henri de Mondeville (AD 1260–1320) was a far-seeing and broad-minded mediaeval scholar at Bologna, Italy, who advised that:

> It is dangerous for a surgeon, who is not of repute, to operate in any way different to that method in common use.

Squabbles over who should be permitted to practice surgery came to a head in the 19th century. In 1826 in Scotland, the Faculty of Physicians and Surgeons of Glasgow obtained an interdiction in the Court of Session preventing the practice of surgery without the faculty examination in a lawsuit that lasted no less than 14 years.

In 1858, the Westminster Parliament in Great Britain gave the General Medical Council the responsibility of deciding who should be permitted to practice.

In 1925, the UK Court of Appeal defined the scope of the criminality of medical mistakes when it stressed that gross negligence had to show such disregard for the life and safety of the patient as to amount to a crime against the state and conduct deserving of punishment.

## 5. National outcome audit in vascular surgery

In an ideal world, it ought to be possible to benchmark a surgeon's clinical performance against a recognised norm. The success of this kind of analytic method depends on the frequency of the procedure, with adjustments for the risk and the frequency of the endpoint, which is usually the mortality of the condition being treated. The methodology is best developed in adult cardiac surgery for the frequently performed operation of coronary artery revascularisation. In a sequential analysis, the actual outcome is compared with the risk-adjusted expected outcome. Comparisons may be made of the individual results of surgeons within a unit and of a unit within a pooled national database.

The London *Times* newspaper has published league tables annually in the last 2 years of inaccurate and misleading raw mortality data following aortic aneurysm operations based on routine workload statistical returns to the Department of Health. The unwelcome publicity has been a powerful stimulus to vascular surgeons to develop a credible alternative. Only the profession can establish this kind of detailed systematic analysis of outcomes.

By November 2003, the national vascular database of the Vascular Surgical Society of Great Britain and Ireland had surveyed the results of 6000 index arterial operations during 2000 and 2001 using data from 181 vascular surgeons. Their reports are available at www.vssgbi.org. Logistic regression models of the results of the index operations of aortic aneurysm repair, carotid endarterectomy and infrainguinal bypass have enabled contributing surgeons to compare their individual results with pooled national figures, thus fulfilling a requirement for professional revalidation [8]. The national society is currently considering how to deal with 'outliers' whose divergent performance causes concern.

## 6. The future

In the UK, statutory provisions are intended to encourage openness in the reporting of adverse events including a duty of candour together with exemption from disciplinary action when reporting incidents with a view to improving patient safety [9]. Legislation is being considered to require all healthcare professionals and managers to inform patients where they become aware of a possible negligent act or omission. Exemption from disciplinary action by employers or professional regulatory bodies is intended for those reporting adverse events, and legal privilege would be provided for reports and information identifying adverse events except where the healthcare professional had committed a criminal offence or it would not be safe for the professional to continue to treat patients.

We live in an age of accountability, in which vascular surgeons have to keep the confidence of patients, relatives, team members and the public. When things go wrong, it is no longer acceptable to remain silent and hope that the trouble dies down. Any shortcomings in care and communication should be addressed with candour, sympathy and humility. Failure to do so can lead to a breakdown in the trust of the patient and the clinical team in the surgeon, which is essential for good clinical care. Once that trust has been lost, it may be difficult or impossible to rebuild it.

## References

[1] R.N. Baird, The vascular patient as a litigant, Ann. R. Coll. Surg. Engl. (Suppl.) 78 (1996) 278–282.
[2] W.B. Campbell, F. France, H.M. Goodwin, Medico legal claims in vascular surgery, Ann. R. Coll. Surg. Engl. 84 (2002) 181–184.
[3] W.E.G. Thomas, et al., Vascular surgical audit—arterial reconstructions and amputations for lower limb ischaemia, Acta Chir. Scand. 149 (1983) 127–132.
[4] J.J. Earnshaw, et al., The importance of vascular surgical audit to surgeons, patients and purchasers, Eur. J. Vasc. Surg. 6 (1992) 540–544.
[5] The Management of Suspensions of Clinical Staff in NHS Hospitals and Ambulance Trusts in England, Report by the Comptroller and Auditor General, The UK Stationery Office, 2003.
[6] J. Holbrook, The criminalization of fatal medical mistakes, BMJ 327 (2003) 1118.
[7] I. Kennedy, The Report of the Public Inquiry into Children's Heart Surgery at the Bristol Royal Infirmary 1984–1995, The UK Stationery Office, 2001.
[8] D.R. Prytherch, et al., A model for national outcome audit in vascular surgery, Eur. J. Vasc. Endovasc. Surg. 21 (2001) 477–483.
[9] Making Amends, A report by the Chief Medical Officer, A consultation paper setting out proposals for reforming the approach to clinical negligence in the NHS, UK Department of Health, 2003.

International Congress Series 1272 (2004) 72–75

www.ics-elsevier.com

# The need for exit examinations for vascular surgeons in the various European countries

Bernhard Nachbur*

*Department of Surgery, University of Berne, Talmoosstrasse 48, Ittigen 3063, Switzerland*

**Abstract.** To answer the question whether an exit examination is needed or not for vascular surgeons in Europe, it is helpful to bear in mind two events that bring considerable influence to bear on the direction in which medicine in general and surgery in particular in Europe are heading. © 2004 Elsevier B.V. All rights reserved.

*Keywords:* Examinations for vascular surgeons

## 1. Ruling (directives) of the European Court of Justice of October 3rd 2000 regarding working hours of clinical doctors in Spain

Judgement was passed by the European Court of Justice regarding a claim lodged by Spanish hospital doctors working for the public service of hospitals in the region of Valencia. The doctors, represented by the labour union Sindaco de Medicos de Assistencia Publica (SIMAP), were required to work without daily, weekly, monthly or annual temporal limitation. In short, these doctors had long, i.e. unlimited weekly working hours, no recompensation for on-call services rendered at night and weekends and insufficient time for recuperation. The court judged that weekly working hours should be limited to 48 and that on-call service was to be considered as working time if the service was provided by a physician on in-house call. The directive went on to define and lay down the adequate time for resting and recuperation (a minimum of 11 h following daily duties, also a 35-h rest period once a week, etc.).

Judgements from the European Court of Justice concern all member states of the European Community, are not subject to a right of appeal, cannot be overruled and are therefore law.

Most European countries have had legislation concerning health and safety at work prior to October 2000, but this had in general not been fully enforced whether for clinical physicians in general or for clinical surgeons (residents) in particular.

* Tel.: +41-31-921-54-82; fax: +41-31-921-55-86.
*E-mail address:* nachbur@bluewin.ch (B. Nachbur).


doi:10.1016/j.ics.2004.04.082

On balance the result of the directives of the European Court of Justice cuts working hours in surgical institutions dramatically; this makes it necessary to sign up additional residents and trainees. As a consequence, given that the caseload in a surgical institution remains constant, the time that a surgeon in training is exposed to surgical practice is shortened. The residents in training are consequently less well experienced, quite probably at the expense of the patients. Wide variation from one country to the other is to be expected and it is questionable whether residents can be provided a sound academic and clinical education within the outlined time frame.

This is one reason why vascular surgeons in every EU country should at the end of their training period be audited by a European institution—a court of assessors drawn equally from all member states of the EU—in the interest of standardisation and harmonisation between countries committed to guarantee freedom of movement and residence to all citizens of the union.

## 2. 10 new countries to join the European Union

In May 2004, 10 Eastern European and Mediterranean countries officially joined the European Union. These are: Estonia, Latvia, Lithuania, Slovenia, Poland, the Czech Republic, Cyprus, Hungary and Malta. Citizens of these countries shall become citizens of the union and will be entitled to freedom of movement and residence within the union. This includes physicians that shall have the right to practice in any one of the 25 member countries, as well as in EFTA countries such as Switzerland. (Switzerland is engaged in bilateral accords with the EU and has accepted the right of free movement.) What does that mean in terms of a need for exit examination of vascular surgeons from countries in Europe?

To be eligible for EBSQ VASC assessment, one of the most important prerequisites has been the Certificate of Completion of Surgical Training (CCST). The examinee is not allowed to outflank the medical authorities of his/her country by applying directly for eligibility to the European Board of Vascular Surgery. The candidate must therefore present evidence of completed and successful surgical training in his/her own country. In Greece, Italy, France, Spain, Portugal, Denmark and Finland, Austria and Luxembourg, the eight countries where vascular surgery has independent specialty status, the national CCST will certify completed training in vascular surgery. In the remaining countries (United Kingdom, Ireland, Iceland, Germany, the Netherlands, Belgium, Sweden, Norway and Switzerland), the CCST is proof of completed and successful training in "general" surgery. It can be expected that vascular surgeons from these nine countries should welcome the EBSQ VASC assessment as an exit examination unless they have specialty examinations of their own which they feel and consider superior or at least equal to the European assessment. This could be all the more so for the 10 new member countries where vascular surgery is probably not a specialty in its own right and where the structure of education and training in vascular surgery no doubt varies widely from one country to the other. Even if freedom of movement of the 10 new countries shall be postponed for a few years because of the threat of gross influx of cheap labour, the right of free movement will be fully implemented in the near future. The need for a defining exit examination ensuring a common denominator for a high standard of vascular surgical practice is obvious.

## 3. What are the advantages of an exit examination carried out by the European board of vascular surgery?

The EBSQ VASC examination is a carefully executed assessment of a wide variety of medical accomplishments of the candidate. All the certified medical records regarding his or her education and training are carefully looked into, clinical cases with a number of questions demanding unequivocal responses are presented, the ability to understand and interpret articles in scientific journals is judged, the overall dedication to vascular surgery and practical expertise is gauged and finally the manual skills and dexterity are measured objectively. Immediately after the examination the assessors, on average two to three eminent vascular surgeons from each member country, sit together and review the achievement of every single candidate, discussing with special care the performance of those examinees that fail by general agreement. There follows a critical review of the execution of the examination itself with an input from representatives from all member states, the consequence of which is a steady improvement of the exam from year to year. It is hardly possible for a national specialty examination to match this kind of progress made by the European Board of Vascular Surgery which keeps close account of developments in the field of vascular disease and which is intimately related to one of the major annual vascular surgical events in Europe.

The EBSQ VASC assessment is a platform of objectivity where favoritism resulting from personal acquaintance—almost inevitable in most countries—can be largely avoided. This enhances the prestige of the examination which has tested candidates from all European member countries, but has been especially popular with Belgium, Greece, Italy, Spain and Switzerland.

## 4. The Swiss experience

At the first of January 2002, vascular surgery in Switzerland was recognized as a surgical specialty equivalent to 'thoracic surgery', 'visceral surgery' and 'general surgery and traumatology' by the Swiss Society of Surgery. It has become the responsibility of the Swiss Society for Vascular Surgery (SSVS) to specify the requirements and to carry out an exit examination at the end of 4 years specialty training. The council of the SSVS decided that the EBSQ VASC assessment should be designated as the official exit or specialty examination in order to qualify for specialty status in Switzerland. A candidate that has not met the remaining preconditions (4 years of specialty training, of which 2 years are to be spent in a university setting) will be advised by the council of the SSVS not to apply for the EBSQ VASC assessment. With very few exceptions all surgeons practicing vascular surgery in Switzerland carry the title EBSQ VASC. Consequently, the contingent of Swiss vascular surgeons taking the EBSQ VASC assessment has become the biggest of all since its introduction in 1996. Of 115 successful candidates for European Board of Surgery Qualification in Vascular Surgery, 27 are Swiss, to which are to be added the assessors from Switzerland (7). There are also those who fail the examination, the yearly average varying between 15% and 25%. In this delicate matter, the EBSQ VASC assessment allows for objective judgement and avoidance of bias and cronyism.

When the impact of a European exit examination is thought of in terms of the European Union it becomes more and more evident that this examination is not the concern of one single country alone, but rather in the interest of the whole, i.e. of all the countries that are members of one union which, slowly but inevitably, shall become stronger from year to year and of which we are all residents.

When more European countries accept the EBSQ VASC assessments as their exit examination a competitive spirit between candidates from the various countries shall evolve which in turn shall strengthen the benchmark function of the assessments themselves.

## 5. Conclusion

There is little doubt that there is a need for an exit examination for vascular surgeons in the European countries which guarantees the desired high standard of training and vascular surgical practice in Europe. Eventually, the EBSQ VASC assessments shall prevail.

International Congress Series 1272 (2004) 76–94

www.ics-elsevier.com

# European Association of Vascular Surgeons in Training (EAVST)

Alexei V. Svetlikov[a,*], Thomas Nyheim[b], Murat Aksoy[c]

[a] *M. Toreza, Avenue 35, P.O. Box 50/50, 194223 St. Petersburg, Russia*
[b] *Norway*
[c] *Turkey*

*Keywords:* EAVST; Vascular surgery; Vascular training

## 1. History of EAVST

During the ESVS Meeting in Berlin in 1994 the European Association for Vascular Surgeons in Training (EAVST) was founded and the initial Executive Committee consisted of Jes Sandermann (Denmark), Alun H. Davies (UK), Domenico Valenti (Italy), Jan Gniadek (Poland), and Albert Verhulst (Belgium). The statutes were ready in April 1995, and later that year the Executive Committee was supplemented with Anders Albäck (Finland) and Luis Mendes Pedro (Portugal).

The idea was that two representatives from each European country should be elected and approved nationally and meet once a year for the EAVST General Assembly during the ESVS Meeting. Here election for the EAVST Executive Committee should take place. To get this idea out to the individual countries was very difficult and was not established during the first years. Keeping and updating an address list of interested trainees was another problem.

EAVST should take an active part in discussing international vascular training matters well founded with national characteristics, should be able to cooperate well with both the UEMS Board and ESVS Council, taking part in the latter's scientific programme, etc.

The EAVST was from the very beginning well received both by the UEMS Division for Vascular Surgery, and a year later by the newly formed European Board for Vascular Surgery (EBVS) and the ESVS Council. EAVST was immediately offered a seat as an observer, and to secure the initial continuity Mr. Jes Sandermann was the representative from 1994 to 1996 in both the division, board and council. From 1996 to 1997 he represented the Permanent Working Group of Junior Doctors (PWG) in the EBVS, a seat with voting rights in the EBVS, and giving the observer post to another EAVST Executive Committee member.

* Corresponding author. Tel.: +7-812-552-0031; fax: +7-812-543-1571.
*E-mail address:* asvetlikov@mail.ru (A.V. Svetlikov).


doi:10.1016/j.ics.2004.04.069

In 1994/1995 Mr. J. Sandermann circulated seven EAVST Newsletters and was in the editing committee in 1996, when Domenico Valenti was the editor. It was a hard task with very few willing to give contributions—but an important tool for providing information and showing the vitality of the association.

## 2. Current aims, projects

EAVST is an organisation that aims

1. to collect information on the training and education of European vascular surgeons, and
2. in cooperation with national or international vascular surgical organisations to perform surveys or research in relation to the training of vascular surgeons.
3. EAVST also wants to promote intra-European exchange programmes for vascular trainees
4. as well as the formation of National Associations of Vascular Surgeons in Training
5. to organize/arrange sessions concerning Training in Vascular Surgery at national or international conferences
6. in cooperation with vascular organizations to arrange congress sessions where vascular surgeons in training can present their papers (Young Vascular surgeons Scientific Session at the ESVS Meeting).

### *2.1. EAVST cooperation with Union of Medical Specialists (UEMS) and European Board of Vascular Surgery (EBVS)*

The EAVST and UEMS/EBVS are both working towards harmonizing vascular training in Europe. This is a challenging task with the existing linguistic, cultural and organizational differences in Europe. Both organizations are working towards a common goal in many areas. The EAVST has been given an observer status on the UEMS/EBVS Board meetings and can provide our members with information on the latest developments in our Newsletter. Trainee views on pertinent issues are promoted in this forum. The EAVST is cooperating with the UEMS/EBVS in some important areas, these will be discussed below.

#### *2.1.1. European logbook*

The purpose of this important logbook, devised by a Committee under the supervision of Dominico Palombo (Italy), is to document candidates vascular clinical and operative experience for the European Board of Surgical Qualification exam in Vascular surgery (EBSQ-vasc). The EAVST has been asked to promote and assess the interest of using this logbook as a supplement to the existing national logbook. The Board finds this to be a useful tool in mapping a candidate's clinical and operative activity. It is also useful for the candidate to see the minimum training requirements needed to sit the EBSQ-vasc exam. If all vascular trainees where required by the national organizations to adopt this logbook, there would be many advantages. A standardized European logbook would allow a comparison of training practices, cross-fertilization of ideas and innovations. Illustrating strengths and weaknesses in training structure could contribute to changes in training practices on a national level. Unless the EBSQ-vasc examination is adopted more widely in Europe, the generalized use of a European logbook will have an uncertain future. We recommend using the logbook if there is a chance that you may take the exam in the future or if you want to keep track of your clinical and operative experience and find the need to supplement the national logbook. It is available on the internet: www.uems-vasc.org/LOGBOOK.doc.

*2.1.2. EuREG-vasc registry*

Jes Sanderman (DK) chairman of this committee is gathering data on both National and Centre levels across Europe. This data specifies the requirements in vascular training in each country, registration of vascular activity with names, vascular training requirements, outpatient and operative activity. Maintaining updated information on the registry is of utmost importance in monitoring development of Vascular Surgery in Europe, aiding in the process of harmonizing vascular activity, particularly with the EU enlargement.

A proposal was presented by the EAVST to the Division and Board of Vascular Surgery to present suggestions of a new trainee registration form in collaboration with EuReg-vasc registry. This registration form will reflect the trainees clinical activity in vascular surgery. This trainee form would give the EAVST the opportunity to provide objective feedback on all aspects of training in each European country and highlight problems in a forum (UEMS and EBVS) which can make recommendations to change training practices. The EAVST could be a stronger advocate for our members and make this information freely available to all. Vascular Centers which do not provide adequate training opportunities may therefore need to change their practices to attract qualified and motivated candidates. The content and mode registration will be presented at the next meeting UEMS/EBVS in April 2004.

## 3. Training system on vascular surgery in different European countries, presented by EAVST members

The current problems of European trainees in vascular surgery

1. There are many hospitals where trainees have very few opportunities to get operative experience, because consultants have their "private" patients and trainees just assist with operations. It must be pointed out and changed.
2. Next year the EU will have 10 more members and the postgraduate training program in new countries is not yet standardized.
3. Funding of courses, congresses, etc. from national bodies in East Europe currently is a hopeless situation, because they are in period of permanent transformation and every trainee must have sponsors for courses, especially abroad. The salary is very low in terms of European standards.

### *3.1. Austria*

The vascular surgical education in Austria takes 3 years. First you have to finish a 6-year training in general surgery by rotating in several departments before starting vascular specialization. Only hospitals with at least two consultant vascular surgeons are qualified for trainees. Now it is recommended to fulfill an operating list with 110 arterial reconstructions, 60 venous operations and 10 endovascular procedures. At this time we are creating a new training model, including an operating list comparable with this for the European Vascular Surgical Examination.

Additionally, training in endovascular procedures and duplex-sonography will be required. After 3 years of vascular surgical training and completion of the operating list an optional final examination can be performed, including knowledge about scientific work.

The time from starting surgical training until gaining the vascular surgical specialty requires at least 9 years.

Dr. Michael Gorlitzer.

### *3.2. Croatia*

The programme of specialisation in vascular surgery was issued in 1994 by the Ministry of Health, Republic of Croatia.

Candidates for training in vascular surgery should first finish the specialisation in general surgery. They continue with a two-year programme, which includes:

- at the Department of Vascular Surgery: 16 months
- at the Vascular Ward of the Department of Internal Medicine: 2 months
- at the Vascular Radiology Ward with intensive diagnostics: 1 month
- at the Transfusion Ward: 1 month
- at the Cardiosurgery Ward: 1 month
- at the Intensive Care Ward: 1 month

At the Department of Vascular Surgery, the specialist is supposed to master theoretical as well as practical part of education. A total of minimum 125 operations should be performed, and the candidate is supposed to carry out 60% of them independently.

Dr. Lidija Erdelez.

### *3.3. Denmark*

Vascular surgery has been a separate surgical speciality in Denmark since 1983. There are 45 vascular surgical specialist and 12 vascular surgical trainee positions in Denmark.

In brief the postgraduate vascular surgical education in Denmark consists, like all other postgraduate medical education, of three parts.

> "Phase 1"—Internship and introduction to general surgery. Besides internship the employment should consist of orthopaedics and gastroenterology (24 months). Having fulfilled the employment and having performed a pre-set number of surgical procedures you are able to apply for phase 2.
>
> "Phase 2"—Rotation on three of the five surgical departments: (Surgical Gastroenterology (obligatory), Urology, Vascular surgery, Thoracic surgery and Plastic Surgery) in a university clinic. Twenty-seven months and obligatory theoretical and practical lectures leading to phase 3.
>
> "Phase 3"—Employment in vascular surgical department at least 2 years in a university clinic and 1 year in another clinic, performing vascular surgery.

There are no formal examinations, but all employed doctors except the consultants have a tutor to guide and evaluate the knowledge and skills of the trainees. During the employment, formulas set up by the health authorities (who should receive a copy), are to be fulfilled.

On applying for specialisation it is mandatory to document your surgical experience by fulfilling a formula regarding your surgical procedures both assisted and personally performed. To become a vascular specialist you have to have performed at least 200 arterial reconstructions. In total the postgraduate surgical education takes approximately 8–12 years.

At the moment we have 10 surgical departments performing vascular surgery, four of them being university departments, and the other surgical departments are in county hospitals, where specialised vascular surgeons perform the operations assisted by junior doctors.

However, this programme is still changing. The newly defined Danish postgraduate training programme in vascular surgery is expected to replace the existing one in 2004. The main objectives of this total revision of the education are improvement in quality, shortening of specialist training and definition of minimum competences. The Danish Vascular Surgical Society's educational committee is presently finalising these vascular surgical competences.

Dr. Franz von Jessen and Dr. Thomas Balezantis.

### 3.4. France

In France, vascular surgical training is split in two parts. The first part lasts 5 years and represents the "basic surgical training". It is made of 10 rotations of 6 months each in different departments. A minimum of 2 years in general surgery (1 year in digestive surgery and 1 year in bone and joint surgery) is mandatory. For vascular surgery, the minimum required during this period is 2 years. The remaining two training rotations are left to the discretion of the trainee (usually people do 6 months in cardiac surgery and 6 in thoracic surgery). Duties of the trainee during this period are care of patients in the ward, with ward rounds twice a day, and presence in theatre, helping and performing basic procedures. At the end of this period the trainee should have passed two degrees: a thesis for the degree of Doctor in Medicine, and a degree in general surgery (that entitles to have a practice in general surgery). The second part of the training is purely vascular and requires an appointment in one department (sometimes two) for a duration of 2–4 years. During this period regular attendance at the meetings of the College of Vascular Surgery (about four meetings per year) is mandatory. During these meetings, the trainee will have to do oral presentations on various topics of vascular surgery and also discuss case presentations. At the end of this period the trainee should be able to perform the usual surgical and endovascular procedures and know about anatomy, physiology and pathology of occlusive and aneurysmal vascular diseases. He should know about the outcome and complications of these procedures as well as patient follow-up. The degree of specialist training in vascular surgery is the final step before becoming consultant surgeon.

The number of training centres in France is currently 44. Vascular surgical training is coordinated by the French College of Vascular Surgery.

Dr. Jean-Noël Albertini.

### 3.5. Italy

There are 31 universities providing training in vascular surgery and granting the certificate of completion of specialist training (CCST). They are spread as follows:

(1) North: Bologna, Ferrara, Genova, Milano I and II, Modena, Padova, Parma, Pavia, Torino, Trieste, Verona.
(2) Centre: Ancona, Chieti, Firenze, L'Aquila, Perugia, Pisa, Roma La Sapienza I and II, Roma Tor Vergata, Roma Catholic University, Siena.
(3) South and Islands: Bari, Cagliari, Catania, Catanzaro, Napoli "Federico II", Napoli II Ateneo, Palermo, Sassari.

There were 98 first year trainees in 1998/1999. Eleven of them financed by local authorities, while 42 are affiliated with non-university hospitals (the Italian term is "convenzionato") and 43 are interns at the universities*.

The high level of alternative financing throughout Italy could be an answer to the shortage of financial resources of the universities in our country. This development surely requires an efficient quality control, since the decentralisation of teaching could increase some problems which are already present in the training in vascular surgery, as there are:

- absence of rotation (Italian law recognises 1 year in general surgery; also, the possibility of spending a certain period abroad or doing research is rarely given);
- difficulty in verifying the number of surgical procedures performed by the student in observance with the European training programme;
- guarantee of the qualification of the affiliated hospitals in terms of number of patient admissions and number of surgery procedures performed;
- absence of a national organisation at the trainee level which would allow comparison of personal experiences and uniform single courses of specialisation.

The organ guaranteeing the standards should be an agency of self-control on European level and should be competent to recall and admonish failure in respecting the European standards.

Once these standards are fulfilled the CCST would automatically be vested with the same significance of the EBSQ-vasc.

Dr. Corrado Cirielli.

### 3.6. Norway

The postgraduate specialisation in vascular surgery in Norway is divided into two phases: Primary phase—the specialisation of General Surgery is 6 years, which includes 1 year of a subspecialty (which may be in any area in medicine). This involves rotating in the surgical specialties of gastroenterology, urology, vascular surgery, orthopaedics and general surgery mainly with other optional areas in surgery. An obligatory number of operations and courses (some with exams) within the above specialties need to be completed within the specified time. One year of pure vascular surgery as an appointed specialist trainee can be included in the 6 years of general surgery and deducted from the next stage. Throughout this a consultant supervisor is appointed in each hospital where the trainee works. At least one and a half years of this training must be carried out in a university hospital. It will then be possible to apply for the specialty of General Surgery. Phase two continues with 2–3 years as an appointed vascular surgical trainee of which one and a half years in a university hospital is necessary. An obligatory operating list must be fulfilled with at least 150 arterial reconstructions, 20 endovascular procedures and 30 venous reconstructions. Obligatory and optional courses in vascular surgery, interventional radiology and congresses will complete the training of vascular surgery. A consultant vascular surgeon is appointed as a supervisor during this training with regular formal meetings. There are currently 20 vascular trainee posts in Norway distributed over 15 vascular surgical centers of which 8 are university hospitals. There are no formal final examinations required to gain the vascular surgical specialty. The time required gaining the specialty after the internship is 8–9 years.

Dr. Thomas Nyheim, Bergen University Hospital.

### *3.7. Portugal*

Vascular surgery is an autonomous and recognised speciality in Portugal since 1977. In order to become a vascular surgeon one has to successfully conclude an internship of 2 years in a central Hospital (which includes Internal Medicine, General Surgery, Paediatrics, Gynaecology and Obstetrics, and Primary Care) and get a high result in a very demanding multiple-choice examination based on the Harrison's *Principles of Internal Medicine*. It then takes 6 years to become a specialist in vascular surgery. It involves 2 years of training in general surgery followed by 4 years of pure vascular surgery (including a 2-month training in a cardiothoracic surgery unit). A vascular surgeon in training has to perform at least 250 major operations. At the moment, only five hospitals are authorised to instruct vascular surgeons, and the number of trainees are around 30.

Dr. Jorge Cruz.

### *3.8. Russia*

Vascular surgeons in Russia have to go through a rigorous training before qualifying. Firstly, they complete a 2-year Internship programme in general surgery. Having fulfilled the post, performed a number of surgical procedures and passed the final exam, a doctor is then allowed to apply for a PhD. The candidate must take two more exams before he can begin a research project and it usually takes 3–5 years before the investigation is completed. Once the final PhD exams are over, the candidate must defend his thesis. Only when a trainee's results have received official confirmation by an independent committee based in Moscow can he start his training in vascular surgery. It then takes about 5–7 years before a trainee is fully qualified to work as a vascular surgeon and able to perform the majority of vascular procedures. The whole process of postgraduate surgical education can take anything from 8 to 14 years to complete. In addition, every vascular surgeon in Russia must have a license approving their ability to work in this field.

The future of vascular surgery in Russia is promising, with the number of procedures set to rise rapidly year after year. One of the main reasons for this increase in vascular activity is the vastly expanding field of carotid and endovascular surgery. The younger generation of vascular surgeons in Russia seems to be the predominant force in the movement to keep abreast of these advances. The foundation of Russian Association of Vascular Surgeons in Training (RAVST), bringing Russian trainees in line with their European counterparts in EAVST, was another inevitable step in the development of Russian vascular surgery.

Russia has much to contribute to the international community of vascular surgery and exchange programmes should also be developed for young surgeons from Western Europe to study at Russian centers of excellence to reciprocate in this learning process.

Dr. Alexei Svetlikov.

### 3.9. *Switzerland*

In Switzerland there was no formal education in vascular surgery until 2002. The only known qualification was the EBSQ-vasc. Recently, a traineeship in vascular surgery has been established. It is regarded as a subspecialisation of the postgraduate education in General or Cardiac Surgery. The candidates shall be already trained either in General or in Cardiac Surgery. The programme of specialisation in vascular surgery takes 4 years and is divided in two parts. The first part takes 2 years and is to be attended before the examination of postgraduate education in General Surgery. After having passed this examination, the candidates complete their programme for another 2 years in a Vascular Surgery Department. At least 2 years of this programme have to be completed in a Hospital having an “A” rating. Hospitals with a Vascular Surgery Department are rated as level “A” or “B”. An “A” Hospital has a Department of Vascular Surgery which is actively involved in science and research and is able to impart the whole educational programme of stationary and ambulatory treatment. The “B” Hospitals cover only some parts of vascular surgery. In order to get the degree in vascular surgery, candidates have to pass an examination and must have performed around 200 operations.

Dr. Tamim Obeid.

### 3.10. *Turkey*

Vascular surgery is not an independent specialty in Turkey at the moment. After having graduated from medical school (6 years), students are capable of practicing as medical doctors in the country. The medical doctors are permitted to examine and treat patients, who do not need any further examinations by specialists. Two times per year, an examination is carried out, which is the basic and only method of residency selection. According to the success at the exam, the doctors are assigned to residency programs. Doctors who are willing to be trained in vascular surgery are assigned to cardiovascular departments. Another method of being trained in vascular surgery is being assigned to general surgery departments. Although not many, some centers of general surgery offer training in vascular surgery. A proper training is usually available after attaining a fellowship state at these centers. Although there are many Cardiovascular Departments in the country, there are only two General Surgery Departments which are capable of training vascular surgeons. One of them is our Medical School in Istanbul University and the other is the Ankara University.

Dr. Murat Aksoy.

### 3.11. UK

At present, after qualification we undertake a year as a pre-registration house officer. Doctors then work for 2–3 years as a senior house officer where basic surgical skills are acquired. It is during this time that surgical trainees are required to pass the MRCS examination. This is a moduled course and examination and has replaced the old style FRCS parts 1 and 2. This is known as Basic Surgical Training (BST). We are interviewed for a Calman number that allows you to proceed as a Higher Surgical Trainee (HST). This requires 6 years of further surgical practise prior to attainment of a CCST. There is of course the minor hurdle of a final examination (year 5/6)! If candidates are unsuccessful in gaining a number, then there are unnumbered locum posts available but this does not count in terms of training towards your final CCST.

I was elected as an EASVT committee member at the ESVS conference held in Copenhagen, Denmark in 1999. I have also been elected as the UK representative of the Rouleaux Club. This Club represents UK vascular trainees and has a voice at the Vascular Surgical Society of Great Britain and Ireland. We encourage as many members as possible to join (free of charge) and hold two meetings a year. There is a winter meeting, which coincides with the Annual Conference of the VSSGBI, and a summer meeting that is more informal and encourages members to bring their families along! This is quite a useful Club and I would encourage you to look at our website: www.rouleaux.org.

Dr. Stella Vig.

### 3.12. Finland

Medical school in Finland is planned to take 6 years. After that we have a 6-year programme of general medicine, general surgery and vascular surgery, of which at least 3 years should be in vascular surgery, including 6 months of cardiothoracic surgery, in order to graduate. In 2001 we started a quality controlled educational programme for trainees in vascular surgery. Currently, five of us are in vascular training and two in general surgery rotation. A senior tutor was appointed for each vascular trainee. The trainee is evaluated every 6 months by the professor, his/her tutor, nurses on wards and by themselves. Not only are the surgical and theoretical skills under evaluation, but also the “softer” values such as coping with patients and their relatives, working together, etc. are under scrutiny. A computer software company (QPR Finland) has provided us with a score card system that we hope will give us a well-documented follow-up of our progression. The number of procedures performed by trainees is increasing and we have a point counting system to ensure the minimal amount of procedures during training. At the moment we are guaranteed to be able to attend two international plus a varying number (2–5) of national educational congresses per year.

Dr. Pirkka Vikatmaa.

## 4. Reforming training in vascular surgery, EAVST point of view

When we discuss the future of training in vascular surgery we should first of all think about the future of vascular surgery and vascular surgeons. Who are they in 20 or 50 years? In terms of our understanding of this issue we should decide where to move the training in the field of vascular surgery.

Currently it is clear that the number of patients with cardiovascular diseases including patients with peripheral vascular diseases will increase every year.

This determines the requirement of the increasing the number of experienced vascular specialists. The first aim of training in vascular surgery is expansion of vascular surgery in medical schools with involvement of students in scientific work and practical skills training in vascular surgery and Vascular Medicine.

Another goal in training vascular surgeons should be profound education on the subjects:

- "Atherosclerosis and Medical Angiology" for both trainees in vascular surgery and medical students.
- The special courses in Vascular Genetics, Immunology and Molecular Biology.
- Research methodology and statistics.
- Special training courses in minimal invasive, endovascular surgery for a long period of time (at least equal to open surgery training).
- Regular technical skills courses (for example, Pontresina Vascular course).

This will attract an additional number of the new, well-educated generation of young doctors, trainees in vascular surgery and provide the new quality level of vascular patient treatment.

There are many factors which will influence future training in vascular surgery. The EAVST does not have any legislative power to influence this process. EAVST membership is increasing (>1300). The role of Board members and National representatives is to provide information on European matters and provide feedback on important trainee issues in relevant forums, such as the UEMS and ESVS meetings. The EAVST presented the trainees perspective on the issue of 'Reforming training in Vascular Surgery' at the UEMS symposium on the 4/9/03 in Dublin. This section will present a summary of the most important views presented at this symposium.

### *4.1. Directive '48-h week' (2000/34/EC)*

European working time directive states that junior medical personnel may not work more than 48 h/week by 2007, before this there will be a gradual reduction in working hours. By August 2004 doctors in training may not work more than 58 h/week (the average being calculated over a 4-month period). Daily and weekly rest breaks and annual leave will also be included. This calls for a break every 6 h (length of break not defined), 11 consecutive hours every 24-h period and 35 h consecutive break every 7 days (not calculated on a weekly basis) [1].

The consequences of this legislation are numerous and have already been tested in the European Court of Justice, as illustrated by the SIMAP judgment. The Spanish doctors union (SIMAP) brought their employers to court over working hours. "Work" was then defined for resident doctors as being at the employer's disposal, even when not performing his/her duties, i.e. asleep in the hospital. Doctors on-call at home are classified as working only when they are actually performing their duties.

This legislation will force us to look critically at what we do and why.

Possible solutions as suggested by Paul Thorp, chairman of the Junior Doctors Committee (UK) were 'more staff, new ways of working and properly negotiated derogation' and 'changing structure within hospitals'.

The costs of implementing these changes are difficult to assess. In the present economic climate (in many countries) of cost cutting in the health care sector, certain clinical activities including training may suffer. Norway, Portugal, Holland and Denmark have already implemented a 48-h working week and there does not appear to be a problem producing qualified Vascular surgeons with the reduced working hours [2]. Reviewing on call/clinical rotations, reducing the non-medical workload, increased junior staffing and centralizing vascular training seem necessary to optimize training with the new time constraints. This comes at an unfortunate time considering the changing landscape of vascular surgery with new evolving technology, expanding knowledge base and the move towards multidisciplinary approach to vascular patients. These latter factors alone could account for the need for creative restructuring of vascular training.

Possible solutions are to intensify and streamline present vascular training, prolong vascular training and/or reduce time spent in general surgical training. In some countries this may lead to vascular training becoming a monospecialty. The need for more junior staff will increase costs and create more competition for operative experience especially in smaller centers. Centralizing vascular training could ensure volume training and may buffer some of the costs of maintaining resident on-call rotation.

Recommending a model for creative restructuring of vascular training is difficult as each country has its own traditions, goals and methods. The author can only present subjective feedback gathered during international meetings, which is at best random. The EAVST is currently looking into ways of gathering more objective data on training. Some restructuring suggestions include:

(a) Choosing an on-call schedule that would optimize operative and other clinical work during daytime hours. This has been discussed at length in the literature and the details will not be dealt with here. However, concentrating all on-call at night for 1-week periods, thus allowing trainees to concentrate on operative and other clinical work during the day in the intervening weeks, is one good suggestion. There are clearly many other solutions with equal merit.
(b) Reducing the non-medical workload would certainly do much to allow the trainee to concentrate on clinical activity. Examples are as follows: secretarial/administrative functions, teaching specialized nursing staff to perform some practical functions.
(c) Restructuring trainee rotation allowing adequate time in the vascular laboratory, radiological department, and other relevant areas. Facilitating exchange programs or

rotations to other hospitals with specialized areas of excellence to ensure volume training and other relevant experience.

Reducing the time spent in the hospital by junior staff may increase the workload of senior staff, in addition to the requirement of an intensified teaching schedule to optimize training with the new time constraints. This may stretch the system further unless meticulously planned.

Quality control and training accreditation are important and may need to be re-evaluated. In Europe practices on awarding Certificates of Completion of Specialist Training (CCST) vary greatly. Authorities awarding CCST are evenly spread between governments (4 countries), professional organizations (5 countries) and universities (6 countries). Assessing and accrediting the quality of the training program is done by site visits (6 of 16 countries), assessing trainees on logbook (13 of 16 countries) and examination (10 of 16 countries). Some countries use all 3. Minimal required number of surgical operations range between 150 and 300, but some countries have not defined a minimum operative requirement [3].

The different training requirements throughout Europe make a consensus of minimum training requirements challenging. The Union of Medical Specialists (UEMS) and European Board of Vascular Surgery (EBVS) have defined these parameters for candidates wishing to take the European Board of Surgical Qualifications in Vascular surgery (EBSQ-vasc) exam. In addition, the EuReg-vasc, a committee under the UEMS, is gathering data in Europe on a national and center level on clinical activity and training requirements. In collaboration with EuReg-vasc, the EAVST is working on developing a Trainee Registration form. The aim is to further balance the data from the National and Center registration forms. This will hopefully allow the UEMS/EBVS/EAVST to follow the progress on reforming training across Europe from a trainee perspective.

Introducing the 48-h week is a challenging task. The need to maintain or increase the vascular units' productivity will increase the need for resources, both personnel and economic, to meet these demands. The reduction of working hours together with an expanding field of vascular surgery, the onslaught of endovascular surgery, may lead to vascular surgery becoming a monospecialty in more countries. There is also the danger that this will increase the workload on senior staff and may reduce the time available for teaching, supervision and research.

Creative restructuring of surgical training is necessary to ensure compliance.

There will be a need for a fundamental change in educational mentality, increased flexibility of clinical rotations and on-call duties, coordinating/tailoring vascular training to fit the individual trainee. A strict yearly schedule with well-defined operative goals and clinical activity should ensure no one falls behind. This requires restructuring of vascular training in many countries with the dramatic reduction in time spent assimilating the required knowledge and skills. There will be a need to focus on effective training programs, to continually update and redefine minimum training standards on a national level. It is important to learn from those countries that have already implemented the 48-h week. It may be necessary to centralize vascular function and training in some countries to ensure adequate operative volume, exposure to other relevant specialties, experience in a vascular lab, and a wide range of vascular clinical exposure.

### 4.2. Endovascular surgery (EVS)

This is an increasingly popular and significant treatment modality which is fuelled by patient demand, its minimally invasive nature and the industry. The status of EVS as an established treatment option in vascular surgery is undisputed, but practices vary. Endovascular training and credentialing of the vascular surgeon continues to be a poorly defined area in many centres and countries. Several pathways, albeit some incomplete, are available for the incorporation of EVS skills into the surgical armamentarium. Different professional groups have laid claim to this 'treatment tool'. EVS is carried out by interventional radiologists, cardiologists, cardiothoracic surgeons, vascular surgeons and/ or other groups across Europe.

The national CCST requirements for endovascular procedures during vascular training is generally small and individual caseloads vary greatly. Feedback from the EAVST members reflects a general dissatisfaction with endovascular training in most countries. Four of sixteen European countries do not require EVS to qualify in vascular surgery [4]. With technological advances and improving skills some predict that this will become 30% of future vascular surgical practices in the USA [5]. This estimate is speculative, but EVS is an established treatment modality throughout Europe. It therefore follows that vascular trainees should spend more time learning the necessary skills required in EVS, in order to ensure its future as a treatment option in vascular surgery. Where other professional groups perform the EVS it is still important for the vascular surgeon to understand the advantages/ limitations of this treatment option. Thus EVS training remains important. Developing hybrid or integrated training programs with other relevant professional groups has been successful and will increase mutual understanding and cooperation. This will facilitate a multidisciplinary approach in treatment of vascular patients and ensure volume training in EVS for vascular trainees [6].

The impact of EVS on open vascular procedures remains unclear and the literature offers many different views. Endovascular treatment techniques have already replaced some vascular operations. The likelihood is that new endovascular techniques involving stents and stented grafts will replace additional vascular operations [7]. Some authors suggested reviewing some index procedures in open surgery, such as fem distal bypass surgery as it is becoming too rare [8]. Others claim EVS has reduced the number of open vascular procedures, except for carotid and femoral–popliteal/tibial interventions [9]. EVS has allowed us to treat high-risk patients who would otherwise not be treated by open surgery. There is undoubtedly truth in all above statements and that EVS will have important implications for the future training of both general and vascular surgeons.

The author's subjective impression from speaking to other trainees across Europe is that too few vascular trainees are gaining adequate exposure and practical experience in EVS and that there is a lack of defined index procedures in the field. The EAVST will strive to find objective criteria to validate this statement. There is also some evidence that there will be a critical shortage of endovascular trained specialists in the future, with expected increase in the aging population and advances in EVS techniques [10].

A review on the definition of competence in catheter-based treatment has been carried out in the USA [11]. Consensus in Europe is being debated and the UEMS/EBVS are currently discussing EVS role in the European Board of Surgical Qualification exam in vascular surgery and the creation of an independent endovascular exam/diploma has been considered. There is agreement that vascular surgeons need to gain experience in EVS and that volume training provides better patient outcomes [12].

In many European countries there is an ongoing turf war on 'ownership' of EVS. It is vital that this does not interfere with vascular trainees exposure to this treatment tool. This exposure will be necessary, even if vascular surgeons do not perform EVS procedures themselves, simply to acquire knowledge of the complexity of treatment options, complications and follow-up. Vascular surgeons are best suited to deal with all aspects of EVS treatment as they often set the indication, are able to treat the complications, are familiar with postoperative care and follow-up [13]. Arguments against are that vascular surgeons are often unfamiliar with catheter-based technology and diagnostic tools such as Duplex scanning, Digital Subtraction Angiography. Should this be the case a multidisciplinary approach is the obvious choice.

Improving EVS training is important for the future. Technology cannot be owned by a specialty. Techniques do not comprise a discipline or specialty—they are simply tools [14]. There are several ways to secure adequate training: defining index procedures where this is lacking and increase minimal training requirements; creating integrated/hybrid training programs with other professional groups carrying out EVS procedures; creating multidisciplinary vascular centres; and national and international exchange programs. EVS will also need to be centralised in some countries to ensure volume training and better patient outcomes [4]. There will also be a need to increase/develop practical hands-on training courses with virtual reality computerized and other models in EVS across Europe to familiarise trainees with catheter-based techniques while ensuring patient safety.

On balance, it is felt that endovascular techniques are crucially important for the vascular surgeon of today and tomorrow. Vascular trainees in many countries should be more aggressively trained in EVS to ensure its place in the future of vascular surgery's armamentarium.

### *4.3. Education*

Increased complexity of vascular surgery and greater skills requirement requires:

- Knowledge of natural history,
- All methods of non-invasive and invasive diagnosis,
- Conservative and medical treatment,
- Open and endovascular treatment,
- Periprocedural care.

With a busier and more complex working schedule, teaching vascular trainees remains one of many duties of the vascular surgeon.

In an era of rapidly emerging technologies, scientific advances, changing societal expectations, focus on surgical competence, patient safety, new management skills' development and education are central pillars. This will transform the practice of vascular surgery in the future and therefore needs to be incorporated into trainee educational programs. This is a formidable challenge for every individual institution and country.

These changes in the vascular surgical curriculum will need to be continually re-assessed and revised. Certification and verification of surgical competency becomes very challenging in this setting.

Europe displays a wide range of practices when it comes to training in vascular surgery. Austria, Denmark, Finland, France, Greece, Norway, Italy, Luxemburg, Portugal and Spain all have vascular surgery as an independent speciality, either as a mono- or a subspecialty [4]. Ireland, Sweden, Switzerland, Netherlands and UK all have vascular surgery as an area of interest within general surgery [14].

Different methods are employed to evaluate quality in training as mentioned above with considerable differences in length of training (Fig. 1). Education is often a time consuming activity with long-term cost benefit. In many European countries there is an economic drive to reduce the cost of running hospitals, making doctors work more for less money. This together with imminent 48-h week may threaten education, teaching and research as these are not measurable in terms of pure economics and are time-consuming.

The legislative role of the EAVST is limited in this area. Working towards supporting the educational process through our educational web page (www.eavst.org), organising and promoting courses/conferences of interest to trainees across Europe and providing feedback from the trainees on all aspects of training/education to relevant forums. We are presently developing a trainee registration form in collaboration with EuReg-vasc to better perform this function.

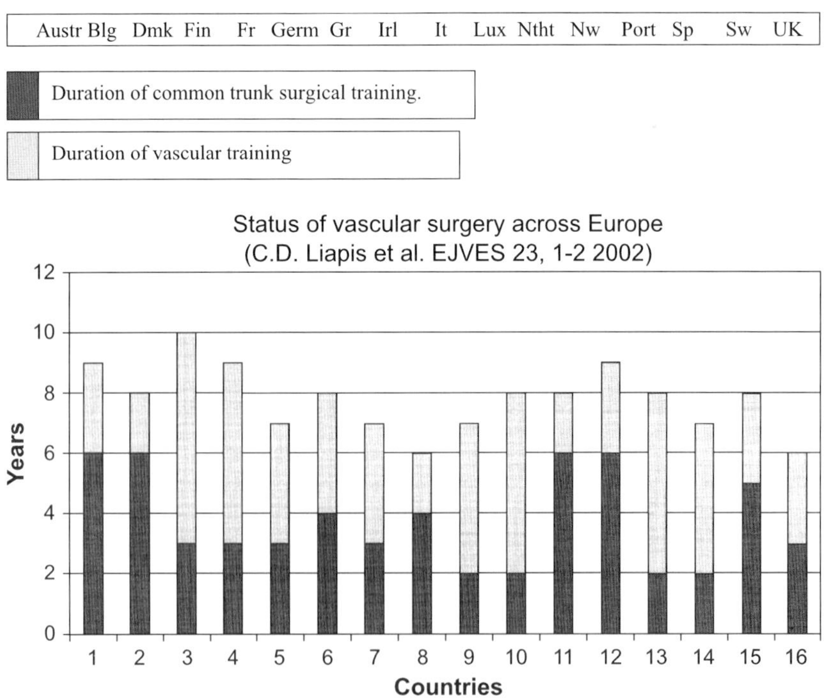


Fig. 1. Variation in length of training in general and vascular surgery.

Hospitals are becoming training centres for advanced technology—endovascular surgery, surgical robotic operations and other advanced surgical techniques. This requires intensive and expensive training of doctors and affiliated staff, the cost of training difficult to measure and is often carried out in cooperation with the industry, who often has a vested interest in the venture.

The development of a 'European Vascular School' is an attractive concept and would be a giant step towards harmonising and setting standards in vascular training. From a trainee point of view this would be appealing if it was an accredited supplement to the existing national curriculum. It would be beneficial if the curriculum was available on the internet with an exam at the end of different teaching modules. Each module could be an area or topic in vascular surgery or relevant affiliated subjects and evolving new fields. Thus, avoiding costly journeys and expensive course fees.

The use of telemedical conferences could also be considered as it has shown to have potential as a teaching tool and clinical aid in smaller centres [15]. This could be tied in with the nomination of European Vascular Centres. The Centres could then be given responsibility for developing European curriculum in certain fields of expertise, hosting courses and exchange programs. European Board of Surgical qualifications in vascular surgery at the end of the training period would be a natural evolution in testing acquired knowledge. The EBSQ-vasc exam would be useful for trainees/newly qualified vascular surgeons, especially if used actively and encouraged by all European countries as a supplement to the existing CCST accreditation. This could ensure harmonization and quality of training on a European level. The challenge is to choose which system is best and who should set the minimal training requirements—countries where vascular surgery as a mono-speciality, subspecialty versus those where vascular surgery is an area of interest. This is a complex issue which cannot be dealt with here.

Developing a standardized European curriculum could be a supplement and an update on current and evolving new fields and developments. Obviously this would be developed by all European countries, amalgamating knowledge and experience, with the creation of a reference and guide for the educational process on a national level. It would be important that courses or teaching modules (either over internet or organized at a European Vascular Centre) be accredited supplement to the national curriculum by all countries in Europe.

## 5. New initiatives and future of EAVST

After the first years with slow progress of EAVST a quiet period followed, but actually there is no doubt that EAVST is fully awake and alert having a strong and generally active Executive Committee working with many new ideas and projects. Currently we are working to change our work in EAVST to intensify the contribution of every member, as the progress of the association is impossible without them. We have increased the number of national representatives (3–4) in the larger European countries because recruitment of new members requires plenty of work. The most active member are awarded with sponsorship to attend the European Vascular Course, Charing Cross Symposium, International Association of Vascular Surgeons Meeting. The Congress travel grants to attend the Annual ESVS Meetings awarding are based on the activity in ESVS, EAVST work. This contribution includes the recommendation of new EAVST, the submission of abstracts to the Young

Vascular Surgeons Scientific Session (YVSSS) at the ESVS Meeting, sending the papers for the Educational section of EAVST Web site (www.eavst.org), attendance of YVSSS and ESVS Junior members, EAVST General Assembly. EAVST promotes exchange programmes and scientific studies within Europe and other continents.

We have established the new EAVST Student Section. The members of Student Section should be students of last 3 years interested in vascular surgery.

This allows us to attract the new, younger generation of future vascular surgeons. We shall sponsor the most active students by recommendation in their application for the ESVS student grant.

### *5.1. Education*

The EAVST should take a lead in promoting and providing educational tools for our members. This can be done by:

- continuing to develop the educational section on our website. Also providing a pointer to important articles with commentaries. We now have the opportunity to ask publishers to include central articles on our web page. Also in the future this may include on-line textbooks for reference and the creation of a journal club.
- promotion of relevant courses, exchange programs and congresses for trainees. I will send a mail to the UEMS to see if they can send us a list of CME accredited courses across Europe. We should promote this on our webpage: www.eurocme.org which has freely available, on-line lectures from different congresses.
- EAVST should place itself as a watchdog on training practices across Europe, thus the promotion of the ‘trainee registration form’ in collaboration for EuReg-vasc. We could also send questionnaires to our members on different issues relevant to training and offer a place on the EVC to a lucky trainee (drawn from a list by us) who fills in the questionnaire.
- promotion of relevant travel grants and our support to active national representatives or other members/students.
- promotion of research opportunities or available jobs. Vascular centres can be offered advertising space if they are looking for personnel to perform research or if they have available jobs in vascular surgery. With the 48-h week there will be a great demand for more trainees in Europe. We need to promote this function of our web page.
- organization of trainee courses. We should try to look into organizing a separate course for vascular trainees once or twice a year to prepare for the EBSQ-vasc exam and also maybe endovascular hands-on training, diagnostic tools, etc.

This could be separate from any other congress or be available on the internet.

Internet courses with relevant lectures on-line on the web page could be an interesting future prospect.

The current aims of EAVST also include establishing a database of vascular training features and vascular surgery trainees in Europe. The comparison of training methods between different countries may be helpful in finding better ways of training. This may also help in finding solutions from different countries, which have already gone through such processes. The EAVST National representatives take an active part in the reforming of vascular surgery in their countries. For example, the main project of the members in Turkey is to improve relationships within the Turkish membership. This might be achieved through exchange programs within the country, and maintaining grants for the international and national courses, subscriptions to medical journals, etc.

EAVST plans to promote exchange programmes and scientific studies within Europe and other continents. By becoming an active member, the trainee has the opportunity of being a part of scientific studies or involved in an exchange programme for vascular surgeons.

### 5.2. Future international cooperation

- Development of an International Vascular Trainees Society across the world between all the continents. For example, currently we already have close relations with trainees of Australia and Canada.
- Development of medical student affiliation (Student Section)
- Develop closer ties with radiological society, angiologists, internal medical specialties relevant to vascular surgery—a multidisciplinary vascular trainee society for trainees with a special interest in vascular patients.

Offer the affiliated membership to the EAVST for trainees from all over the world. This can spearhead the concept of a multidisciplinary cooperation for the future.

### 5.3. Monitoring function of the EAVST

- The EAVST should have an updated overview of the training structure in all of Europe.
- Create a questionnaire on the impact of training with the 48-h week and distribute it to all national representatives to provide feedback on a yearly basis. Focus on trainee problems so we can provide feedback on the UEMS and or ESVS meetings.
- Monitor the progress of endovascular training in Europe. This can be included in the trainee registration form.
- Monitor the trainees operative and practical experience in Europe (trainee registration form).
- Trainee travelling opportunities and exchange/elective cross-border opportunities.

## Acknowledgements

We acknowledge the contribution of Dr. Jorge Cruz (Senhora Hora, Portugal), Past EAVST Secretary General, EAVST Executive Committee member Dr. Peter Mondek (Trnava, Slovakia), Professor Jes Sandermann Consultant Vascular Surgeon, former EAVST member (Denmark) and all EAVST members.

## Appendix A. List of EAVST Executive Committee members (2003–2004)

- Alexei Svetlikov (St-Petersburg, Russia), Secretary General, asvetlikov@mail.ru
- Murat Aksoy (Istanbul, Turkey), maksoy@turk.net

- Grzegorz Biolik (Katowice, Poland), grzegorz.biolik@eth.pl
- Jorge Cruz (Senhora Hora, Portugal) Past Secretary General, jorgecruz36@hotmail.com
- Rafael Manvelyan (Erevan, Armenia), rafaelmanv@yahoo.com
- Peter Mondek (Trnava, Slovakia), mondo@pobox.sk
- Thomas Nyheim (Bergen, Norway), thomasnyheim1@yahoo.com.

## References

[1] R. MacDonald, BMJ (2002 May) 23–24.
[2] J. Sandermann, EJVES (2002 April) 45–47.
[3] J. Buth, et al., Cardiovasc. Surg. (2000 March) 74–77.
[4] C.D. Liapis, EJVES 28 (2002) 63–67.
[5] V. Kashyap, et al., J. Endovascular Ther. (2002 Oct.) 31–33.
[6] L.M. Messina, et al., Ann. Surg. (2002 Oct.) 57–59.
[7] F.J. Veith, Semin. Vasc. Surg. (1997 Dec.) 78–81.
[8] M.K. Nasr, EJVES (2003 Feb.) 34–36.
[9] T.M. Sullivan, J. Vasc. Surg. (2002 Sep.) 21–25.
[10] C.K. Wieslander, J. Vasc. Surg. (2001 June) 98–101.
[11] S.P. Woratyla, Vasc. Endovasc. Surg. (2003 Jan.–Feb.) 71–75.
[12] W.H. Pearce, J. Vasc. Surg. (1999 May) 111–115.
[13] C.K. Zarins, J. Vasc. Surg. (2000 Feb.) 43–45.
[14] J. Sandermann, EJVES 23 (2002) 91–94.
[15] M.A. Ricci, Telemed. J. (1998 Winter).

International Congress Series 1272 (2004) 95–101
www.ics-elsevier.com

# Funding of research in vascular surgery-related topics

Yannis Skalkidis*, Fotios Papadopoulos

*Department of Surgery, Athens University Medical School, Ellanikou 32 Street, 11635 Athens, Greece*

**Abstract.** Medicine, at an increasing pace and to a great degree, owes its impressively rapid progress to extensive research both in the basic as well as in the clinical domain. Funding for research and development is undoubtedly a crucial contributing factor for the advancement of sciences, especially those that rely more on rapidly evolving and expensive new technologies, like medicine and biomedical sciences in general. 

*Keywords:* Vascular surgery; Medicine; Funding

At the beginning of the century, most research in medicine was undertaken by universities and other academic bodies. Gradually, the private sector has started playing a more active role. On the same line, although funding was initially a public sector activity, the private sector is seen nowadays to support some types of biomedical research. In domains of medicine, like clinical applications in vascular surgery in which the presence of technology is more apparent, related industry seems to be more willing to fund relevant research activities.

However, few studies have been published in regard to the degree and sources of funding in biomedical research. This is even truer for specific research related to vascular surgery (clinical applications, as well as related to basic research) where very poor results were yielded. It is also rather difficult to get data on key information about this funding, like the amount of funding. Nevertheless, the importance of publicising relevant information on the degree and sources of funding in vascular surgery related research is undoubtedly pertinent and useful. To this end, a critical assessment of the situation is considered that can effectively facilitate constructive policies in this domain by all involved, relevant organisations.

Despite the abovementioned difficulties in searching for appropriate, relevant data, an effort was made to identify sources in the European Union's Directorate for Biomedical

* Corresponding author. Tel.: +30-210-729-7350; fax: +30-210-729-7351.
*E-mail address:* helcohop@ath.forthnet.gr (Y. Skalkidis).

0531-5131/ 
doi:10.1016/j.ics.2004.04.091

Research and focus specifically on all supported projects in vascular surgery the last few years.

Generic RTD activities and research infrastructure projects of "Community funded projects 1998–2002" were studied. The projects selected for funding under the action lines "Research and Technological Development Activities of a Generic Nature" and "Support for Research Infrastructures" of the programme on "Quality of Life and Management of Living Resources" (QoL) within the Fifth Framework Programme (1998–2002) were identified. A complementary Internet search was conducted, through the CORDIS website, for projects funded under the Fifth Framework Programme by the "Quality of Life". Initially, the keywords "vascular surgery" were used, but only two projects were indicated. That meant that projects very strictly defined as "vascular surgery" related were narrowing the scope of this survey too much. Consequently, the search was broadened by entering only the keyword "vascular" and selecting one-by-one the most relevant projects from the total of 40 returning ones.

Having completed the above survey, thirty projects funded by the EU were identified for the time period of December 1999 to February 2003 (date of project start). Classifying the projects according to research organisation, a slight excess for university organisations (53%) was revealed. Focusing on the coordinator country of origin, only four EU countries (UK, Italy, France and the Netherlands) were responsible for over 60% of the projects. As far as the type of study is concerned, the majority dealt with basic research (70%) (Table 1).

Information on the total amount of the EU funding was made possible only for thirteen of the projects. Out of them, EU contribution in funding was 1,698,258 per project coordinated by university organisation and € 2,071,264 per project coordinated by other than university organisation. Accordingly, the EU share in funding was € 1,674,464 per project concerning basic research and € 2,018,311 per project concerning clinical research.

In parallel to this search, an additional and complementary method was recruited relying on all the published work in two renowned peer review journals, The European

Table 1
Research Projects in vascular surgery related topics funded by the European Union from 1998 up to now

| Coordinator country | Total projects | Research organization | |
|---|---|---|---|
| | *N*, % | University | Other |
| Italy | 6 (20.0%) | 3 (50.0%) | 3 (50.0%) |
| UK | 6 (20.0%) | 4 (66.7%) | 2 (33.3%) |
| France | 4 (13.3%) | (0%) | 4 (100.0%) |
| The Netherlands | 3 (10.0%) | 1 (33.3%) | 2 (66.7%) |
| Belgium | 2 (6.7%) | (0%) | 2 (100%) |
| Finland | 2 (6.7%) | 2 (100.0%) | (0%) |
| Germany | 2 (6.7%) | 2 (100.0%) | (0%) |
| Greece | 2 (6.7%) | 2 (100.0%) | (0%) |
| Denmark | 1 (3.3%) | (0%) | 1 (100.0%) |
| Hungary | 1 (3.3%) | 1 (100.0%) | (0, 0%) |
| Spain | 1 (3.3%) | 1 (100.0%) | (0, 0%) |
| Total | 30 (100%) | 16 (53.3%) | 14 (46.7%) |

Journal of Vascular Surgery and the Journal of Vascular Surgery. The published research work from 2001 up to now was identified and the acknowledgement of potential funding was recorded, originating either from one or more funding sources. A number of concrete, identifiable, important parameters of the published work was also recorded and taken into account, like research organisation (alone or in collaboration with others), type of organisation (university, public and non-profit organisations, for profit or private for profit organisations), country of origin of those organisations, funding organisations (one or more) and its type (likewise with the types of research organisations), type of research (basic or clinical) and in the published work of one of the two journals that were available, key words for the categorisation of the research were also taken into account. All those parameters and their relationships were considered important to be communicated to the academic community, to all health related organisations, to responsible public authorities and to relevant industrial companies that are actively, directly or indirectly involved in the delivery of medical services in the domain of vascular surgery.

A total number of 1453 publications have been identified in the abovementioned journals since the year 2001. It was found that 413 (28.4%) were funded.

Further breakdown of the type of research organisation and the degree of their financial support reveals substantial differences. Nine hundred forty (64%) of those publications originated only from university sources, namely the one or all involved research organisations were universities. Out of those, 302 altogether (32.1%) were funded. The source of funding was exclusively from governmental/non-profit organizations in 65.9% of the cases, 12.3% from university and governmental funds and another 5.3% only from universities. The private sector was involved as an exclusive (12.9%) or contributing source for 3.6% of funding (Table 2).

Table 2
Source of funding and type of research organisations for research related to vascular surgery and published in selected peer review journals

| Research organization | *N* (%) | *N* (%) funded | Source of funding |
|---|---|---|---|
| University only | 940 (64%) | 302 (32.1%) | 65.9% exclusively from governmental/non-profit organizations<br>12.3% from university and governmental funds<br>12.9% exclusively from private sector<br>3.6% from private sector and other sources<br>5.3% exclusively from universities |
| University participation | 156 (11%) | 60 (38.5%) | 70.0% exclusively from governmental/non-profit organizations<br>10.0% from university and governmental funds<br>10.0% exclusively from private sector<br>3.4% from private sector and other sources<br>6.7% exclusively from universities |
| Other than university | 357 (24%) | 51 (14.3%) | 54.9% exclusively from governmental/non-profit organizations<br>7.8% from university and governmental funds<br>25.5% exclusively from private sector<br>9.8% from private sector and other sources<br>2.0% exclusively from universities |

An additional number of 156 published papers originated from universities in collaboration with other organizations and out of them 60 (38.5%) were funded. The origin of funding was mainly from public sources in 86.7% (governmental/non-profit organizations in 70.0%, university and governmental funds 10%, 6.7% from universities only) and the remaining 13.4% (10% exclusively from industry) private sector funds had supported the published research (Table 2).

On the contrary, the 357 papers originated only from other than university sources and only 51 (14.3%) were funded. Out of them, 64.7% were funded by public organisations (54.9% were exclusively funded from governmental/non-profit organizations, 7.8% were funded from university and governmental funds and 2.0 % were funded from university organizations only). The remaining 35.3% of the research was supported by private sector, either exclusively (25.5%) or in combination with governmental/non-profit and company funds (9.8%) (Table 2).

The analysis of the research publications from the year 2000 onwards and in regard to the geographical origin of the research organisations revealed that 688 (47.4%) came from European Union countries, 619 (42.6%) from the USA, 39 (2.7%) from Japan, 22 (1.5%) from Australia and New Zealand, 19 (1.3%) from Canada and the remaining 64 (4.4%) originated from other countries. Funding of the research though, broken down by geographical region, showed that in the USA 31.2% of the published work was funded, in EU countries funding was granted to 27.8% and in Japan 20.5% was funded. On the other hand, research that originated from Canadian organisations was funded in 47.4% of the cases and in Australia and New Zealand the funding reached 59.1% of the cases. In the rest of the countries, the percentage of funding was a mere 4.7%.

A further analysis of the type of funding organisations demonstrated that all over the world the organisations most commonly supporting research, at least in the field of vascular surgery, are governmental/non-profit organisations. Even the variation of this funding among geographical regions as the proportion of the total funding provided for research is rather minimal ranging from a high 100% in Japan to 53.8% in Australia and New Zealand (65.3% in the USA and 62.8% in the EU). It becomes more striking to the above figures when all public funding organisations are added, leaving the private sector's funding to a minimum of 15.2% in Europe, 14.5% in the USA, 7.7% in Australia and New Zealand and no funding at all in Canada and Japan. The exception to this observation is that in the category "other countries," there are only three research publications funded, out of which one is funded 33% by private company but this figure lacks any statistical significance (Table 3).

A more detailed analysis of the proportion of funding of the published research work inside the European Union showed that research from Scandinavian countries was funded in 49% of the cases, followed by Germany in which 37.9% of the work was funded. In the Netherlands the funding reached 27.3%, in France 23.5%, in the UK 22.5% and in Italy a mere 14% of the cases were funded. In all EU countries, like in all other geographical areas, the public sector was the most commonly funding source leaving the private sector to fall within 2–33% of financial support for the research field under scrutiny (Table 4).

In regard to the type of study that was published, basic research studies accounted for one-fourth of all published studies. Basic research studies originating from universities alone or

Table 3
Source of funding for research related to vascular surgery and published in selected peer review journals

| Geographical origin of research organization | *N* (%) | *N* (%) funded | Source of funding |
|---|---|---|---|
| EU | 688 (47.4%) | 191 (27.8%) | 62.8% exclusively from governmental/non-profit organizations<br>8.9% from university and governmental funds<br>15.2% exclusively from private sector<br>4.7% from private sector and other sources<br>8.4% exclusively from universities |
| USA | 619 (42.7%) | 193 (31.2%) | 65.3% exclusively from governmental/non-profit organizations<br>14.5% from university and governmental funds<br>14.5% exclusively from private sector<br>3.6% from private sector and other sources<br>2.1% exclusively from universities |
| Japan | 39 (2.7%) | 8 (20.5%) | 100.0% exclusively from governmental/non-profit organizations<br>0.0% from university and governmental funds<br>0.0% exclusively from private sector<br>0.0% from private sector and other sources<br>0.0% exclusively from universities |
| Australia and New Zealand | 22 (1.5%) | 13 (59.1%) | 53.8% exclusively from governmental/non-profit organizations<br>7.7% from university and governmental funds<br>7.7% exclusively from private sector<br>15.4% from private sector and other sources<br>15.4% exclusively from universities |
| Canada | 19 (1.3%) | 9 (47.4%) | 77.8% exclusively from governmental/non-profit organizations<br>11.1% from university and governmental funds<br>0.0% exclusively from private sector<br>0.0% from private sector and other sources<br>11.1% exclusively from universities |
| Other countries | 64 (4.4%) | 3 (4.7%) | 66.7% exclusively from governmental/non-profit organizations<br>0.0% from university and governmental funds<br>33.3% exclusively from private sector<br>0.0% from private sector and other sources<br>0.0% exclusively from universities |

in collaboration with other institutions reached 84% of cases, leaving the remaining 16% for other types of organisations or institutions. Similarly, clinical studies that originated from universities alone or in collaboration were around 77% of the cases. In terms of the origin of the funding organisation in relation to the type of research, it was shown that the majority of

Table 4
Source of funding in regard to the geographical origin of the research organisations within the EU and for topics related to vascular surgery

| Geographical origin of research organization within European Union | N (%) | N (%) funded | Source of funding |
|---|---|---|---|
| UK | 262 (38.1%) | 59 (22.5%) | 52.5% exclusively from governmental/non-profit organizations<br>13.6% from university and governmental funds<br>16.9% exclusively from private sector<br>5.1% from private sector and other sources<br>11.9% exclusively from universities |
| Scandinavian | 104 (15.1%) | 51 (49.0%) | 80.4% exclusively from governmental/non-profit organizations<br>9.8% from university and governmental funds<br>2.0% exclusively from private sector<br>5.9% from private sector and other sources<br>2.0% exclusively from universities |
| The Netherlands | 88 (12.8%) | 24 (27.3%) | 79.2% exclusively from governmental/non-profit organizations<br>8.3% from university and governmental funds<br>8.3% exclusively from private sector<br>4.2% from private sector and other sources<br>0.0% exclusively from universities |
| Germany | 58 (8.4%) | 22 (37.9%) | 50.0% exclusively from governmental/non-profit organizations<br>0.0% from university and governmental funds<br>27.3% exclusively from private sector<br>9.0% from private sector and other sources<br>13.6% exclusively from universities |
| France | 51 (7.4%) | 12 (23.5%) | 58.3% exclusively from governmental/non-profit organizations<br>8.3% from university and governmental funds<br>33.3% exclusively from private sector<br>0.0% from private sector and other sources<br>0.0% exclusively from universities |
| Italy | 43 (6.3%) | 6 (14.0%) | 66.7% exclusively from governmental/non-profit organizations<br>0.0% from university and governmental funds<br>33.3% exclusively from private sector<br>0.0% from private sector and other sources<br>0.0% exclusively from universities |

the basic research was funded from public organisations in 92.3% (governmental organisations exclusively in 69.8%), leaving a mere 7.7% for private sector funding for basic research. For clinical research though, funding of research from the public sector was 72.5% and from the private sector it reached 27.5% of the cases (Table 5).

The correlation between the type of published research and the type of scientific organisations that undertook the work demonstrated a significant difference showing that universities alone are responsible for 65% of the research.

Table 5
Type of research organisation and type of funding source in relation to the type of research in the domain of vascular surgery

| Type of study | Research organisation | | Source of funding | |
|---|---|---|---|---|
| | University alone or in collaboration (%) | Other (%) | Public (%) | Private (%) |
| Basic | 84.4 | 16 | 92.3 | 7.7 |
| Clinical | 76.8 | 23.2 | 72.5 | 27.5 |
| Other | 49.4 | 50.6 | 72.3 | 27.7 |

Concerning the type of research based on the identified key words that were chosen by the researchers in the publications of the European Journal of Vascular Surgery, it was shown that 14.3% of the articles referred to aortic related topics, 9.5% carotid arteries, 8.5% arterial occlusive diseases, followed by aneurysms (except aortic and carotid), venous related disorders, etc. (Table 6).

Finally, an interesting search would be to correlate the number of published works originating from different countries to the number of medical doctors or the total health budget in the respective country. Of course, it goes without saying that in order for such a correlation to be accurate, valid and reliable, all research work in those countries should be taken into consideration. However, a first glimpse of the relevant figures (number of publications, number of medical doctors and health budget) from the countries that have most commonly published their research in the two journals that were used in this work shows that the UK, Scandinavian countries and the Netherlands are the most proliferate in this respect. It should be highlighted again, though, that further and detailed analysis is imperative before we can reach more definite, but maybe quite interesting, results.

In conclusion, despite the considerable limitations of this effort, some of which were unavoidable and others needing further and more elaborate and extensive search to additional parameters, it is thought that the outcome concisely described above offers important information about vascular surgery related research, in terms of the extent and sources of its funding.

Table 6
Source of funding in relation to topic-specific research in the domain of vascular surgery

| Keywords | *N* (%) | Source of funding | |
|---|---|---|---|
| | | Public (%) | Private (%) |
| Aortic related Aneurisms | 71 (14.3%) | 75 | 25 |
| Carotid related | 47 (9.5%) | 100 | 0 |
| Arterial occlusive | 42 (8.5%) | 76.9 | 23.1 |
| Aneurysms, except for aortic | 25 (5.0%) | 100 | 0 |
| Venous related | 25 (5.0%) | 62.5 | 37.5 |
| Exam related | 23 (4.6%) | 100 | 0 |
| Therapeutic related | 22 (4.4%) | 75 | 25 |
| Stents-grafts | 19 (3.8%) | 50 | 50 |
| Other | 223 (44.9%) | 75.3 | 24.7 |

International Congress Series 1272 (2004) 102–108

www.ics-elsevier.com

# Endovascular surgery in Europe

Piergiorgio Cao*, Paola De Rango

*Struttura Complessa di Chirurgia Vascolare, Policlinico Monteluce, Via Brunamonti, 06122 Perugia, Italy*

*Keywords:* Endovascular practice; Randomized controlled trials; Vascular registries

## 1. Introduction

The diminishing invasiveness of therapeutic procedures is a natural and desirable consequence of medical research. In this perspective, catheter-based endovascular techniques have advanced significantly over the past three decades. Vascular surgeons have become more interested in these developments involving an increasing number of vascular diseases, and are now rapidly gaining in training widening practice opportunities. However, technology improvements will substantially diminish the need to perform open vascular reconstructions. Surgeons are being confronted with a variety of specialty groups (e.g., cardiologists, interventional radiologists, etc.) who intend to provide independent vascular services.

Europe showed great enthusiasm and immediate suitability for endovascular innovations. Although there is a growing body of evidence suggesting that this new treatment modality is associated with less trauma to the patient, providing outcomes competitive with open vascular surgery, concerns about the evaluation, applicability and long-term durability of new technology with respect to the traditional gold standard remain. Furthermore, there may be a tendency for economic and ego gratification to guide decisions, that may outweigh the quality of patient care.

## 2. Specialists involved

The development of endovascular techniques has forced vascular specialists to collaborate and interact. Cardiologists, vascular surgeons, interventional radiologists and angiologists involved in this field, consider the endovascular procedure as their task and conflicts may develop. In some vascular centers, a partnership between vascular surgeons and radiologists has been developed since the era of abdominal aortic aneurysm (AAA) endoluminal repair. The cooperation between radiologists and surgeons is becoming stronger than between surgeons and cardiologists, there are several reasons

* Corresponding author. Tel.: +39-75-573-2876; fax: +39-75-578-3194.
*E-mail address:* pcao@unipg.it (P. Cao).


doi:10.1016/j.ics.2004.04.079

to explain this: the most important is based on the fact that radiologists, compared with the cardiologists, are less directly involved in patient clinical care and consequently the professional competition with vascular surgeons is less pronounced. In theory, collaboration among specialists is realistic in Europe because in the majority of cases, physicians are not directly paid by the patients but receive a salary, the main obstacle to teamwork being represented by the wish of the single physician for visibility and prestige.

Nevertheless, there are an increasing number of vascular surgeons who acquired all the skills necessary to perform endovascular procedures and are working independently.

Cooperation between vascular specialists in Europe was implemented by the organization of collaborative bodies. In 1985, the Cardiovascular and Interventional Radiological Society of Europe (CIRSE) was founded by the joining of forces of two formerly independent European societies: the European College of Angiography (ECA) and the European Society of Cardiovascular and Interventional Radiology (ESCVIR). Today CIRSE has 1400 members from about 50 countries. The objectives of the Society, which meets regularly, are principally to provide education and an exchange of scientific information for all physicians practicing or interested in cardiovascular and interventional radiology, to implement the role of cardiovascular and interventional radiology as a subspecialty.

## 3. The problem of training

An important issue in endovascular practice is the lack of a formal program of training or accreditation in endovascular techniques. In Europe, quality assurance of vascular surgical training is not the responsibility of a centralized European authority, but is a matter in which the different countries have autonomous regulations. Consequently, different targets for duration, contents, and general principles for training in vascular surgery have been set. These differences are more pronounced for endovascular practice. The unification of countries into the European Union (EU) has changed this perspective because there is an increasing impetus towards a mutual recognition of education between member states.

Currently, all the physicians involved in endovascular procedures have undergone formal training and are certified in their respective specialties but they are not certified in the associated specialties: surgeons are usually not trained in interventional radiology and radiologists and cardiologists are not trained in vascular surgery care. However, it has to be acknowledged that many European countries are developing cross-specialty training and accreditation [1]. Most physicians presently acquire additional knowledge and skills by visiting other centers or by attending one or more training courses available throughout Europe. The problem is that the nature, aims, and quality of such courses are variable, ranging from single-day device-specific workshops to comprehensive diploma courses that offer theoretical and practical training in all aspects of a particular technique.

Recently, new initiatives and foundations have been promoted to support education and collaboration in these fields throughout Europe. The European Vascular and Interventional Training Academy (EVITA) was promoted as a joint initiative of CIRSE, ESVS (European Society of Vascular Surgery) and FIRE (the Foundation for Research and Education of CIRSE), in order to strengthen the joint forces of both vascular surgeons and interventional radiologists in the treatment of vascular diseases. The format of EVITA, conceived as a purely educational annual meeting, is based on workshops including hands-on training, panel discussions, live case transmission, and state-of-the-art lectures. Results of these recently established initiatives are under observation.

In Europe, as in the United States, industries have a key role in the research of new technologies for endovascular treatment of arterial diseases. Their contribution is performed either through research projects directly managed by industries, or by financial support to single institutions for conducting clinical studies. The downside is that, as the market changes, economic pressure in specific departments and among individuals will increase.

Ideally, funding for research should come from official bodies, such as Local Government Authorities and European Union Administration. This type of funding is largely insufficient because of bureaucratic difficulties and scarcity of available grants, therefore industries may have a fundamental role in supporting vascular research. In general, industries respect the independent role of the researcher and an optimal balance between innovation, patient care, and business can be achieved.

Recently, CIRSE supported the creation of FIRE, an independent research and education foundation, a non-profit organization, which promotes and supports research and education in diagnosis and treatment in Cardiovascular and Interventional Radiology. Sponsoring of basic research, pilot studies, large multicenter randomized trials, endovascular registries and educational development are the principal objectives of FIRE.

## 4. Regulatory bodies

Industry pressure and financial reward may lead to uncontrolled adoption of endovascular techniques available with possible scant evaluation causing improper patient care. Medical device regulation generates divergent criticism: Food and Drug Administration (FDA) in the United States is more often regarded as too restrictive. In contrast, the general opinion of EU device regulation is usually considered too lax.

In the United States, there are different types of stents and endografts with different characteristics, and more than a dozen companies are actively marketing these in different stages of clinical use or investigating them for FDA approval. On the other hand, throughout Europe, regulations exist to prevent the use of new devices until their safety and effectiveness have been proved.

On 1 January 1995, a new European directive covering implantable medical devices became effective. This requires all medical devices to bear a CE mark from 14 June 1998. The CE marking, which is the abbreviation for 'European Conformity', indicates that the device meets all the essential requirements and other applicable provisions that have been imposed upon it by means of European directives, and that the product has been subject to the appropriate conformity assessment procedures. The CE marking system has the requirement to demonstrate safety of the medical device for an intended use, prior to commercialization.

Many countries in the European Union have implemented these directives. CE marking is not a quality-mark. First, it refers to the safety rather than the quality of a product, secondly CE marking is mandatory for the product that applies, whereas most quality markings are voluntary.

The CE marking is a kind of trade passport for the European marketplace: it allows the manufacturer to freely circulate their product throughout the 18 countries of the European Economic Area (EEA). The advantage of this policy is that there is only one set of requirements and procedures to comply with the designing and manufacturing of a product within the entire EEA. The various and conflicting national regulations are eliminated.

Differently from FDA approval that implies Phase I and Phase II studies, the European directive covers only safety, not efficacy, and concern remains about the uniformity of safety standards imposed by individual countries.

## 5. Online surveys, vascular registries and randomized trials

Economic forces are certainly driving towards the less invasive modes, which are presumed to be less expensive. Patients and physicians are contributing to the impression that endovascular procedures should be preferred because of their perception that less is better. Outcome studies and cost analysis need to be done before the attractive conclusion that 'less invasive' is 'cheaper' as well as 'better' can be drawn.

In the last years, the Industries supported a proposal made by the Editorial Board of the journal *Vascular News* to conduct a survey to monitor vascular and endovascular activity in Europe: the European Vascular and Endovascular Monitor (EVEM), updated quarterly by online questionnaires. The main objective of EVEM is to regularly inform and advise members on changes in vascular and endovascular practice in Europe, via updated reports. Data from EVEM 2003 showed that endovascular procedures in Europe are mostly performed by vascular surgeons and radiologists together (67%) or by vascular surgeons alone (29%). EVEM showed that endovascular procedures have increased in the last 2 years and constitute about 12% of all aortic or carotid repairs, and about 55% of infrainguinal vascular procedures. Interesting changes and trends in endovascular applications can be expected in further EVEM reports. Limitations of EVEM reports are that data are given on a retrospective basis and that there is no effective control on information reliability. However, the numbers are periodically matched with the numbers of devices sold by the different companies operating in any single European country. Recent figures from EVEM are reported in Table 1.

Dedicated Vascular Registries have been established in European countries to ensure that evolving endovascular techniques can be monitored [2–4]. Several vascular registries (see Table 2) have been in use for many years, the Swedish Vascular Registry (SwedVasc) is the oldest and the Eurostar the most widely known.

Table 1
Procedures in Western Europe[a]

| Procedures | Total no. | Endovascular | (%) | Open repair | (%) |
|---|---|---|---|---|---|
| Carotid | 100,728 | 11,142 | 11 | 89,586 | 89 |
| AAA | 74,467 | 9645 | 13 | 65,002 | 87 |
| Thoracic aneurysm and dissection | 9841 | 3342 | 40 | 6499 | 60 |
| Infrainguinal | 169,245 | 93,192 | 55 | 76,053 | 45 |

[a] Based on EVEM report, September 2003.

In general the voluntary nature of all the registries raises questions about the completeness and accuracy of the returned data [5]. Furthermore, when compared with Randomized Controlled Trials (RCTs), vascular registries show lower levels of evidence and lack of monitoring for patient data. However, registries seem extremely useful to answer pertinent questions regarding the 'real world' of clinical practice and have the advantage to provide information faster than RCTs. These clinical questions may relate to the mortality associated to the endovascular procedure, complications, and the risk of conversion to open repair. In addition, the risk of systemic, arterial and device-related complications can be assessed in a large study population [6,7]. Reports from recent dedicated vascular registries have been found extremely useful for identifying anatomic and patient-related risk factors and device failures [8,9].

The cost-effectiveness of a registry is difficult to define in strict economical terms; however, the cost per registered case appears negligible compared with the overall cost of treating a vascular patient, and definitely less than costs associated with RCTs. More detailed information on this issue can be found in another chapter of this book.

RCTs remain the 'gold-standard' for the assessment of any new intervention. Randomizing a new technology against conventional treatment may jeopardize the results if carried out too early. However, delaying the start of randomization may cause risk of loss of clinical equipoise, i.e. the surgeon or the patient will no longer accept conventional treatment.

After some initial logistic delays, different RCTs comparing efficacy of endovascular repair of AAA with open surgery are now well underway in Europe. Trials organizers have in general made great efforts to ensure that centers involved are proficient so there is little or no learning curve effect about which to be concerned. Countries with ongoing trials on aortic repair include the UK EVAR 1 (Endovascular Abdominal Aortic Aneurysm Repair) trial and EVAR 2 trial (evaluating high-risk patients), the French Aneurysme Chirurgie de l'aorte contre Endoprothèse (ACE) trial, the Dutch Randomised Endovascular Aneurysm Management (DREAM) trial (Table 3) [10–12], and recently trials on endoluminal treatment of small aneurysms have been planned.

Ongoing RCTs in Europe on carotid stenting include: in the United Kingdom, the CAVATAS II/ICSS (International Carotid Stenting Study); in France the EVA 3S, and in Germany the SPACE (Stent-protected Percutaneous Angioplasty of the Carotid Artery with Endarterectomy) trial.

Table 2
Vascular registries in Europe

| | Registry | Country | Procedures |
|---|---|---|---|
| National | Swedvasc | Sweden | vasc and endovasc |
| | Hellenic Angio | Greece | vasc and endovasc |
| | Spanish hospital, Karbase | Spain, Denmark | vasc and endovasc, vasc and endovasc |
| | Swiss National | Switzerland | vasc and endovasc |
| | RETA | UK | aortic endograft |
| International | EUROCAST | European | carotid |
| | EUROSTAR | European | aortic endograft |
| | EVEM | European | vasc and endovasc |

Table 3
Randomized clinical trials on endovascular surgery in Europe

| | Trial | Country | Status |
|---|---|---|---|
| Carotid | CAVATAS | UK | completed |
| | Leicester | UK | stopped |
| | CAVATAS II/ICSS | UK | ongoing |
| | EVA 3S | France | ongoing |
| | SPACE | Germany | ongoing |
| Aortic | DREAM | The Netherlands | ongoing |
| | EVAR 1 | UK | ongoing |
| | EVAR 2 | UK | ongoing |

## 6. Conclusions

The multidisciplinary approach and the relatively easy CE marking process led to a widespread endovascular surgery in Europe. Endovascular specialists collaboration in Europe is somewhat encouraged by the perception of a faster learning curve in performing the procedure; organization of collaborative societies and multidisciplinary meetings sponsored by manufacturers can contribute to this.

Online surveys as well as dedicated registries have an important role in gathering data, testing new techniques, and monitoring outcomes of endovascular procedures in Europe, while waiting for the results of the ongoing RCT trials.

Constant and accurate control on endovascular practice is essential to ensure balance between patient benefit and industrial pressure.

## References

[1] P. Cao, F. Verzini, P. De Rango, Endovascular surgery in Europe, in: P. Glovitzky (Ed.), Perspectives in Vascular Surgery, vol. 15, No. 1,Westminster Publications, 2003, pp. 15–22.

[2] P. Harris, Eurostar: the need to audit new generations devices separately, in: R.M. Greenhalgh, J.T. Powell, A.W. Mitchell (Eds.), Vascular and Endovascular Opportunities, Saunders, London, 2000, pp. 237–247.

[3] S.M. Thomas, et al., on behalf of the Vascular Surgical Society of Great Britain and Ireland and the British Society of Interventional Radiologists, Short-term (30 day) outcome of endovascular treatment of abdominal aortic aneurysm: results from a prospective Registry of Endovascular Treatment of Aneurysms (RETA), Eur. J. Vasc. Endovasc. Surg. 21 (2001) 57–64.

[4] M.R.H.M. Van Sambeek, on behalf of the EUROCAST Registry Steering Committee, The EUROCAST Registry of carotid stenting, in: R.M. Greenhalgh, J.T Powell, A.W. Mitchell (Eds.), Vascular and Endovascular Opportunities, Saunders, London, 2000, pp. 123–127.

[5] L.P. Jensen, T. Troeng, Vascular registries—are they worth the effort? Eur. J. Vasc. Endovasc. Surg. 20 (2000) 225–226.

[6] J. Buth, et al., on behalf of the Eurostar Collaborators: early complications and endoleaks after endovascular abdominal aortic aneurysm repair, Report of a multicentre study, J. Vasc. Surg. 31 (2000) 134–146.

[7] P.L. Harris, et al., Incidence and risk factors of late rupture, conversion and death after endovascular repair of infrarenal aortic aneurysms: the EUROSTAR experience, J. Vasc. Surg. 32 (2000) 739–749.

[8] J. Buth, et al. (on behalf of the EUROSTAR Collaborators), Outcome of endovascular abdominal aortic aneurysm repair in patients considered unfit for an open procedure: a report on the EUROSTAR experience, J. Vasc. Surg. 35 (2002) 211–221.

[9] C. van Marriewijk, et al., Significance of endoleaks after endovascular repair of abdominal aortic aneurysms: the EUROSTAR experience, J. Vasc. Surg. 35 (2002) 461–473.

[10] R.M. Greenhalgh, et al., for the UK EVAR Trial Participants, The UK EndoVascular Aneurysm Repair

(EVAR) trials: background and methodology, in: R.M. Greenhalgh, J.T. Powell, A.W. Mitchell (Eds.), Vascular and Endovascular Opportunities, Saunders, London, 2000, pp. 215–227.
[11] J.-P. Becquemin, et al., for the ACE trialists, Abdominal aortic aneurysms—surgical versus endoluminal repair: the French prospective randomized (ACE) trial, in: R.M. Greenhalgh, J.T. Powell, A.W. Mitchell (Eds.), Vascular and Endovascular Opportunities, Saunders, London, 2000, pp. 234–236.
[12] M. Prinssen, E. Buskens, J.D. Blankesteijn, The Dutch Randomised Endovascular Aneurysm Management (DREAM) trial, J. Cardiovasc. Surg. 43 (2002) 379–384.

International Congress Series 1272 (2004) 109–115

www.ics-elsevier.com

# Postgraduate training in endovascular surgery for vascular surgeons

Giorgio M. Biasi [a,*], Claudia Piazzoni [b]

[a] *Department of Surgical Sciences and Intensive Care, University of Milan, Bicocca, Italy*
[b] *Vascular Surgery-Bassini/S. Gerardo Teaching Hospital, Milan, Italy*

**Abstract.** Vascular Surgery began in the period between the first and second world wars, as the need to treat arterial war injuries arose. Vascular operations were performed by general surgeons and often ended in major amputations. Between the second world war and the Vietnam war, Norman Rich published his volume entitled "Vascular Trauma" and Drs. DeBakey and Simeone defined guidelines in vascular surgery. A new vision of this specialty commenced, but it was always considered as a branch of general surgery and was performed by surgeons with varying backgrounds. Few vascular operations were performed by surgeons who restricted their practice exclusively to the vascular field. The necessity of certification came with the modern concept of vascular surgery in Europe in the 1960s, with a new specialist in surgery with vascular competence. The Board of Vascular Surgery came into existence, recognizing the independent figure of the vascular surgeon. 

*Keywords:* Vascular surgery

During the last 15 years, we have witnessed incredible progress in technology with the advent of endovascular procedures, which represented a real revolution (Table 1).

Although the first catheter was introduced in the 1960s by a vascular surgeon, Tom Fogarty [1], vascular surgeons had not had an active participation in the initial steps in the development of endovascular techniques. Pioneers of this revolution were cardiologists Dotter and Judkins [2], who introduced percutaneous transluminal angioplasty (PTA) in 1964 and radiologists Gruntzig [3] and Kumpe, who improved this procedure by introducing non-compliant balloon catheters several years later. With increasing evidence that endovascular procedures could be effective, vascular surgeons began to approach and use this technique. In the 1990s, the introduction of the endovascular stent grafts completely revolutionized the treatment of vascular diseases. Today, endovascular proce-

* Corresponding author. Universita delgi studi di Milano Bicocca, Vascular Surgery Unit, 3rd floor, Bassini Teaching Hospital, Via M Gorki 50, Cinisello Balsamo, Milan 20092, Italy. Tel.: +39-2617-4928; fax: +39-2660-12568.

*E-mail address:* giorgio.biasi@unimib.it (G.M. Biasi).


doi:10.1016/j.ics.2004.04.083

Table 1
Status of vascular surgery across Europe

| Country | Vascular surgery independent specialty | | Duration of vascular training | Duration of common training | No. of vascular surgeons | Endovascular procedures during training | |
|---|---|---|---|---|---|---|---|
| | Yes | No | | | | No | Yes |
| Austria | + | | 3 | 6 | 120 | + | |
| Belgium | | + | 2 | 6 | 150 | + | |
| Denmark | + | | 7(4) | 3 | 45 | | + |
| Finland | + | | 6 | 3 | 120 | + | |
| France | + | | 4 | 3 | 500 | + | |
| Germany | | + | 4 | 4 | 800 | + | |
| Greece | + | | 4 | 3 | 90 | + | |
| Ireland | | + | 2 | 4 | 20(6) | | + |
| Italy | + | | 5 | 1–2 | 600 | + | |
| Luxembourg | + | | 6 | – | 12 | + | |

dures are the treatment of choice for many arterial diseases, both obstructive and aneurysmal, in most vascular territories (Fig. 1).

With the rapid, progressive increase in the number of peripheral endovascular procedures performed (100,000 in the year 2000 alone), it was inevitable that the question would arise as to which specialist was most qualified to treat these cases: vascular surgeons, interventional cardiologists, interventional radiologists or neuroradiologists? These four specialties were the most prominent to become involved in the late 1980s, whereas today vascular medicine physicians, cardiac surgeons and general surgeons would not mind stepping onto the stage, too [4] (Fig. 2).

Each of the four main specialists has some characteristics and skills missing in the others, which puts them in an attractive and privileged position. The vascular surgeon, for

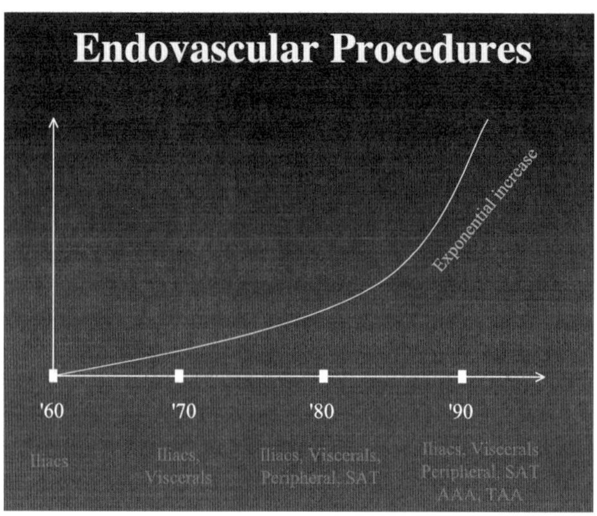


Fig. 1. Increase of endovascular procedures in last 40 years.

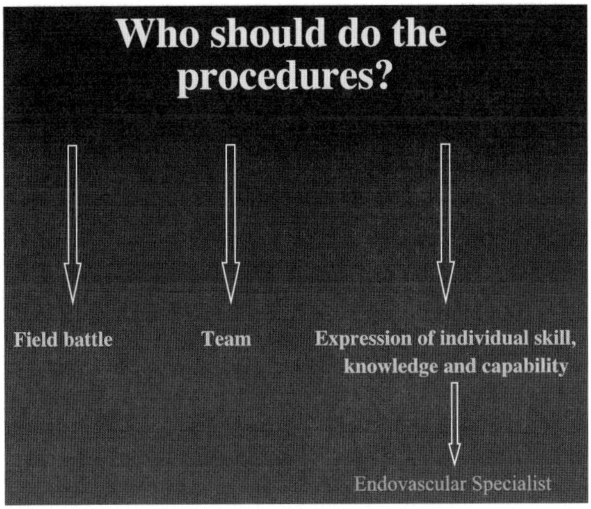


Fig. 2. Who should do endovascular procedures?

example, has good experience in the ward, in the operating theatre and in both elective and emergency surgery. He/she is familiar with peripheral arterial plaques and lesions, has an excellent concept of three-dimensional anatomy, and is aware of the importance of sterility. Probably to a greater degree than the other specialists, the vascular surgeon has the capability to resolve procedural complications, which has become a discriminating factor in favor of the surgeon's fundamental importance in the debate.

The interventional cardiologist has equally good clinical experience on the ward, less surgical experience and less familiarity with peripheral plaques; however, the cardiologist has a much wider experience in coronary angioplasties. Both vascular surgeons and interventional cardiologists have little practical knowledge in the use of radiological apparatus and "imaging".

Interventional radiologists and interventional neuroradiologists are those who have the most experience in navigating and maneuvering guidewires and catheters in the vascular territories but, compared with interventional cardiologists and especially vascular surgeons, they have the least experience in elective surgery, in emergency situations and in patient follow-up.

In the interest of the patient and to maintain the standard of care, it is now preferable that at least two or more of the above-mentioned specialists be present and consulted in each center where endovascular procedures are performed. This situation may not always be possible and could cause conflict among fellow members of an endovascular team, since it is quite clear that only one person can be considered ultimately responsible for each procedure. Other potential drawbacks of the team approach are patient referral and, last but not least, the increase in costs.

As a consequence of these considerations, The Monza Medical School of the University of Milan-Bicocca, in accordance with its Post-Graduate Medical Education (PGME) Programs, has established a Master in Endovascular Techniques (MET). The program seeks to train a new type of endovascular specialist who would acquire the knowledge base and skills representative of all the qualified specialties currently involved in endovascular interventions.

To start with, the task of constructing such a program appeared particularly arduous and ambitious considering that (1) there are no definitions of what an endovascular specialist should do and where (2) it is not clear if there is a need for such a specialist, and (3) competition and professional and academic rivalries characterize this peculiar field of practice in such a way that the "actors" often assume a more contentious than collaborative attitude, ending ultimately in a dreadful turf battle.

Clearly, answers to the following questions were mandatory: Are vascular surgeons today receiving sufficient instruction in endovascular procedures during their training program? Are specialists in interventional radiology, neuroradiology, and cardiology likewise sufficiently trained? The answer to these questions is probably no!

The MET is open to physicians who have completed a certified training program in vascular surgery, interventional radiology, interventional cardiology, or neuroradiology or to those who have received the appropriate Certificate of Completion of Specialist Training (CCST) in their respective country of origin Fig. 3. The centres listed in Fig. 4 are presently participating in the educational programme. After presenting his/her curriculum vitae, the prospective candidate is selected, once the eligibility criteria have been fulfilled.

The aims of the MET are (1) to master catheter skills; (2) to be exposed to a relevant number of cases (100 diagnostic angiograms, >100 balloon/stenting procedures and from 30 to 50 aortic stent-grafts) as an assistant and operator, under the tuition of trained doctors, nurses, and technicians; (3) to learn how to select patients appropriately; (4) to learn how to foresee and avoid problems, but if they occur, to find the best, most efficient, durable, and least invasive solutions; and (5) to be skilled in the performance of endovascular procedures.

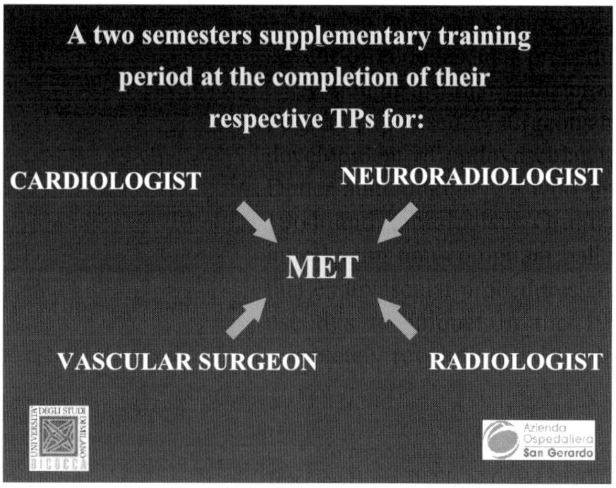


Fig. 3. Organization of MET.

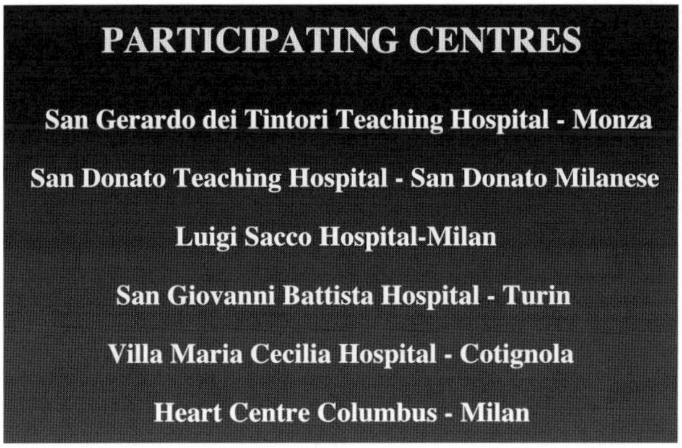
PARTICIPATING CENTRES
San Gerardo dei Tintori Teaching Hospital - Monza
San Donato Teaching Hospital - San Donato Milanese
Luigi Sacco Hospital-Milan
San Giovanni Battista Hospital - Turin
Villa Maria Cecilia Hospital - Cotignola
Heart Centre Columbus - Milan

Fig. 4. Participating centres.

Three didactic programmes have been constructed on the basis of the specialty background of the trainee. A faculty of lecturers and recognized experts in diagnosis, indications, and practice of endovascular procedures from the Milan-Bicocca University and other national and international institutions, has been formed to conduct didactic activities, such as seminars, lectures, master classes, workshops, etc. in Italian and English, providing a high level of specialization and education.

The 1-year MET Programme is divided into two semesters starting on the 15th of November and the 15th of May. Trainees are required to attend the institutions connected to the MET full-time for 1500 hours, comprising 900 hours of clinical practice, 300 hours of seminars, master classes, interactive lectures, workshops and courses with live-case demonstrations and 300 hours of individual study. The minimum attendance has been established at 80% of the total hours required. An assessment of progress is made at the end of the first semester and upon the successful completion of the final oral examination, when 60 university credit points are assigned. Those who complete their training period receive official certification, awarded by the University of Milan-Bicocca and are credited by the Italian Health Department.

The 3rd edition of the MET for the academic year 2003/2004 received 10 applications for the three posts available.

Since November 2003 the Master in Endovascular Techniques of the Department of Surgical Sciences and I.C. of the University of Milan-Bicocca, is listed as a recognized endovascular training Centre with the UEMS, Division and Board of Vascular Surgery.

The University of Milan-Bicocca, with the endorsement of the Italian Ministry of University and Research (MIUR), has recently approved a 4-year International PhD in Translational and Molecular Medicine with the aim of covering the entire educational programme from "the benchside to the bedside" (Fig. 5). The first 3 years of this programme is a Doctorate. The 4th year is represented by Masters, among which is the MET, which has a strong professional structure. The programme has been devised to comply with the European Community requirements for International PhDs.

MET represents a philosophical approach to the need of creating a hybrid specialist through professional training from highly qualified tutors. We are well aware that we are in

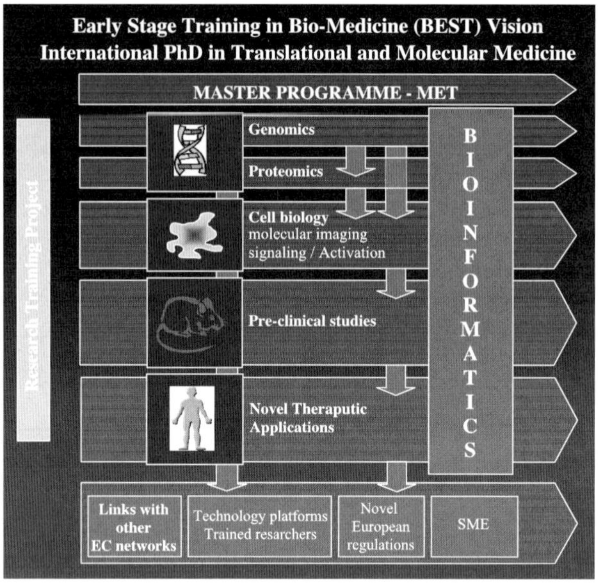


Fig. 5. International PhD in Translational and Molecular Medicine.

a transitional period in peripheral endovascular interventions and that a solution has to be provided now. The problems that we are presently experiencing did not exist in the past and will not exist in the future. To our knowledge, MET is the only endovascular educational program open to different specialties (Fig. 6).

As Veith wrote in 1997: "As Darwin noted, the death of a species is a consequence of non-adaptation to changing circumstances".

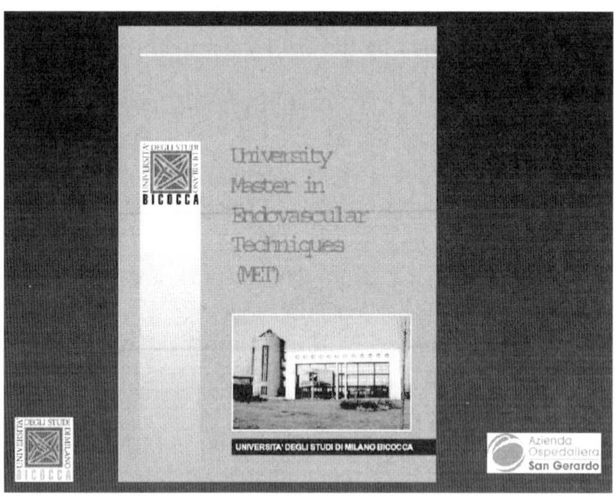


Fig. 6. MET brochure.

## References

[1] T.J. Fogarty, et al., A method for extraction of arterial emboli and trombi, Surg. Gynecol. Obstet. 116 (1963) 241–245.
[2] C.T. Dotter, M.P. Judkins, Transluminal treatment of arteriosclerotic obstruction: description of a new technique and a preliminary report of its application, Circulation 30 (1964) 654–670.
[3] A. Gruntzig, Die perkutane rekanalisation chronischer arterieller Verschlusse mit einem doppellumigen dilatations-katheter, Fortscher. Rontgenstr. 124 (1976) 80–86.
[4] C.J. Kwolek, Endovascular qualification for practicing surgeons, Semin. Vasc. Surg. 15 (2002) 174–177.

International Congress Series 1272 (2004) 116–129

www.ics-elsevier.com

# National vascular registries

Thomas Troëng[a,*], Martin Björck[b]

[a] *Department of Surgery, Blekinge Hospital, Karlskrona S-371-85, Sweden*
[b] *Department of Surgery, University Hospital, Uppsala, Sweden*

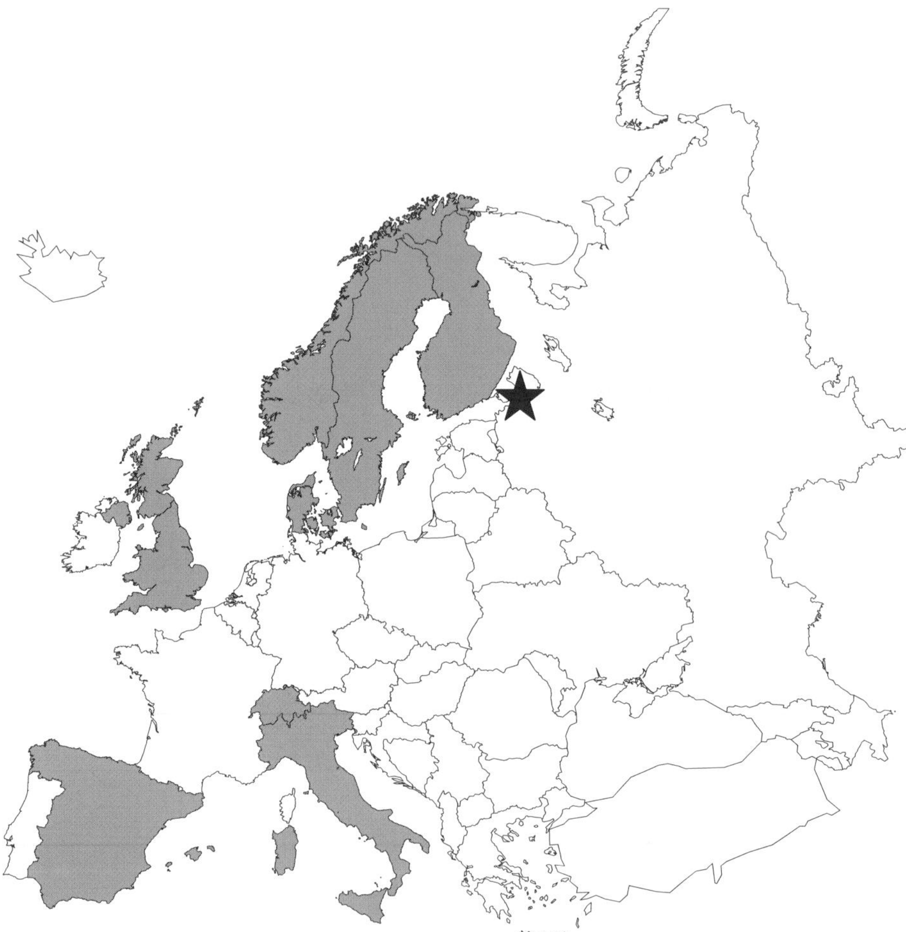

* Corresponding author. Tel.: +46-455-734-482; fax: +46-455-734-483.
*E-mail address:* thomas.troeng@ltblekinge.se (T. Troëng).


doi:10.1016/j.ics.2004.05.028

## 1. The rationale and controversies of national vascular registries—open audit

Centres of excellence in vascular surgery in North America developed vascular registries early and impressive retrospective series were published. The European Health Systems were neither as centralized, nor as commercialized, and it was difficult to produce such large series in our context. Some presentations and published reports of extremely good results from centres in North America were not always credible. The importance of prospective studies was recognized but the scientific issues often emerged late in the process and thus the idea of prospective registration of vascular surgical intervention and its complications emerged. European vascular surgeons also became more aware of epidemiological issues and the importance of studying the whole population at risk of an event became evident.

Some of the aims of the national vascular registries emerging in the late 1980s were:

- To register population-based interventions and results.
- To initiate an intercollegial discussion on indications for surgery and on complication rates.
- To initiate a process where surgeons with extreme indications or inferior results will take actions towards change.
- To improve healthcare for patients with peripheral vascular disease.
- To create a base for scientific projects where analyses are made based on register data and are leading to specific questions where the registry, with potential additions, could be used as an instrument for prospective scientific studies.

Thus, the idea of creating national vascular registries developed. This process is described below, specifically and in more detail regarding different countries. However, as results emerged and were analyzed, a series of issues or controversies had to be addressed:

- Are the results valid, are adverse events reported? What kinds of mechanisms could bias the registries?
- What techniques are most appropriate to validate the registries?
- If and how can differences in case–mix be controlled for when results are compared?
- How can the results be used in a structured process to improve outcome?
- In the issue of transparency, should hospital and/or surgeon-specific results be available to the public? If so, what are the consequences of transparency, both negative and positive?

These will be discussed in the following texts. It must be recognized, however, that these issues are complex and have been addressed differently at different times and in different countries.

## 2. The development of vascular registries

The early North American publications on vascular registries in the late 1970s were a stimulus and provided the first prompting to organize vascular registries in Europe [1–4].

The choice of variables to register is not an easy matter. There is a tendency in many professionals to prefer detail and completeness to what is practical and possible in clinical practice. It can take long and heated discussions to agree on a minimal data set, focused on the individual vascular procedure not on the individual patient [5]. Many useful suggestions are found in Karmody's original paper [3].

*Patient*, *Procedure* and *Postoperative follow-up* are the three 'Ps' of a registry for vascular procedures including endovascular procedures (Table 1).

Data on the patient are rather self-evident: patient ID, indication, which also may be the degree of disease (claudication or critical ischaemia, elective or emergency AAA), ankle index, other diseases and the patient's level of care.

The procedure is specified by where, by whom and when the operation is performed. It has been useful not to use a list of specific operative procedures, like fem-pop, crossover-bypass and others, but rather the Karmody inflow–outflow–vessel specification. This, combined with right and left and other technical details, led to the feeling that most conceivable reconstructions could be registered, as indeed they have (Table 2).

A postoperative follow-up at 30 days and 1 year is a reasonable compromise to give data on short- and long-term clinical outcome. Postoperative events include general complications, like myocardial infarction or pneumonia, separated from the surgical complications like thrombosis, hemorrhage or infection. Reoperations and amputations unfortunately also accompany surgery and should be carefully recorded.

Table 1
An example of a set of variables in a vascular registry

| | | |
|---|---|---|
| *Patient* | | |
| Patient ID | | |
| Indication | | |
| Ankle index | | |
| Comorbidities | | |
| Level of care | | |
| | | |
| *Procedure* | | |
| Hospital | | |
| Dates of admission, -discharge | | |
| Surgeon's ID, assistant | | |
| Choice of technique, procedure code | | |
| Inflow–outflow/side | | |
| Type of graft/brand, technical details | | |
| | | |
| *Postoperative follow-up* | | |
| Events | General complications | |
| | Surgical complications | |
| | Reoperations | |
| | Amputations | |
| Outcome | Vessel | Method |
| | Limb | Function |
| | Patient | Level of care |
| Interval | 30 days | |
| | One year | |

Table 2
An example of possible standards for process and outcome of vascular surgery

| |
|---|
| *Carotid endarterectomy* |
| Asymptomatic stenosis as indication in less than 10% |
| Stroke and/or death within 30 days should be below 5% |
| All cases with stroke/death should be investigated by a commission of inquiry |
| |
| *Abdominal aortic aneurysm repair* |
| More than 10 procedures/centre/year |
| Mortality after elective procedure within 30 days below 6% |
| Reoperation within 30 days below 3–4% |
| Zero % amputation within 30 days |
| |
| *Femoro-popliteo-distal-bypass* |
| More than 25 procedures/centre/year |
| Amputation within 30 days below 5% |
| Patency within 30 days above 90% |
| Mortality within 30 days below 6% |

The recording of ankle index, the function of the limb and the patient's whereabouts can define outcome of the reconstruction at 30 days and at 1 year. In some countries, it is impossible to go beyond a 30-day follow-up.

A very basic definition of clinical outcome is the Karmody classification of "patent/worse", "occluded/better", etc., at the follow-up [2,6]. It may sound a primitive way of assessing outcome; nevertheless, it includes both the conditions of the vessel and of the patient.

## 3. National vascular registries in Europe—the present situation

Vascular registries are increasingly becoming a part of the everyday work of many vascular surgeons in Europe. During the last 15 years, a number of European countries have seen the establishment of population-based vascular registries. The Scandinavian countries were early starters followed by Northern Ireland. United Kingdom, Spain, Italy and Switzerland have organised theirs more recently. In the metropolitan area of St Petersburg, data are collected from a population of close to five million. These registries are population-based and intend to record all peripheral arterial surgery, except in the UK where the national initiative is restricted to carotid endarterectomy, AAA and femoro-popliteo-distal (fem-pop-distal) bypasses. Multicentre international registries have also been established for the new techniques of endovascular stentgrafts for aortic aneurysms and carotid stenoses.

### *3.1. Denmark (1989)*

The Danish national vascular registry, Karbase (a pun, "karbase" can be understood both as "vascular base" and "cane"!), is now Internet-based but the process has been troublesome and the reporting tools are still under development. Legal problems with informed consent for registration have been solved by the political system and it is now not needed for registration. English language annual reports are available for downloading from the Karbase website.

### 3.2. Finland (1989)

The Finnvasc registry, although limited to a 30-day follow-up, has been very active publishing a number of papers on various aspects of vascular surgery [7–12]. Unfortunately, legal restrictions for the use of patient ID-codes have made later follow-up impossible and registration cease by the end of 1999. At present, representatives from the surgical profession and national authorities are negotiating a possible resuming of registration.

### 3.3. Italy (2001)

An Italian Vascular Registry has been established but further details are not available at the time of writing. Contacts and addresses are given in the Appendix A.

### 3.4. New Zealand

New Zealand has been represented for several years in the European registry cooperation. The three centres that perform the vast majority of the vascular procedures in New Zealand report their cases to the NZVASC registry. Two audits have been performed using registry data: Stroke and mortality rates for CEA were compared with the ECST data, and mortality after AAA surgery was correlated with surgeon volume. A recent paper illustrates the rewarding combination of registry and national health statistics data [13]. Further details about the New Zealand registry and audit experiences can be found on the registry web site.

### 3.5. Northern Ireland (1995)

The Northern Ireland registry used automatic reading of mailed paper forms early on, enhancing reporting and national coverage. The experience of this national registry has been presented at several national and international meetings.

### 3.6. Norway (1996)

The Norwegian Vascular registry—NORKAR—was established in 1996 with the intention of recording all vascular surgical activity including complications and follow-up at 1 month and 1 year. Two main problems have been incomplete: reporting to the registry and limited feedback information to participants.

A standardized form is used, much following the Swedvasc protocol: recording risk factors, main symptoms, aneurysm size, whether critical ischaemia, whether emergency or elective, etc. Procedure data include date, surgeon and procedure codes and type/brand of graft. Endovascular procedures are also recorded.

Postoperative data are recorded on the same form and includes procedure-related and general complications and the immediate outcome (and ABI). Four weeks and 1-year follow-ups are registered as well, however, not always complete.

Most vascular centres are members of NORKAR and they mail their records each year to the registry centre in Trondheim. Possibly 80–95% of all procedures are registered, no validation studies have been done. In 2000, 13 of 21 hospitals reported their data, one more in 2001.

NORKAR is the property of the Norwegian Vascular Society and is managed by a board and a halftime secretary. Member hospitals pay a fee, and some funds are also given by national authorities. Yearly reports are given to the general assembly of the society. Previous rules allowed only the presentation of aggregated national data, but now, hospital level data are also made official. Individual surgeon data are known only within each individual centre.

Future plans include standardized reports on a website and using web technique for the registering of data.

### *3.7. Poland*

In 2001, an attempt to organize a "Polvasc" unfortunately did not succeed because of lack of funds. However, there is an annual questionnaire collecting national data on the number of procedures and treated patients in vascular centres.

### *3.8. Russia (1998)*

In Russia, 110 centres are reported to perform vascular surgery. The number of procedures is increasing by 10% annually. In 2002, 24 arterial reconstructions per 100,000 inhabitants were performed. In the St. Petersburg region, with 4,5 million inhabitants, approximately 200 CEA and 400 aortoiliac procedures are performed per year. Ten vascular centres cooperate in a vascular registry, Petr–Vasc. The frequency of operations for AAA and peripheral bypasses is increasing and is now more than 100 and 600/year, respectively.

### *3.9. Spain (2000)*

The number of centres participating in the Spanish vascular registry is steadily increasing. At present, 50 of 68 Spanish vascular surgery centres participate, of which 23 are teaching institutions (Fig. 1). During 2002, more than 33,000 hospital admissions (43% urgent) and 11,945 arterial surgical procedures were registered, 9384 open and 2561 endovascular. The Spanish registry also includes venous open (13,879, mainly varicose vein surgery) and endovascular (209) procedures.

### *3.10. Sweden (1987)*

From the start in 1986, the Swedish registration has been based on hand-filled paper sheets which were sent by post to one centre, data being fed into the computer of the South Sweden regional oncological centre. By 1994, all vascular centres were participants (Fig. 2). Gradually, an increasing number of centres have sent their data as computer files. The practical aspects of establishing a registry and the early experiences of running a vascular database have previously been reported [14–16]. Data from Swedvasc have been used for

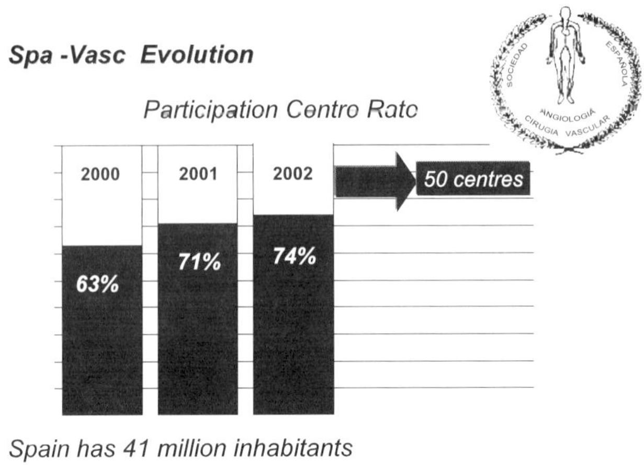


Fig. 1. In the more recently developed Spanish registry, the number of participating centres is still increasing.

various analyses and reports [17–19], for observational studies [20–28] and for organizing randomized studies [29].

The Swedvasc registry is now in the process of converting into a web-based system within the UCR (Uppsala Clinical Research Centre) together with other registries on cardiovascular diseases and treatments. The advantage is immediate registration and above all, having online access to one's own data in comparison to those of the whole national registry. Thus, it will no longer be necessary to wait for the yearly reports which, because of follow-up and data processing, are delayed for about 1 year. The new system will hopefully increase compliance and stimulate good registration. It can also easily be adapted for use in other countries.

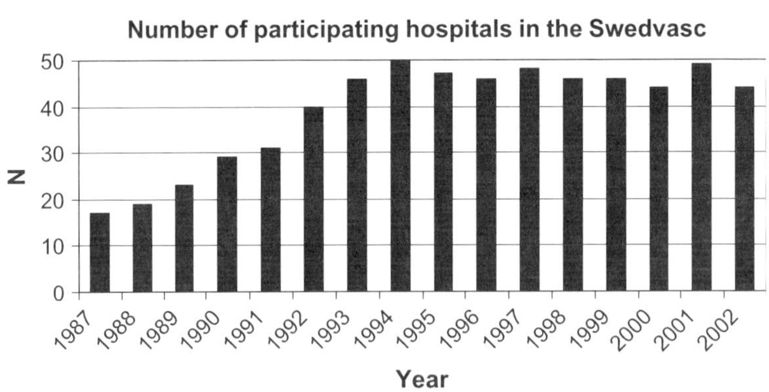


Fig. 2. The different national registries are in different phases of development. In Sweden, the registry reached national coverage in 1994 and the number of participating centres has been stable since.

Indicators of quality have been established [34] and after long discussions and meticulous preparations, it has been decided to publish hospital-specific results in 2004.

### 3.11. Switzerland (2003)

The Swissvasc Registry is a common project of the Swiss Society of Vascular Surgery and the Swiss Society of Cardio-, Thoracic- and Vascular Surgery. A pilot phase with seven hospitals was run from May to August 2003. After revision of the questionnaire, routine registration will start in January 2004. This national registry will be open to all hospitals performing vascular surgery in Switzerland but the participation is mandatory for teaching hospitals only.

It is an Internet-based solution, with access to the registry (protected by username with password) from any personal computer connected to the Internet. Alternatively, it is also possible to fill out the questionnaire and scan the form. Every participating department has access to its own data but not the data of other hospitals. The department can import its own data at any time. All data are stored in the central server.

As there are very strict regulations, data are stored only in an anonymous form (year of birth, sex and unique patient number) so that no one but the home hospital can identify the patient via the patient identity number given by the hospital information system. Hopefully, in early 2005, the first national report with the 2004 data will be published.

### 3.12. United Kingdom (1998)

The UK national database focused from the beginning on the three core vascular surgical procedures and aortic aneurysmectomy, carotid endatherectomy and distal bypass. There are 217 surgeons from 84 centres that participate in the work on risk stratification using the National Vascular Database of the VSSGBI. It is managed by a special audit and research committee and has resulted in a number of scientific publications [30–35]. A total of 5930 procedures have been registered since the start in 1999. After having explored VPOSSUM and Bayesian risk models, the group is now working with a new system called V-BHOM (which is not an explosive but the abbreviation of Vascular Biochemical and Hematological Outcome Modelling). The interesting and well-designed annual reports for 2001 and 2002 are available for downloading from the vascular society website.

## 4. The utility of a vascular registry

Population-based data on vascular interventions and treatment results (i.e., clinical epidemiology) cannot be derived from administrative databases because they do not provide any detailed medical information. A professional registry, on the other hand, is designed for collecting specific data on technical details, type of implants, various outcome measurements or exact test values. A number of clinically important issues can only be studied through the use of such data. The occurrence of redo surgery [8,24], the possible importance of case load for outcome [9] or the effectiveness of different techniques in routine care [12,18] are examples of such practical medical care issues.

Usually not anticipated, the intercollegial discussion needed for the organizing and design of a registry can prove very useful in promoting professional and interdepartmental cooperation. The development of university to county to district hospital contacts may result in new joint studies [29] and the exchange of experience and staff between health care institutions, where previously collaboration was limited.

Quality development is the order of the day. Inferior outcomes in some centres or individual providers call for action, new treatment modalities should be monitored to reveal possible adverse effects [20], a sufficient case load must be provided to satisfy educational demands [36], are but some of the many aspects of quality in vascular surgical care. Registry data are necessary prerequisite to identify and monitor quality deficiencies [27,30]; there is no other way. Possible future accreditation of centres will have to rely on some kind of monitoring of the processes and outcomes of care.

It has not yet been shown that the use of scarce resources to acquire a more detailed knowledge of surgical practice also will lead to improved health for the vascular patient. However, most people will believe that more knowledge could be followed by better decisions and better use of resources which in the end will be of benefit to our patients. As has been said..."if you consider knowledge too costly, try ignorance!"

Observational studies, often carried out in relation with registries, do have a limited value as scientific evidence. That value can be improved by specific study designs such as the often very cost-effective case–control technique (Fig. 4) [23]. Preliminary and hypotheses-generating observational data can be of great value for planning before embarking on an expensive and complex randomized clinical trial. These different methods of research are not conflicting but complementary [38].

Vascular surgeons all over Europe agree that audit of vascular surgery through registries is a commendable practice. The issue of open audit was scrutinized at the 2003 Charing Cross Vascular Conference in London during the session "Open audit is a waste of time", with speakers for and against the motion [37,38]. Among the more than one thousand head audience of international vascular specialists, 80% voted for open audit and the utility of vascular registries.

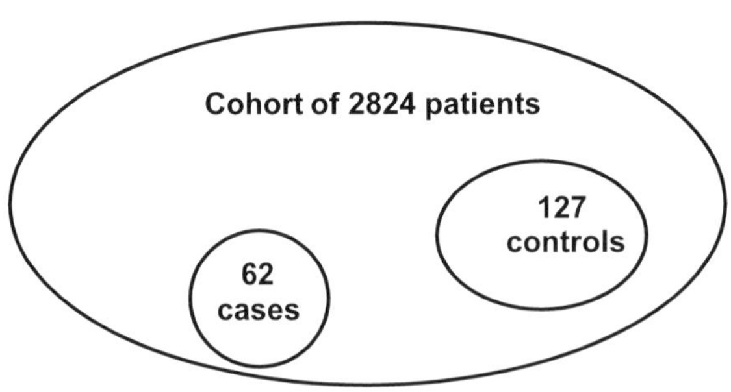


Fig. 4. A case–control study nested in the cohort of a national registry is an appropriate method to study complications and other adverse events after vascular surgery [26].

## Appendix A. Addresses, contacts for European National Vascular Registries

| | | | |
|---|---|---|---|
| Denmark | Karbase | Leif Panduro Jensen | www.karbase.dk |
| Finland | Finnvasc | Maarit Heikkinen | |
| Italy | Italian Vascular Registry | Flavio Peinetti, Michel Rollandin | fpeinetti@netvallee.it mrollandin@uslaosta.com |
| New Zealand | NZVASC | Ian Thompson | http://www.otago.ac.nz/surgery/9audit.html |
| Northern Ireland | NIVASC | Aires Barros D'Sa | |
| Norway | NORKAR | Ola Saether | www.legeforeningen.no |
| Poland | | Arkadiusz Jawien | ajawien@ceti.com.pl |
| Russia | Petr-vasc | Alexei V. Svetlikov | asvetlikov@mail.ru |
| Spain | Spa-Vasc | Rosa M. Moreno Carriles | www.seacv.org/ |
| Sweden | Swedvasc | Martin Björck | www.ssvs.se |
| Switzerland | Swissvasc | Pius Wigger | p.wigger@ksw.ch http://www.rehabnet.ch/SWISSVASC/ |
| United Kingdom | National Vascular Database | Chris Gibbons Simon Ashley | www.vssgbi.org simon.ashley@phnt.swest.nhs.uk |

## Appendix B. Vascular registries—the future

Vascular registries are often started by a group of enthusiastic vascular surgeons, With time, however, the interest among their colleagues tends to decrease and a certain fatigue over the surplus work associated with registering the patients is noted. To maintain the interest, a series of problems have to be addressed.

### *B.1. How do we address validity?*

One of the fundamental problems of an open audit, how to validate data in our registries, is to be addressed at a symposium arranged by the VascuNet, the collaboration of vascular registries in Europe, at the ESVS meeting in Innsbruck 2004. Hopefully, this symposium entitled, "Validation—the Achilles heel of open audit?" will result in a systematic review of the different experiences of validation throughout Europe. We do not yet have a full picture of the European experience in this field but within the Swedvasc, the following techniques of validation were performed:

- Double registration of a sample of registered interventions where the second registration was based on a retrospective analysis of the case-records.
- The Vascular Registry was cross-checked against the National In-Patient Registry [16] (Fig. 3). The fact that every Swedish citizen has a personal unique code, facilitates comparisons between different registries containing the personal code. Recent legislation, however, has created some administrative problems in performing such comparisons.

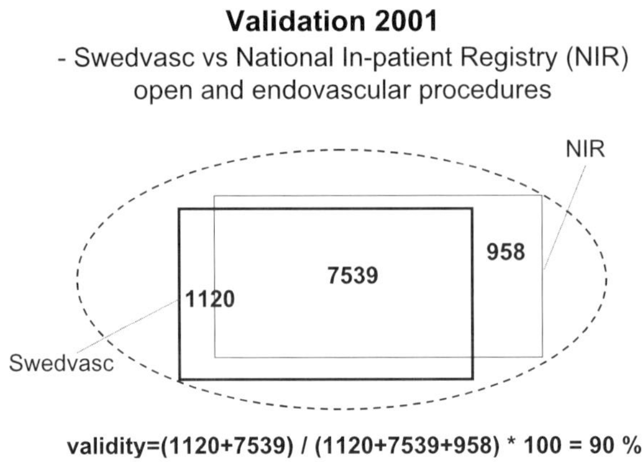


Fig. 3. Principle of a validation procedure. The dotted oval indicates a possible totality of vascular procedures. The National In-Patient Registry and The Swedvasc overlap and both record the majority of cases, but each also record some cases not identified by the other; that is, there is no "gold standard", only "defective standards" with various degrees of overlap.

- In-depth analysis of specific patient groups. We have validated the registry for femoro-popliteal reconstructions [14], adverse events after chronic leg ischaemia [17,20], amputations [21,25], complications after carotid surgery [26,27], colonic ischaemia after aortoiliac surgery [22,23], mesenteric revascularisation [28] and reoperations in general [24].
- Triangular inspections where hospital A inspects hospital B which inspects hospital C which inspects hospital A. The inspections scrutinize validity by cross-checking data against the local operation/anaesthesiology and radiological registries to evaluate inclusion of patients into the vascular registry. Perioperative deaths are analysed. Indications for surgery are compared and questioned.

### *B.2. Can we compare our results?*

Even if validity can be reasonably well documented, the issue of case–mix has to be addressed. In the Swedvasc, different in-depth analyses have shown that complications after carotid and aortoiliac [22] surgery were more frequent when the patient was operated on at a regional hospital than when the patient was operated on at a district hospital. This was not found in lower limb reconstructions [17,20]. Referral and differences in case–mix may explain this difference, but the Swedvasc registry with its basic set of variables does not permit in-depth analysis of case–mix. The National Vascular Database of the VSSGBI in the United Kingdom has focused on different risk stratification systems and on only three standard procedures. Few patients are registered but every patient is described meticulously. The rest of Europe is very interested in following the results of this experience. Will it be possible to correct for case–mix and compare results more correctly by these procedures? Will it be possible to motivate vascular surgeons in general to participate in such an extensive registration for a prolonged time period?

*B.3. How can results be improved?*

It is virtually impossible to distinguish the possible effect of the vascular registries from other factors that contribute to improvement in results. Even if it is understood from common sense that the analyses of results and the intercollegial discussion does play an important role in the process of improvement, it is not easy to evaluate the specific value of the registry. We are only in the beginning of exploring different techniques of quality improvement, and in this respect, it seems that other sectors of society than the Health Care can inspire us. We also believe that the VascuNet collaboration can be important to spread ideas and experiences among vascular surgeons in different countries.

*B.4. How to handle differences in results between centres, which fall outside reasonable confidence limits, and therefore may reflect true differences in quality of care?*

This is a professional challenge that has to be approached. The cultural and administrative diversity of European countries precludes generalized answers, but there is a motion towards opening the societies, which brings us to the next controversial issue.

*B.5. How shall we deal with demands of transparency?*

Many surgeons have good reasons to feel threatened by demands from journalists, often with personal ambitions to make a "scoop", who are eager to get hold of hospital-specific outcome data. If we gather data and compare results, we will sooner or later be confronted with demands to reveal our secrets. There is a movement towards open audit as a demand from healthcare authorities and increasingly, also from patients. Before this will be forced upon us, it is better to build the system ourselves. We ought to show that it works and be prepared to analyze and handle the problems, rather than becoming the victims of a political or administrative playground [39,40]. We believe that it is preferable that we ourselves present our results, together with a professional and scientifically based interpretation. Within the Swedvasc, we have identified 12 indicators of hospital-specific quality assessment that are to be publicly available beginning in 2004. We believe that this movement towards transparency will enhance the quality improvement process, in the interest of our patients and our own professional development.

In summary, evidence is accumulating that an open audit can be used as a tool in many ways, with its advantages but also with awareness of its problems. "Surgeons who don't count, don't count..."

## References

[1] J.C. Avellone, et al., A Regional Speciality Society as a model to monitor surgical care, JAMA 240 (1978) 2177–2180.

[2] F.R. Plecha, et al., A computerized vascular registry: experience of the Cleveland Vascular Society, Surgery 86 (1979) 826–835.

[3] A.M. Karmody, R.M. Blumenberg, C.A. Wall, Preliminary experience with a large scale vascular registry, Am. J. Surg. 146 (1983) 162–163.

[4] F.R. Plecha, et al., The early results of vascular surgery in patients 75 years of age and older: an analysis of 3259 cases, J. Vasc. Surg. 2 (1985) 769–774.

[5] A.M. Karmody, et al., Development of a computerized vascular registry for large-scale use, J. Vasc. Surg. 1 (1984) 594–600.
[6] T. Troëng, D. Bergqvist, J. Elfström, B. Hedberg, K.-G. Ljungström, L. Norgren, et al., VRISS (Vascular Registry in Southern Sweden): the Vascular Registry—A responsibility for all vascular surgeons? Eur. J. Vasc. Surg. 1 (1987) 219–226.
[7] M. Lepantalo, et al., Introduction of a population-based vascular registry: validity of data and limitations of registration. The Finnvasc Study Group, Br. J. Surg. 81 (1994) 979–981.
[8] M. Lepäntalo, et al., Frequency of repeated vascular surgery, Eur. J. Surg. 162 (1996) 279–285.
[9] I. Kantonen, et al., Influence of surgical experience on the results of carotid surgery. The Finnvasc Study Group, Eur. J. Vasc. Endovasc. Surg. 15 (1998) 155–160.
[10] I. Kantonen, et al., Factors affecting the results of surgery for chronic critical leg ischemia—A nationwide survey. Finnvasc Study Group, J. Vasc. Surg. 27 (1998) 940–947.
[11] I. Kantonen, et al., Mortality in ruptured abdominal aortic aneurysms. The Finnvasc Study Group, Eur. J. Vasc. Endovasc. Surg. 17 (1999) 208–212.
[12] M. Luther, et al., Arterial intervention and reduction in amputation for chronic critical leg ischaemia, Br. J. Surg. 87 (2000) 454–458.
[13] J.I. Rossaak, et al., Abdominal aortic aneurysms in the New Zealand Maori population, Br. J. Surg. 90 (2003) 1361–1366.
[14] J. Elfström, A. Stubberöd, T. Troëng, Adjusting outcome measurements for casemix in a vascular registry—Is it possible and desirable? Eur. J. Vasc. Endovasc. Surg. 12 (1996) 459–463.
[15] J. Elfström, A. Stubberöd, T. Troëng, Patients not included in medical audit have a worse outcome than those included, Int. J. Qual. Assur. 8 (1996) 153–157.
[16] D. Bergqvist, et al., Auditing surgical outcome. Ten years with the Swedish Vascular Registry—Swedvasc, Eur. J. Surg. 164 (1998) 581 (Suppl.).
[17] T. Troëng, L. Janzon, D. Bergqvist, Adverse outcomes in surgery for chronic leg ischaemia—Risk factors and risk prediction when using different statistical methods, Eur. J. Vasc. Surg. 6 (1992) 628–635.
[18] T. Troëng, et al., The choice of strategy in the treatment of intermittent claudication—A decision tree approach, Eur. J. Vasc. Surg. 7 (1993) 438–443.
[19] T. Troëng, et al., Decisions about treatment of aortoiliac claudication—The current practice among Swedish vascular surgeons, Eur. J. Surg. 163 (1997) 643–650.
[20] T. Troëng, D. Bergqvist, L. Janzon, The incidence and causes of adverse outcomes of operation for chronic ischemia of the leg, Eur. J. Surg. 160 (1994) 17–25.
[21] M. Eneroth, et al., Operations, inhospital length of stay and costs in 321 patients with critical leg ischaemia. A population-based longitudinal outcome study, Acta Orthop. Scand. 67 (1996) 459–465.
[22] M. Bjorck, D. Bergqvist, T. Troëng, Incidence and clinical presentation of bowel ischaemia after aortoiliac surgery—2930 operations from a population-based registry in Sweden, Eur. J. Vasc. Endovasc. Surg. 12 (2) (1996) 139–144.
[23] M. Björck, D. Bergqvist, T. Troëng, Risk-factors for postoperative intestinal ischaemia after aortoiliac surgery. A combined cohort and case–control study of 2824 operations, Eur. J. Vasc. Endovasc. Surg. 13 (1997) 531–539.
[24] T. Troëng, et al., Reoperations, redo surgery and other site interventions constitute more than one third of vascular surgery. A study from Swedvasc—The Swedish Vascular Registry, Eur. J. Vasc. Endovasc. Surg. 14 (1997) 244–251.
[25] Z. Zdanowski, T. Troëng, L. Norren, Outcome and influence of age after infrainguinal revascularisation in critical limb ischaemia, Eur. J. Vasc. Endovasc. Surg. 16 (1998) 137–141.
[26] A. Ahari, et al., Diabetes mellitus as a risk factor for early outcome after carotid endarterectomy—A population-based study, Eur. J. Vasc. Endovasc. Surg. 18 (1999) 122–126.
[27] T. Troëng, et al., Complications after carotid endarterectomy are related to surgical errors in less than one fifth of cases, Eur. J. Vasc. Endovasc. Surg. 18 (1999) 59–64.
[28] M. Björck, et al., Revascularisation of the superior mesenteric artery after acute thromboembolic occlusion, Br. J. Surg. 89 (7) (2002) 923–927.
[29] K. Logason, D. Bergqvist, Low molecular weight heaprin(enaoxparin) versus dextran in the prevention of

early occlusion following arterial bypass surgery distal to the groin, Eur. J. Vasc. Endovasc. Surg. 21 (2001) 261–265.

[30] P.T. McCollum, et al., Carotid endarterectomy in the UK and Ireland: audit of 30-day outcome. Committee for the Vascular Surgical Society, Eur. J. Vasc. Endovasc. Surg. 14 (5) (1997) 386–391.

[31] A.F. da Silva, et al., The management and outcome of critical limb ischaemia in diabetic patients: a national survey. Audit Committee of the Vascular Surgical Society of Great Britain and Ireland, Diabet. Med. 13 (8) (1996) 726–728.

[32] Audit committee of The Vascular Surgical Society of Great Britain and Ireland. Recommendations for the management of chronic critical lower limb ischaemia, Eur. J. Vasc. Endovasc. Surg. 12 (2) (1996) 131–135.

[33] T.A. Lees, J.D. Beard, B.M. Ridler, A survey of the current management of varicose veins by members of the Vascular Surgical Society, Ann. R. Coll. Surg. Engl. 81 (6) (1999) 407–417.

[34] W.B. Campbell, B.M. Ridler, T.H. Szymanska, Two year follow-up after thromboembolic limb ischaemia: the importance of anticoagulation, Eur. J. Vasc. Endovasc. Surg. 19 (2) (2000) 169–173.

[35] D.R. Prytherch, et al., The Audit and Research Committee of the Vascular Surgical Society of Great Britain and Ireland. A model for national outcome audit in vascular surgery, Eur. J. Vasc. Endovasc. Surg. 21 (6) (2001) 477–483.

[36] J. Sandermann, L. Panduro Jensen, The Danish specialist training in vascular surgery, Eur. J. Vasc. Endovasc. Surg. 23 (2002) 353–357.

[37] J. Powell, Open audit is a waste of time. For the motion, in: R. Greenhalgh (Ed.), Vascular and Endovascular Controveries, Biba Publ., London, 2003, pp. 1–8.

[38] P. Harris, Open audit is a waste of time. Against the motion, in: R. Greenhalgh (Ed.), Vascular and Endovascular Controveries, Biba Publ., London, 2003, pp. 9–16.

[39] N.R. Hertzer, Presidential address: outcome assessment in vascular surgery—Results mean everything, J. Vasc. Surg. 21 (1995) 6–15.

[40] J.J. Earnshaw, Clinical outcomes audit in vascular surgery: a shield for our profession, Ann. R. Coll. Surg. Engl. 85 (2003) 256–259.

International Congress Series 1272 (2004) 130–136

www.ics-elsevier.com

# European vascular registries: Vascunet and Eurovasc

Leif Panduro Jensen[a,*], Jesper Laustsen[b]

[a] *Department for Vascular Surgery B, Gentofte University Hospital, Hellerup DK-2900, Denmark*
[b] *Department of Cardiothoracic & Vascular Surgery T, Aarhus University Hospital, Skejby Sygehus, Denmark*

*Keywords:* Vascular surgery

## 1. Introduction

Vascunet is a forum for vascular registries, mainly European. It has until now been an informal forum for exchange of experiences between the existing vascular registries, and has served as inspiration for colleagues involved in the creation of new registries. Recently, Vascunet became a more formal and permanent body under the Vascular Society.

The concept of vascular registries began in Europe in the mid-1980s. The purpose of a vascular registry is provision of data on everyday performance, providing the basis for promotion of advances in the treatment of vascular diseases, research, statistical purposes and surgical audit. The strength of a vascular registry is that data reflect results and complications of everyday practice more realistically than a series published in the medical literature. At the same time, this is the weakness of a registry that data collection and validity are less controlled and the case mix of patients often leads to difficulties in interpretation of data. If used the right way and with proper caution to these aspects, registries have proven to be valuable sources of information over the last decade.

## 2. The history and organisation of Vascunet

Vascunet was founded in 1996, at an informal meeting between a few European registries, at the ESVS meeting in Lisbon. It has since then grown in size; in 2003 more than 10 countries contributed actively to the content of the meeting. The Vascunet meetings have always been in connection with the yearly meeting of the European Society for Vascular Surgery. At first, the Vascunet meetings only took place as small lunch meetings, but in recent years with more extensive meetings and even scientific symposiums on matters related to vascular registries. This development will probably continue to grow and extend in the future.

Up till 2003, there was no formal leadership of Vascunet. *Thomas Troëng* from *Sweedvasc* chaired the first meetings, which later on continued with *Leif Panduro*

* Corresponding author. Tel.: +45-3977-3403; fax: +45-3977-7674.
*E-mail address:* lpj@dadlnet.dk (L.P. Jensen).


doi:10.1016/j.ics.2004.05.079

*Jensen* from the *Danish Vascular Registry* (*Karbase*), who also arranged the first symposiums. In 2003, at the meeting in Dublin, it was decided to create a more formal organisation with a steering group and a spokesman. *Martin Björck* (spokesman, Sweden), *Leif Panduro Jensen* (Denmark), *Jesper Laustsen* (Denmark), *Rosa M. Moreno Carriles* (Spain) and *Simon Ashley* (UK) were elected. The purpose of this group was to further develop the concept of Vascunet into a more permanent group or committee under the ESVS, and to further strengthen the cooperation between the existing and developing vascular registries.

## 3. Eurovasc

Along with the creation of Vascunet, Prof. W. Paaske did some work on collecting information regarding vascular surgery in Europe from volunteering registries. These data were published in the *Journal of Vascular and Endovascular Surgery* as the Eurovasc Report. The Eurovasc Report only contained figures on number of procedures for each of the defined index procedures [1] (Table 1), and not any other parameters.

Even with this limited information, the figures showed remarkable differences in practice among the different countries, thus raising interesting questions on the basis of differences in how often various procedures were performed and the proportion of endovascular to surgical procedures, etc. There has been a pause in these publications since 2001, where the figures from 1999 were published. Their continuation will be a task for the reorganised Vascunet in the future.

## 4. Why is Vascunet needed?

The world is getting smaller, Europe as well, and also in the field of Vascular Surgery. At the same time, as the professional organisations are becoming increasingly important, the patients are becoming increasingly alert to the conditions and possibilities

Table 1
Eurovasc index procedures

| | |
|---|---|
| *Open surgical procedures* | |
| A | Carotid Artery disease |
| B | Abdominal Aortic Aneurysm |
| C | Central Arterial Occlusive disease |
| D | Peripheral Arterial Occlusive disease above knee |
| E | Peripheral Arterial Occlusive disease below knee |
| *Endovascular procedures* | |
| F | Central PTA ± stent |
| G | Peripheral PTA ± stent |
| H | Stent graft for Abdominal Aortic Aneurysm |
| I | Stent graft for central Arterial Occlusive disease |
| J | Stent graft for peripheral Arterial Occlusive disease |
| *Others* | |
| K | Arterial trauma |
| L | Angio access for dialysis |

in other neighbouring countries, demanding the same good treatment all over Europe. Since patient outcome reflects the provided quality of care and treatment, the tools of outcome research are increasingly being utilised to evaluate this. So, even if the first purpose of the registries is to support professional knowledge, development and rising quality, we have the patients supporting the same purposes, together with the wish for extensive public transparency.

Vascunet is, and will only be, for a long time, a forum for discussions. We are still far from the demand of common European standards for treatment. That is not to say that there is not already a need for some European standardisation in collection and reporting of data to enable comparison of results, exactly as is the case for reporting of randomised trials. Since vascular surgery is based on a scientific basis all over Europe, we of course also must acknowledge the need for proper, uniform methodology in reporting standards from the registries. Much work is still needed in this area to accomplish the task, stressing the need for the work done in Vascunet, and stressing the need for tight bonds to the scientific organisation.

One obvious need is to establish a minimum data set (MDS) to be included in all the European registries. The MDS should indeed be a minimum data set, a set of core variables, but most registries would choose to include more variables. First of all, the MDS should describe the vascular procedures and indications, but in time also include basic quality parameters, e.g. result and complication parameters, especially in areas where the scientific basis for setting limits is present. Discussions should, of course, not be limited to the minimum data set, but also exchange of views and evidence for suitable parameters for different vascular procedures is important.

Another very important question is regarding validation of data, where common ground and development are needed. See below for further details. Only with valid data it is possible to have reliable reporting.

Vascunet can play an important role in defining minimum standards for reporting of results. Until now, the only fairly reliable reports for comparison across Europe have been the number of certain index procedures, but this will surely be extended in the future with the increasing demand of transparency in the health sector. There is an obligation to monitor results and quality, and to make data available to the public to some extent. In several countries, e.g. Denmark, patients have the right to freely choose the place of treatment. In this respect, patients are asking for information on "best quality," and the politicians are moving along the same line in demanding the same information. This demand is not without problems. If reliable reporting is to be achieved, the whole chain of information should be of high quality as discussed below, that is, in the areas of data collection, data validation and case mix correction.

From a political point of view, this focus on transparency also seems a little narrow. The goal for all countries should be to deliver health service of high quality at every place to every citizen. The best way for a registry to serve this purpose would be as the foundation for scientific discussion and development among colleagues, not by publishing "top 10" lists of best and worst. It is to be remembered, that for any quality parameter, half of the departments/surgeons will always be below average and half above! If too much emphasis is put on public presentation of individual results, the consequence could be defensive surgeons protecting their statistics rather than accepting the challenge of especially weak patients. The balance of public presentation with the need for collecting data for quality improvement will be one of the major challenges in the coming years in Europe.

## 5. Establishing and maintaining a vascular registry

As mentioned, there are huge differences in the different European countries regarding vascular registries. Some have had registries for many years, and some have not even started yet, but everyone recognises the need for them (see the chapter by Troeng et al. in this book for an overview of the current status of each country). Several issues need to be addressed to "do it right" when establishing a vascular registry, and the same issues need to be repeated from time to time to maintain a well-handled and reliable registry.

## 6. The data set

The proper set of data to include in the registry provides a foundation, and should be given a lot of attention. Some countries, like the Nordic ones, have a lot of experience, as well as knowledge that can be drawn from the literature. Some general lessons have been learned by the existing registries:

- Keep it simple! It is easy to be excited with the possibilities of having an extensive amount of data for analysis, but remember that the data should be collected in the busy, everyday practise of each surgeon. Keep the amount of data as low as possible, but still enough to allow case mix correction and risk adjustment of the patients' "health profile," together with information on procedures, results, complications and follow-up. Also, keep each data entry point as simple as possible, easy to fill in, and robust to inter-observer variations. So, try to keep it as close to "yes/no" questions as possible and try to pose self-explanatory questions [2].
- Always have a patient ID, if at all possible. Some countries have huge difficulties in this matter (e.g. Finland and Switzerland), but if even a 30-day follow-up on results and complications shall be possible, there is need for proper ID. The patient ID is also the basis for validation of completeness of data towards other registries, operation protocols etc.

Another question is whether to include all of the vascular procedures of limiting the registration to a few index procedures [3]. The latter is naturally not as time consuming as the former, but then leaves the question if the index procedures are the right ones to evaluate overall performance.

## 7. The collection of data

The technology is so advanced today that one should aim for electronic transferral of data to the registry, but there are still huge differences in this matter in Europe. Some still use paper forms sent by ordinary mail and fed to the computer by a secretary and a few, like the Danish Vascular Registry, have for years had internet-based software with the database placed on a national server.

A vascular registry is probably often seen as a continuous collection of data, but this need not be the case as one can choose to collect data at certain intervals as samples. The advantage is, of course, that less time and effort is needed, but the disadvantages are that the same organisation is needed for both solutions, the same training and maintenance, and most importantly, changes over time will be more difficult to detect due to pauses and reduced amount of data in a given time period.

Another important question is who is going to type the data into the computer. The best quality is obviously obtained by the surgeons doing it themselves, but this is also time consuming. Combining data, with incorporation from various electronic sources and the possibility for automated, continuous check and filtration by the software, will ensure adequate quality for some of the data, while others will be dependent on clinical judgement and honesty. Especially in the USA, it is common to have trained nurses do the registration with the help from the surgeons, thereby securing complete and accurate data, but this is costly [4]. One of the difficulties for the registries is that it is still very little recognised that there should be money and resources allocated also in the health sector for this task, as it has been for many years in the private business sector.

## 8. Validation of data

This is probably the most difficult of all the problems of maintaining a registry [2,5]. Many reports are published without addressing the question of completeness and the quality of data [3]. This task is very time-consuming and takes a lot of resources, which is often used as the reason for not prioritising this in the end [3]. The problem is obvious: if you do not catch, for example, data on complications, the results will seem fine but will, in fact, be unreliable. Several validation questions should be addressed:

- Completeness of data. If at all possible, data should be checked with other sources to see if all patients are included as intended. If not, efforts should be made to include the remaining parts or to verify that the inclusion/exclusion is random and not an important source of bias [6]. The question of completeness has always been related to how difficult it has been to obtain data—the nearer to the source, e.g. filling in operation data right after leaving the operation theatre, the easier it is to include all the data and to check if it is done. By sending forms by mail to another address, completeness is seldom above 90%.
- Reliable and reproducible data. The first factor to obtain this goal is, of course, to design the data set properly, to avoid any misunderstanding of which data to include and how to fill in the forms. The next is to have extensive validation built into the software itself, especially in the case of direct typing into the software by the surgeons, instead of by a dedicated person. There are three levels of validation by the software here: the first and most basic, that only correct values are allowed and you are warned in case of empty required fields. Second is validation across the different fields in a form, e.g. that time for end of operation is after time for start of operation. Third is validation across forms, e.g. that dates are correctly ordered or status for limb amputation affects questions about ankle blood pressure in future forms. Finally, it is important to secure that each surgeon/department uses the same criterions for putting data into the registry. To obtain this goal, there is a need for external review of the practice, something that should be done on a regular basis [2].

## 9. Reporting from the registry

Feedback to the surgeons and departments is, by far, the most motivating factor in keeping a healthy and reliable registry. The main purpose of a vascular registry should always be to promote discussions and dissimilation of principles for best practise and, only to a lesser extent, to provide data to the public. If focus is primarily on the latter and not the former, engagement will rapidly drop and reports will become unreliable.

The basic reporting is not much different from basic scientific reporting. It should include figures on number of procedures, demographic data, results (including standard deviation), and complication rate. The methods used should also be the best scientific and proven ones with emphasis on the very robust ones, since lesser-controlled data create greater risk of bias [6]. It is extremely important that reporting from a registry is standardised and collected on a regular basis to serve the surgeons in the best possible way. Since data in a registry are often collected continuously over a long period of time, this allows both for cross-sectional analysis, e.g. benchmarking, of results, with comparison between different clinics or surgeons, and for time series analysis, where fluctuation over time for each clinic or surgeon is presented. For the latter, much development has taken place in the industry, creating control charts with fixed rules for alarming and reducing the risk of false alarms due to statistical uncertainty, but that the alarm is sounded if suspicious trends are evolving [7]. These methods are currently tested by the Danish Vascular Registry, but many other methods are tested by others too at the moment [3] (Fig. 1).

It is often said that reporting can only be fair if it is risk-adjusted for differences in case mix. The basic assumption is that some surgeons or departments handle the very difficult cases, and thereby may accept a higher complication rate and poorer result than those handling the more fit patients. This is, of course, true and risk-adjusted data should be generated under most circumstances, especially if the aim is publication or benchmarking. However, it is not always the whole truth; there is a range of problems when trying to interpret even valid and well-adjusted data. It is crucial to accept that an outcome better

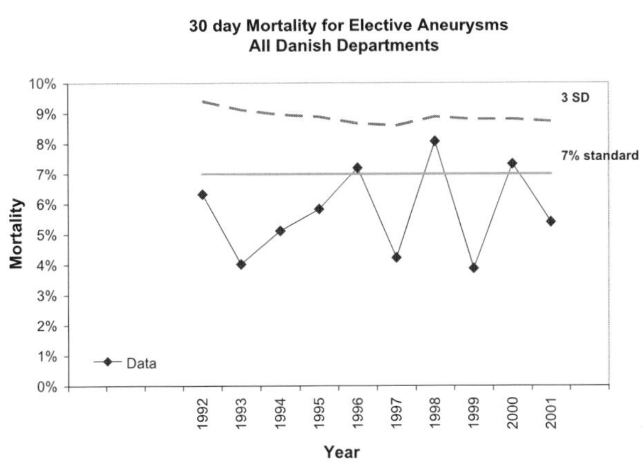


Fig. 1. Control Chart from the Danish Vascular Registry, showing mortality after elective aneurysm repair.

than an accepted standard does not necessarily reflect a better performance [8]. Another problem is that one department may have risk-adjusted mortality at an average level for elective aneurysms with a crude rate triple the average, then revealing that very ill patients are offered surgery despite the fact that there may be an unfavourable outcome compared to the natural history. So, crude rates are equally important as the basis for discussion among colleagues, but may not be fit for publication in a broader sense.

Reporting in itself is not enough; it should be scrutinised through an audit process in order to draw learning from the reports and implement it back into the system. Also, in the border between science and quality improvement, the reports can be used as tools for generating theses on different "seem to be" problems, to be tested later in a randomised, controlled trial. Lastly, but equally important, reports can be used for specialist training, as a tool for documenting training in different surgical procedures [9].

## 10. The future of Vascunet

The coming years will emphasise the need for documentation of results, for standardisation of treatment as an instrument for improvement and for transparency to the public. All these goals can be achieved by vascular registries among other tools, and Vascunet will play an important role in connecting the different national initiatives and discussions, promoting even faster development. The process is already running, along with the increasing awareness in the scientific society.

## References

[1] W. Paaske, EUROVASC report 1999, Eur. J. Vasc. Endovasc. Surg. 22 (3) (2001 Sep.) 282.

[2] J. Laustsen, L.P. Jensen, A.K. Hansen, Accuracy of Clinical Data in a Population Based Vascular Registry, Eur. J. Vasc. Endovasc. Surg. 27 (2004) 216–219.

[3] S. Ashley, B. Ridler, National Vascular Database Report 2002, The Vascular Surgical Society of Great Britain and Ireland, Report published by Dendrite Clinical Systems, publishing@e-dendrite.com.

[4] A.S. Fink, et al., The National Surgical Quality Improvement Program in non-Veteran Administration Hospitals, Ann. Surg. 236 (3) (2002) 344–354.

[5] L.G. Fine, et al., How to evaluate and improve the quality and credibility of an outcomes database: validation and feedback study on the UK Cardiac Surgery Experience, BMJ 326 (2003) 25–28.

[6] L.P. Jensen, O.M. Nielsen, T.V. Schroeder, The importance of complete follow-up for results after Femoro-infrapopliteal vascular surgery, Eur. J. Vasc. Endovasc. Surg. 12 (3) (1996) 282–286.

[7] J.C. Benneyan, Number-Between g-Type Statistical Quality Control Charts for Monitoring Adverse Events, Health Care Manage. Sci. 4 (2001) 305–318.

[8] P.S. Basnyat, et al., Mortality from ruptured abdominal aortic aneurysm in Wales, Br. J. Surg. 86 (1999) 765–770.

[9] J. Sandermann, L. Panduro Jensen, The Danish Specialist Training in Vascular Surgery, Eur. J. Vasc. Endovasc. Surg. 23 (2002) 353–357.

International Congress Series 1272 (2004) 137–142

www.ics-elsevier.com

# Vascular registries and databases in arterial disease: the EUROSTAR registry

Jaap Buth*, Peter Harris

*Department of Vascular Surgery, Catharina Hospital Eindhoven, The Netherlands and Royal Liverpool University Hospital, Liverpool, UK*

*Keywords:* Vascular registries

Registries on vascular interventions and surgical procedures experience a big time interest. Satellite symposia about vascular registries have been organised regularly by the Vascunet Organisation, EUROSTAR Registry on Endovascular Treatment of Abdominal Aortic Aneurysms within the annual ESVS programs.

Vascular registries have already existed for many years. SwedVasc and FinnVasc in Scandinavia are among the earliest initiatives, while Eurovasc was organised more recently [1–3]. Why do vascular registries enjoy so much attention? What is the role of registries in the current provision of information and improving knowledge? Can their impact be compared with that of clinical trials or are VRs supplementary to these trials?

## 1. Types of registries

Registration of performed medical and surgical procedures has been in use for many years. For example, in the Netherlands the SIG (Foundation of Information on Health Care) is a nationwide database, involved with medical procedures and diagnoses since 1972. This registry includes only data of hospital admissions and crude outcome events such as mortality. With regard to vascular disease, surveys of postoperative mortality after AAAs were performed on the basis of SIG-data. Trends in incidence of abdominal aortic aneurysm (AAA) were indicated, and the results in different categories of hospitals compared [4,5]. In the United States similar databases are often organised statewide [6,7]. The "Dartmouth Atlas of Vascular Health Care" draws from US Medicare database and analyses variation in rates of procedures as well as type of providers [8]. In the United Kingdom data often are collated in counties or regions. Responsible bodies for these registries usually are governmental or regional administrations. Funding is from tax payers' money, and outcomes are intended to be used mainly for steering the demand and the provision of health care resources. More recently, individual, free-standing groups of

* Corresponding author. Tel.: +31-402-12-1121.
*E-mail address:* buth@iae.nl (J. Buth).


doi:10.1016/j.ics.2004.04.084

vascular surgeons have taken initiatives of organising databases on new minimally invasive treatments of specific disorders, such as aortic aneurysms and carotid artery obstructive disease (EUROSTAR, RETA, Eurocast and the Endovascular Aortic Aneurysm Registry of the SVS Lifeline Foundation in the US).

## 2. Organisation of a vascular registry

The EUROSTAR collaborators project demonstrates a typical example of a registry organised by a large group of vascular surgeons [9–12]. This database was established for the purpose of collecting data on endovascular AAA-repair (EVAR). It was established in 1996, and as of today, 110 European centers regularly contribute their patient data to the registry. Meanwhile, the council of the European Society for Vascular Surgery decided during its meeting in Lucerne in September 2001 to formally recognise and endorse the EUROSTAR Data Registry in its future activities.

A policy and decision making Steering Committee is responsible for: (1) proposing or approving necessary changes in the registry protocol; (2) supervising and directing the Data Registry Center; (3) organising meetings of the collaborators group; (4) developing or supervising study reports and papers for publication on behalf of the collaborators group; and (5) approving applications from new participating centers. Data are enrolled of patients treated with any CE-approved endovascular device. Data managers have the responsibility for maintaining the database, and most importantly for ensuring that accurate follow-up data are retrieved and entered on time. As of September 2001 the data of almost 4000 patients had been enrolled. This number represents only a proportion of all endovascular AAA devices that have been implanted in recent years. The steering group intends the database to be representative, but not comprehensive, of the European experience.

Financial support for the EUROSTAR organisation is received on the basis of contracted reports on the results obtained with the devices of different commercial companies involved with stent-grafts used for endovascular treatment. Whereas this arrangement may constitute a cause of concern with regard to scientific independence, the individual agreements include explicit clauses regarding scientific integrity. Although, ideally, funding from scientific grants should come from official bodies, such as the European Union administration, grant allocation for clinical vascular topics has been consistently associated with difficulty.

Finally, the technicalities of data retrieval are key for a registry to be useful. Case Record Forms (CRFs) should not be complex or time-consuming to complete. The co-operation between EUROSTAR and KIKA, a dedicated Website building and maintaining company with extensive experience in online clinical data retrieval, has been a considerable step forward (Fig. 1). Data handling has been simplified, the system is more user-friendly and, as a consequence, the compliance of participants has improved. On the other hand, actual and updated registry outcome can be assessed at any time by the involved participants, i.e. medical institutions, industrial companies, and other parties with an interest in this field.

## 3. Responsibilities of registry organisers

The uncontrolled introduction of new technology without proper evaluation has caused serious concerns in the past. The complications associated with the hasty adoption of

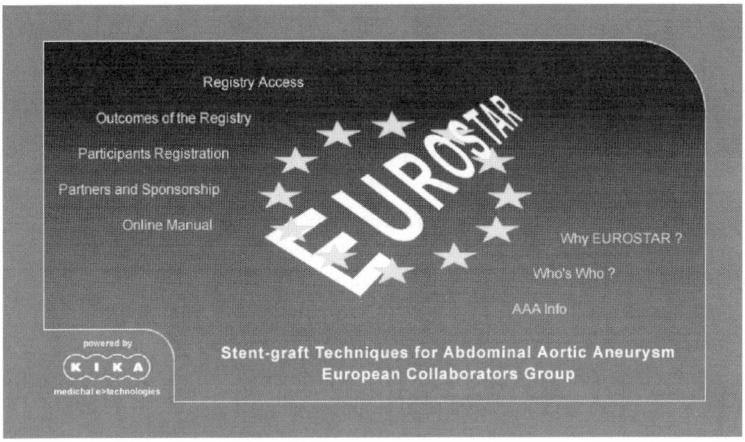


Fig. 1. Portal to website of www.eurostar-online.org providing the entree to an electronic Record Form, patient listing per institution and to processed data overviews, graphs arranged by institution, country, or specific endograft label.

laparoscopic cholecystectomy have led to much adverse publicity [13]. Since 1995, a new European directive covering implantable medical devices has become effective. This required all medical devices to acquire the CE mark from June 1998. The CE mark indicates that the device meets the essential safety requirements. Many countries in the European Union have reorganised their Ministries of Health to implement these directives. However, the European directive covers only safety, not efficacy, and long-term durability of implantable devices. At this point, data registries may fulfil a useful role.

There is little doubt that large databases in vascular registries contain valuable information for the profession as well as for the device industry. Lumped data of outcome of a variety of devices may be of great value, if the data are stratified for different devices. However, caution is needed with regard to distribution of case severity and factors known to affect outcome when differences in performance in device specific groups are observed. Nevertheless, it is the responsibility of vascular registries that real differences or increased rates of adverse events or device failures are reported without delay [14]. Patient safety is the central consideration here. It has appeared that these points are well accepted by the companies who are responsible for endovascular device manufacturing [15].

## 4. Often heard criticism on vascular registries

(1) "The level of evidence of a registry is less than of a randomised trial". For many new treatments it is impossible to organise an RCT at an arbitrary time to compare the results with those of the existing gold standard. Once a method has proven to be safe and efficacious, and expectations are justified that it will perform as well as the gold standard, then an RCT may be planned. This would imply that in the initial phase the new, often less invasive, treatment is justified only in patients, who are unsuitable for the classic method because of poor health. In practice, many doctors and patients are not willing to wait until the results of an RCT are reported and some uncertainties associated with the new method are accepted. Registries seem extremely useful to answer pertinent questions of clinical interest quickly. These

clinical questions may relate to the mortality of the procedure, complications, and in case of EVAR, the risk of conversion to open repair. In addition, the risk of systemic, arterial and device-related complications can be assessed in a large study population.

(2) "There is no monitoring of patient data in VRs" [16]. Owing to the large number of patients that are typically enrolled in a vascular registry, site visits including checks of source data can be performed only to a limited extent. In comparison, monitoring in RCTs is often not comprehensive as well. Core laboratories for checks on imaging studies are customary in company-organised studies. It has occurred that even the opinions of the experts of core laboratories sometimes demonstrate disparate outcomes. Thus, the difference regarding the monitoring of data between a VR and an RCT remains somewhat unclear.

(3) "Adverse events are underreported and follow-up is incomplete in VRs". This criticism is contradicted by the tenor of a recent editorial, published in the British Journal of Surgery [17]. In this editorial, EVAR was characterised as a "failed experiment". This personal opinion was based primarily on publications from EUROSTAR. Although these negative views on EVAR are not shared at all by the EUROSTAR management, the editorial demonstrates great reliance on the registry data even by critical observers. Good registries use prospective patient registration as their main source of data analysis. There is little reason to believe that poor outcome will be concealed from a VR. In fact, an honest appraisal is more likely in larger surveys. It was demonstrated that multicenter studies and national surveys report higher incidences of mortality and complications than single-center studies [18]. In assessments of smaller numbers of patients, those with significant risk factors or even slightly adverse anatomy may be excluded from participation. In addition, reporting methods are perhaps less rigorously checked. In this regard, VRs may reflect existing general practise patterns better than some of the controlled studies.

It is accepted that complete retrieval of follow-up data always is a challenge for registries. Patients move from one area to another. The paperwork involved with registration of follow-up data may cause organisational problems during busy outpatient clinical work. Regular reminders of the registry management to participating centers are usually effective in obtaining follow-up data of sufficient patient numbers for a useful analysis of late treatment outcome.

## 5. Discussion

EUROSTAR is an example of open audit that exemplifies the virtues of this type of study. While tracking the performance of EVAR technology during a critical period of its evolution, EUROSTAR has provided vital evidence about what works and what does not and has thereby contributed beneficially to the process. The data generated has informed the manufacturers of endografts in their quest for optimal design specification and technical refinement and clinicians in their need to select and treat patients for optimal outcomes (Table 1).

The cumulative rate of late rupture of first generation devices registered with EUROSTAR rose to a staggering 12.2% after 6 years. Careful analysis showed evidence that two device-related factors were, in the main, responsible for these failures of treatment, type 3 endoleak (breach of integrity of the device) and migration (Table 2). Appropriate lessons have been learned from this experience. Modern devices are constructed with more robust materials and most have effective mechanisms to prevent migration. The latest results from EUROSTAR confirm the effectiveness of these measures.

Table 1
Total number of different makes of endovascular devices included in latest analysis of aggregated EUROSTAR data (July 2003)

| | Number of patients | Percentage of patients (%) |
|---|---|---|
| AneuRx | 958 | 22.6 |
| EVT | 66 | 1.6 |
| Excluder | 528 | 12.4 |
| Talent | 1108 | 26.1 |
| Zenith | 1372 | 32.3 |
| Other | 181 | 4.3 |

Because of concerns about the long-term durability of EVAR, many clinicians initially elected to treat patients who were at high risk of death or other serious complications associated with conventional treatment of their aneurysm. Subsequently, the wisdom of this approach has been challenged and it has been suggested that the ‘gain’ for high-risk patients may be minimal or nonexistent. EUROSTAR has examined this question and concluded that ‘high-risk’ patients do benefit from EVAR provided that they do not die from the effects of their co-morbid condition within 1 year of treatment. Patients with terminal cancer generally did not benefit in terms of increased longevity whereas those with severe chronic obstructive respiratory disease usually did [19]. Because EUROSTAR did not have access to a valid control group of untreated patients for comparison, these conclusions depended upon certain basic assumptions about the rupture risk of untreated aneurysms.

Recently, EUROSTAR has examined the outcomes from EVAR in patients at the other end of the scale, i.e. ‘good risk’ patients with small aneurysms. Comparison of this group with others (with larger aneurysms) shows that they fare better not only in the short term but also later in terms of the durability of AAA repair [20]. These data are supportive of arguments in favour of offering EVAR to patients with early aneurysmal disease. Linked to programs for population screening, this approach has potential to change radically the impact of aortic aneurysmal disease in our communities.

## 6. Conclusions

Several vascular registries have been in use for many years, of which the Swedish Vascular Registry (SwedVasc) the longest. These registries have increased insight considerably in developments, change in treatment patterns and surgical outcomes. More recently, dedicated registries involved with the outcome of minimally invasive treatments, notably endovascular AAA-repair and carotid artery stenting, have become popular. Their reports have been found extremely useful for identifying anatomic and patient-related risk factors and device failures as well. The cost-effectiveness of a registry is difficult to define in strict economical terms. However, the cost per registered case is negligible compared with the

Table 2
Univariate analysis: factors statistically associated with late rupture of AAA after endovascular repair

| | *P* value | Relative hazard ratio (95% CI) |
|---|---|---|
| Prox. type 1 endoleak | 0.001 | 7.6 (2.1–27.6) |
| Midgraft (type 3) endoleak | 0.001 | 8.9 (2.9–27.5) |
| Endograft migration | 0.001 | 4.5 (1.2–16.7) |
| Kinked endograft | 0.001 | 3.1 (1.4–11.5) |

overall cost of treating a vascular patient. On a community scale, it may be expected that improved assessment and decision making by surgeons, supported by registries, will compensate quickly for the expenses. The EUROSTAR database has recently come up with a number of remarkable observations that would not have been known without this mega database.

## References

[1] D. Bergqvist, et al., Auditing surgical outcome: 10 years with the Swedish Vascular Registry-SwedVasc, Eur. J. Surg. (suppl. 581) (1998) 3–8.
[2] J.P. Salenius, et al., and the FinnVasc study group, Ann. Chir. Gynaecol. 87 (1998) 131–134.
[3] W.P. Paaske, EUROVASC report 1998: vascular and endovascular surgical activity in Denmark, New Zealand, Northern-Ireland, Slovakia, Sweden and St. Petersburg region, Russia, Eur. J. Vasc. Endovasc. Surg. 20 (2000) 233–234.
[4] G.J.M. Akkersdijk, et al., Mortality rates associates with operative treatment of infrarenal abdominal aortic aneurysm in the Netherlands, Br. J. Surg. 81 (1994) 706–709.
[5] J.B. Reitsma, et al., Increasing incidence of aneurysms of the abdominal aorta in the Netherlands, Eur. J. Vasc. Endovasc. Surg. 12 (1996) 446–451.
[6] D.J. Katz, J.C. Stanley, G.B. Zelenock, Operative mortality rates for intact and ruptured abdominal aortic aneurysms in Michigan: an eleven-year statewide experience, J. Vasc. Surg. 19 (1994) 804–817.
[7] A. Dardik, et al., Surgical repair of ruptured abdominal aortic aneurysms in the state of Maryland: factors influencing outcome among 527 recent cases, J. Vasc. Surg. 28 (1998) 413–421.
[8] J. Cronenwett, J. Birkmeyer (Eds.), The Dartmouth Atlas of Vascular Health Care, AHA Press, Chicago, 2000.
[9] P.L. Harris, et al., Incidence and risk factors of late rupture, conversion, and death after endovascular repair of infrarenal aortic aneurysms: the EUROSTAR experience, J. Vasc. Surg. 32 (2000) 739–749.
[10] R.J.F. Laheij, et al., Need for secondary interventions after endovascular repair of abdominal aortic aneurysms. Intermediate-term follow-up results of a European collaborative registry (EUROSTAR), Br. J. Surg. 87 (2000) 166–173.
[11] P. Berg, et al., Spinal cord ischemia after strent-graft treatment for infra-renal abdominal aortic aneurysms. Analysis of the EUROSTAR database, EJVES 22 (2001) 342–347.
[12] V. Riambau, et al., The association between co-morbidity and mortality after abdominal aortic aneurysm endografting in patients ineligible for elective open surgery, Eur. J. Vasc. Endovasc. Surg. 22 (2001) 265–271.
[13] J.D. Beard, How can be introduce new technology safely and actively? Eur. J. Vasc. Endovasc. Surg. 21 (2001) 3–5.
[14] R.B. Rutherford, Problems with the dissemination of up-to-date information on the results of endograft repair for abdominal aortic aneurysm, J. Vasc. Surg. 29 (1999) 1167–1169.
[15] P.L. Harris, J. Buth, Reply on letter by RB Rutherford, J. Vasc. Surg. 30 (1999) 767–768.
[16] L.P. Jensen, T. Troëng, Vascular registries—Are they worth the effort? (Editorial), Eur. J. Vasc. Endovasc. Surg. 20 (2000) 225–226.
[17] J. Collins, J.A. Murie, Endovascular treatment of abdominal aortic aneurysm: a failed experiment, Br. J. Surg. 88 (2001) 1281–1282.
[18] J.D. Blankensteijn, et al., Influence of study design on reported mortality and morbidity rates after abdominal aortic aneurysm repair, Br. J. Surg. 85 (1998) 1624–1630.
[19] J. Buth, et al., Outcome of endovascular abdominal aortic aneurysm repair in patients with conditions considered unfit for an open procedure: a report on the EUROSTAR experience, J. Vasc. Surg. 35 (2002) 616–620.
[20] N. Peppelenbosch, et al., Diameter of AAA and outcome of EVAR: does size matter? A report from EUROSTAR, J. Vasc. Surg. 39 (2004) 288–297.

International Congress Series 1272 (2004) 143–283
www.ics-elsevier.com

# Future prospects and developments in the workings and activities of the European Division and Board of Vascular Surgery (EDBVS) of the UEMS

Christos D. Liapis*

*UEMS Division and Board of Vascular Surgery, Vascular Surgery Clinic, Athens University Medical School, Athens, Greece*

*Keywords:* Vascular surgery; Training; Examinations; Logbook; Vascular centres

## 1. Introduction

The European Division and Board of Vascular Surgery (EDBVS) of the Union Européenne des Médecins Spécialistes (UEMS) has, since its inception in 1993, rapidly developed into one of the most active divisions within the UEMS. The route to this prominent status has been through the establishment of its own examination—the annual EBSQ-VASC Assessments—now in the 9th year of rapid progression [1] (Figs. 1–3); the EuReg-Vasc registry of vascular training centres and practitioners; and the European Vascular Continuing Medical Education (EVCME) Committee that accredits European meetings, courses and workshops by awarding credit hours on the scientific content of the programme and participation on such. All this was achieved through the hard work of the EDBVS pioneers Peter Harris and Jaap Buth, first President and first Secretary, respectively, and Bernhard Nachbur, first Chairman of the EBSQ-VASC Committee, with the help of the members of the Division and Board of Vascular Surgery.

## 2. Current problems

Since vascular surgery is a highly dynamic, ever-evolving specialty, particularly with the advent of endovascular therapies, the EDBVS felt it necessary to address the challenges of the new environment for vascular surgeons through changes in the structure of training to meet the needs of the future vascular "specialist."

* Tel.: +30-210-7456128; fax: +30-210-7456130.
*E-mail addresses:* liapivas@panafonet.gr, liapis@hol.gr (C.D. Liapis).
*URL:* http://www.uems-vasc.org.


doi:10.1016/j.ics.2004.05.118

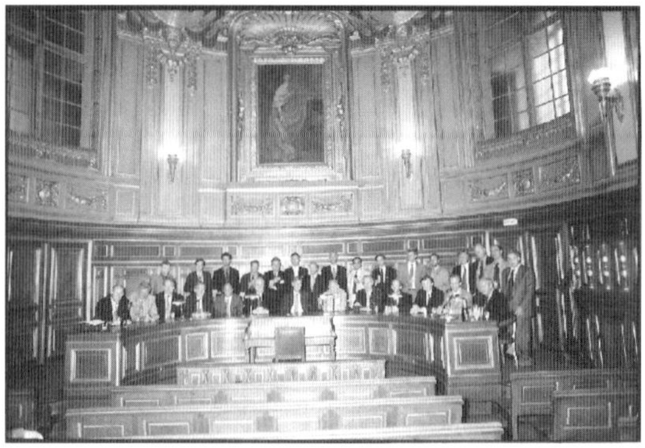

Fig. 1. 3rd Annual EBSQ-VASC Assessments 1998, Salle Authoritee et Liard, Sorbonne University, 29 September 1998, Paris, France.

The changes in the curricula required to encompass the new techniques are vast and difficult to achieve across the European continent because of the varying differences in training from country to country. This task is becoming even greater with the entry of 10 new EU members as of 1 May 2004; and although enlargement is desirable, for there is strength in numbers, it is imperative to be in the position of welcoming our new counterparts with guidelines in training that will ease the process of harmonization across Europe. The new guidelines should be based on the expert knowledge and experience of respected members of the EDBVS who are well acquainted with the training requirements of their own countries and thus able to assist in modifying the curricula to confront the new era. It is imperative to formulate collaboration between the EBSQ-VASC Examination

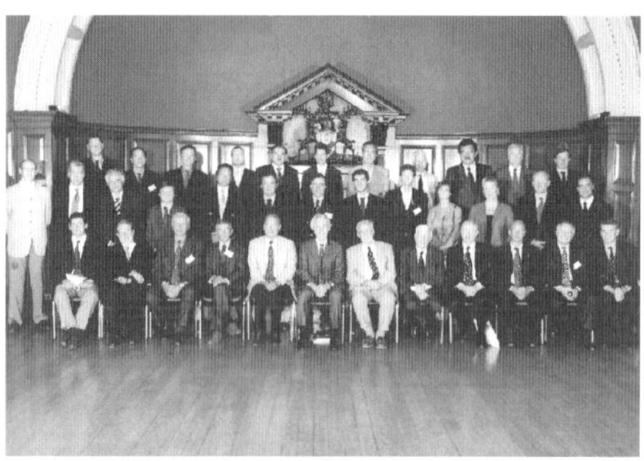

Fig. 2. 8th Annual EBSQ-VASC Assessments 2003, The Royal College of Surgeons in Ireland 2–4 September, Dublin, Ireland.

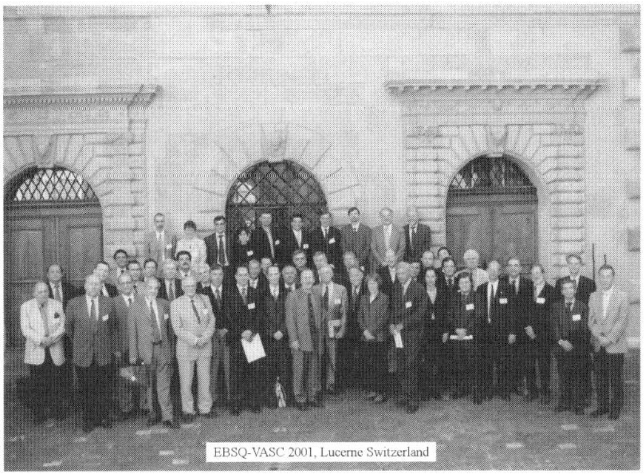


Fig. 3. 6th Annual EBSQ-VASC Assessments 2001, Rathaus Council Hall, 26 September 2001, Lucerne, Switzerland.

Committee and the working group on endovascular therapy and techniques under a new structure such as a Committee on Education and Training.

Endovascular treatment requires the use of various devices that bear the CE mark. Up to now, however, the involvement of vascular specialists in this area and of other representatives within the EDBVS is very limited and certification of such devices is particularly obscure in the countries of Europe. Currently, the implantation of these devices is conducted under the sole responsibility of the physician in charge, who, unfortunately, has little knowledge of the possible dangers or the durability of the mechanisms. As a result, Europe has not yet experienced any control through the withdrawal of inadequately tested or potentially hazardous contrivances from the market, by scientific/administrative bodies such

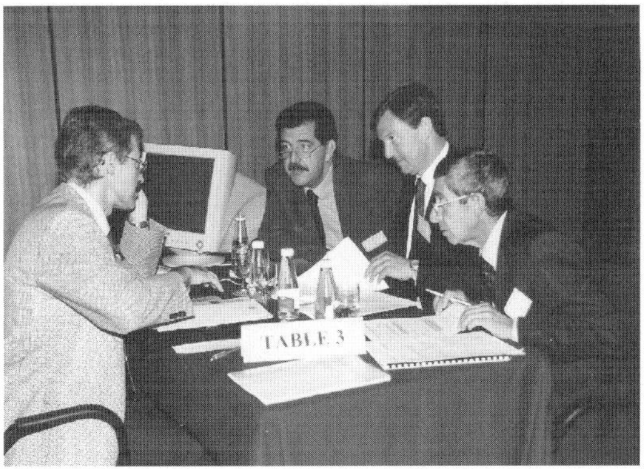


Fig. 4. Viva Voce Examination during the 8th Annual EBSQ-VASC Assessments, September 2003, Dublin.

as the FDA, who are exercising rigid control in the U.S. It is therefore of utmost importance that the EDBVS involves itself in the development of quality control over these devices.

Despite the demanding requirements of the EBSQ-VASC Assessments, it is doubtful that this examination conducted for the purpose of verifying the theoretical knowledge and practical ability of candidates in vascular surgery will ever fully replace national exit examinations; however, the attempt to raise the standard even higher by incorporating endovascular procedures in the theoretical and practical parts of the examination will enhance its profile. The demands of this extensive examination [2] both theoretically and through practical exercise could provide an incentive for countries that do not have their own exit examination to utilize this, or even to duplicate it, for their vascular surgeons, thus accelerating the harmonization process in the various European countries (Fig. 4).

## 3. Developments

A recent move by the EDBVS in the direction of harmonization has been the establishment of a logbook that can be downloaded from the Web site on http://www.uems-vasc.org. The logbook can serve as a helpful tool for both the trainee [3] and the trainer, not only as a daily/weekly/yearly record of procedures performed, but also as a means of ensuring eligibility for the title of Fellow of the European Board of Vascular Surgery (FEBVS).

The Technical Skills Examination, initially conducted as a pilot programme over the last 2 years, will now be an integral part of the examination and is an effective way of comparing logbook data with the practical ability of the candidate [4] (Figs. 5 and 6).

EVCME accreditation has been based on carefully planned criteria evolved to maintain the fine balance between event organizers and industry support, which plays an instrumental role in the realization of such events. The new guidelines [5] will shortly be available on the Web site. The accumulation of credit hours through EVCME accreditation of the Division and Board of Vascular Surgery can be useful in gauging continuous professional development and serving towards recertification,

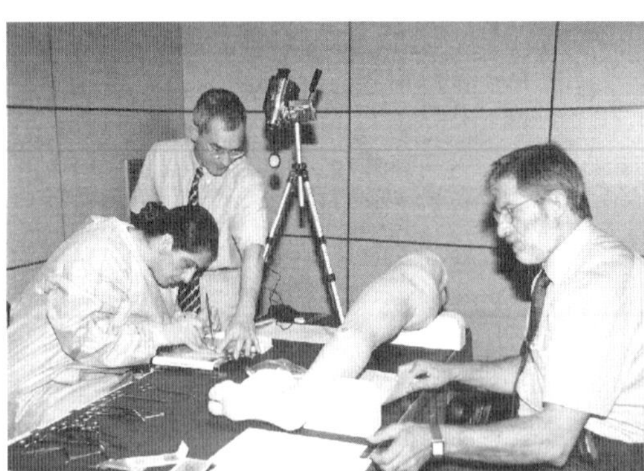

Fig. 5. Technical skills exercise during 7th Annual EBSQ-VASC Assessments, September 2002, Istanbul.

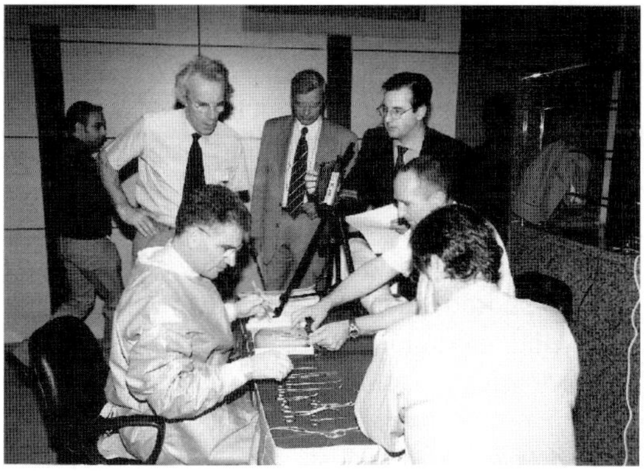

Fig. 6. Technical skills exercise during 7th Annual EBSQ-VASC Assessments, September 2002, Istanbul.

which will probably become mandatory throughout Europe. It is already in force in some European states and in most of the U.S. The EVCME Committee can continue to play a major role in approving meetings, and collaboration should be encouraged with national CME. An indication of the workings of the EVCME Committee under Chairman J. Hajo van Bockel can be found in the annex to this chapter, with particular emphasis on the sound evaluation of European events such as courses, workshops and other meeting proceedings.

## 4. Future direction

An issue that needs to be urgently addressed is the reduction in working hours as stipulated in the Directive 2000/34/EC on the 48-h week, starting with 58 h weekly on 1 August 2004 and, over a transitional period up to 2009, finally being cut down to 48 h total weekly working time including overtime. This also entails a minimum rest period of 11 h per 24-h period, a minimum weekly rest period of 24 h and a maximum of 8 working hours during the night [6]. There is a pressing need for guidelines on training and doctors' duties and proper job descriptions that will enable the trainee to successfully complete the course within the stipulated time and to avoid any drawback of having to extend the training period. Existing models such as Denmark should be looked at, where the reduced working week has been functional for the last two decades. A joint effort, for a possible formula by the Division and Board of Vascular Surgery, has been made in the form of a questionnaire on the 48-h week devised by John Wolfe, President of the Board of Vascular Surgery, and painstakingly filled in by the National Representative Members. A full report can be found as an annex to this chapter.

The day-to-day practice of vascular surgery in Europe is another area that could benefit substantially from a joint collaboration between the EDBVS and the ESVS. Studies should be developed on the prevention of vascular diseases through screening programmes for aneurysms and carotid stenosis detection. Guidelines for the acceptable level of complication rates that are representative of European standards could thus be made available to the medical community. Increasing social awareness of the dangers of vascular diseases should also be on the priority list of actions for the prevention of life-damaging disorders. A textbook on vascular diseases by the members of the EDBVS with regular revisions is already in process.

A top priority project of the EDBVS should be the establishment of vascular centres. A single specialist alone cannot perform the management of patients with vascular disease(s); therefore, this should involve experts from other disciplines such as radiology, endocrinology and cardiology based on rules governing the composition, organization and function of such centres. In this way, total care of the vascular patient will be ensured by a team of multidisciplinary experts working together for the good of the profession. The future vascular specialist, however, should be capable of not only performing surgery, but also be in the position of treating the origin of disease(s) as a whole [7].

It is through such activities, focusing in particular on research, and prevention of vascular diseases, that we can justify our role as vascular specialists aiming to dethrone vascular diseases as the number one killer of the human race.

In order to be able to fulfill the scope of these activities successfully, it is mandatory that the Vascular Surgery specialty be fully recognized throughout Europe. The Division and Board of Vascular Surgery have indeed laid the foundation towards this end. Still, there are several areas of dispute with other specialties and turf wars that, although best avoided and solved by negotiations, should be fought from a position of strength for Vascular Surgery. The creation of a Section of Vascular Surgery working alongside the other major surgical specialties in the form of a federation is imperative in giving Vascular Surgery the negotiating power and recognition it deserves. I am happy that the creation of the Section of Vascular Surgery is becoming a reality.

## References

[1] D. Bergqvist, C. Liapis, J. Wolfe, The Developing European Board Vascular Examination. Eur. J. Vasc. Endovasc. Surg. 27 (4) (2004 Apr.) 339–340.

[2] C.D. Liapis, W.P. Paaske, Training in vascular surgery in Europe—the impact of endovascular therapy, Eur. J. Vasc. Endovasc. Surg. 23 (1) (2002 Jan.) 1–2.

[3] D. Palombo, et al., The value of a logbook for young vascular surgeons in training: the UEMS experience. Int. Angiol. (2004 March) (in press).

[4] V.A. Pandey, et al., European Board of Vascular Surgery. Validity of an exam assessment in surgical skill: EBSQ-VASC pilot study, Eur. J. Vasc. Endovasc. Surg. 27 (2004) 341–348.

[5] J.H. Van Bockel, et al., Guidelines for CME Activities accredited by the EBVS, Eur. J. Vasc. Endovasc. Surg. 27 (2004) 534–536.

[6] C. Liapis, Effects of limited work hours on surgical training, J. Am. Coll. Surg. 196 (4) (2003 Apr.) 662–663.

[7] A.N. Sidawy, et al., Basic science curriculum in vascular surgery residency, J. Vasc. Surg. 33 (2001) 854–860.

## Questionnaires

The European Board of Vascular Surgery
Surgical Training and Working Time in Europe Questionnaire

| | |
|---|---|
| Name and Title | A. Nevelsteen, MD, PhD |
| Country | Belgium |
| Contact Telephone number | 0032-16346850 |
| Date working time directive introduced | DD MM YYYY<br>□□/□□/□□□□ |

**1) Length of Training**

In the UK surgical training is divided into two blocks following graduation. Years 1-5 (Intern/House Officer and Senior House Officer) include a different specialty every six months; years 6-11 (Registrar) are spent in the single career specialty. Supervised training generally finishes by year 12 (when Consultant/independent practitioner status is achieved).

Please specify the structure of the post-graduate surgical training scheme in your country and please indicate qualifications/achievements that must be made before progressing to the next stage. When do the trainees specialize? *(Please indicate stage next to relevant number of years).*

1 - 5
The first Five years of training in general surgery are divided over alle surgical departments (abdominal, vascular, thoracic, cardial, urology, orthopaedics, traumatology) in local and university hospitals

6
The last year of training is mostly done in one specific surgical area

After 6 years they become general surgeons and may operate independently

7 – 8
Most of the young surgeons do 1 or 2 years of extra training in one field (e.g. Cardial surgery, vascular surgery, Abdominal Surgery)

**2) Leave**

In your country, how much time is allowed for

| | |
|---|---|
| a) Vacations and national or religious (e.g. weeks per year) | 20 days |
| b) External training or conferences (e.g. weeks per year) | 5 days |
| c) Internal educational meetings (e.g. hours per week) | Approximately 5 hours/week |
| d) Private study time (e.g. hours per week) | Approximately 5 hours/week |

**3) Assessment**

Please describe how trainees are monitored and assessed during their training in your country.

Every 6 month by their trainer based on their
- techniques, surgical skills,
- social capacities
- administrative capacities
- scientific activities
- general style

At the end of their second year of training they have to do an exam concerning anatomy and pathology (books of Ellis and Way)

At the end of their last year of training they have to do another exam concerning practical knowledge (a case study, an interview concerning general skills, a theoretical examination and a review of an article

**4) Hours of work**

a) When does the normal working day start and finish? (e.g. 8 am - 6 pm) — 7.30 am – 7 pm

b) What is the length (in hours) of the longest shift allowed? — 24 h

c) Night working

How often are surgical trainees on duty at 9 pm? 1 night in 4

How often are surgical trainees on duty at 3 am? 1 night in 4

Does the trainee work the day after a night on duty? Yes ☐ No ☒

d) How long are surgical trainees at work for each week? (please indicate the number of hours per week) — 50 - 55

e) Does the time include training and private study? Yes ☐ No ☒

f) What percentage of your country's surgical trainees currently conform to the Working Time Directive, including the 48-hour week?

Approximately 10 %

**5) Team organization**

In UK hospitals a team of doctors consists of one consultant/specialist, one registrar, one senior house officer and maybe a house officer too. That team cares for 10-30 patients. Each patient is cared for only by doctors of that team.

a) How are the teams organized in your country?

A/ In university hospitals
1 staff member for 2 trainees
1 medical student for 1 trainee

B/ In regional hospitals
2 staff members for 1 trainee
1 medical student for 1 trainee

b) How many consultants/specialists are responsible for each patient?

1 for 10 patients

c) How many consultants/specialists supervise each trainee doctor?

1 for 2 trainees

**6) Specialty cover at night**

a) At night, do surgeons cover just their own specialty or more than one surgical specialty or subspecialty?

| | | | |
|---|---|---|---|
| Year 1-5 | Own ☐ | Several ☒ | e.g.: |
| Year 6 onwards | Own ☒ | Several ☐ | e.g.: |
| Consultant/specialist | Own ☒ | Several ☐ | e.g.: |

b) Do surgical trainees cover any non-surgical specialties? Yes ☐ No ☒

c) Are emergency surgical patients admitted straight to the specialty ward or to a general admissions ward? Specialty ward ☐ Admissions ward ☒

d) In a hospital receiving emergency patients in *general surgery, vascular surgery, urology and orthopaedics*

- How many surgical doctors will be in the hospital to cover these specialties at 3 am?

  4

- How many surgical doctors will be on duty from home to cover these specialties at 3 am?

  4

Please go back to Question 1 and mark * which levels of doctors (including consultants) would be in the hospital at 3 am.

e) Are non-medical staff used to decrease the workload of trainee doctors in any of the following areas?

| | | | | | |
|---|---|---|---|---|---|
| Clerical Work | Yes ☒ | No ☐ | Admitting patients | Yes ☒ | No ☐ |
| Venepuncture | Yes ☒ | No ☐ | Clinics | Yes ☐ | No ☒ |
| ECGs | Yes ☒ | No ☐ | Endoscopy | Yes ☐ | No ☒ |
| Prescribing drugs | Yes ☐ | No ☒ | Catheters | Yes ☐ | No ☒ |
| First operator | Yes ☐ | No ☒ | Assistant Operator | Yes ☒ | No ☐ |

**7) Further information**

The Board would be very grateful if you could provide further information on the organization of surgical training and the service provided by junior doctors and the way in which this has been affected by the requirements of the working time directive. Please provide details of any measures that have been taken which have helped surgical training to adapt to the shorter working week (e.g. greater use of nurses to reduce junior doctors' workload).

Thank you very much for your cooperation.

The 48-hour week has not yet been implemented in Belgium!!

The European Board of Vascular Surgery
Surgical Training and Working Time in Europe Questionnaire

Name and Title Tomislav Sosa, professor of Surgery and Vascular surgery

The European Board of Vascular Surgery

Surgical Training and Working Time in Europe Questionnaire
Country Croatia

Contact Telephone number +385-1- 243-1394

Date working time directive introduced DD MM YYYY
01 / 01 / 1973

**1) Length of Training**

In the UK surgical training is divided into two blocks following graduation. Years 1-5 (Intern/House Officer and Senior House Officer) include a different specialty every six months; years 6-11 (Registrar) are spent in the single career specialty. Supervised training generally finishes by year 12 (when Consultant/independent practitioner status is achieved).

Please specify the structure of the post-graduate surgical training scheme in your country and please indicate qualifications/achievements that must be made before progressing to the next stage. When do the trainees specialize? *(Please indicate stage next to relevant number of years).*

| | |
|---|---|
| 1 Internship | 12 Independent Consultant in Vasculars. |
| 2 General surgery specialization all specialities | 13 |
| 3 " " | 14 |
| 4 " " | 15 |
| 5 " " | 16 |
| 6 General surgery + examination | 17 |
| 7 Supervised training as General surgeon | 18 |
| 8 " " | 19 |
| 9 Independent specialization i.e. Vascular surgery | 20 |
| 10 Vascular surgery + examination | |
| 11 Supervised training as Vascular surgeon | |

**2) Leave**

In your country, how much time is allowed for

| | |
|---|---|
| a) Vacations and national or religious (e.g. weeks per year) | 6 weeks |
| b) External training or conferences (e.g. weeks per year) | 1 week |
| c) Internal educational meetings (e.g. hours per week) | 1 hr/week |
| d) Private study time (e.g. hours per week) | not specified |

**3) Assessment**

Please describe how trainees are monitored and assessed during their training in your country.

General surgery - monitored by mentor
Assessment in General surgery by the Board of Assessors appointed by Minister of Health
Supervised training in General surgery monitored by the Head of the Department where surgeon is appointed
Vascular surgery - monitored by mentor
Assessment in Vascular surgery by the Board of Assessors appointed by Minister of Health
Supervised training in Vascular surgery monitored by the Head of Vascular dept. where vascular surgeon is appointed

Assessments in General and Vascular surgery:

1. Operative procedure done by the candidate in front of the assessors
2. Review of patients in front of the assessors
3. Theoretical part in front of the Board of Assessors which is covering all parts of General/Vascular surgery

**4) Hours of work**

a) When does the normal working day start and finish? 8 a.m. - 4 p.m.
(e.g. 8 am - 6 pm)

b) What is the length (in hours) of the longest shift allowed? 32 hours

c) Night working

How often are surgical trainees on duty at 9 pm? 1 night in 4 days

How often are surgical trainees on duty at 3 am? 1 night in 4 days

(Duty is 24 hrs averagely 8 times per month )

Does the trainee work the day after a night on duty? Yes ☒ No ☐

d) How long are surgical trainees at work for each week? 84 hrs/week
(please indicate the number of hours per week)

e) Does the time include training and private study? Yes ☒ No ☐
yes for the training, private study is not specified

f) What percentage of your country's surgical trainees currently conform to the Working Time Directive, including the 48-hour week?

Approximately 0 %

**5) Team organization**

In UK hospitals a team of doctors consists of one consultant/specialist, one registrar, one senior house officer and maybe a house officer too. That team cares for 10-30 patients. Each patient is cared for only by doctors of that team.

a) How are the teams organized in your country?

The team is the same as in UK. The number of patients cared by the team averages from 35-50 per week. The outpatient clinic is not included in this number. The number represent only the bed ridden surgical patients.

b) How many consultants/specialists are responsible for each patient?

2

c) How many consultants/specialists supervise each trainee doctor?

2 to 5

**6) Specialty cover at night**

a) At night, do surgeons cover just their own specialty or more than one surgical specialty or subspecialty?

| | | | |
|---|---|---|---|
| Year 1-5 | Own ☒ | Several ☐ | e.g.:all branches of General surgery |
| Year 6 onwards | Own ☒ | Several ☐ | e.g.: " " |
| Consultant/specialist | Own ☒ | Several ☐ | e.g.: " " |

b) Do surgical trainees cover any non-surgical specialties? Yes ☐ No ☒

c) Are emergency surgical patients admitted straight to the specialty ward or to a general admissions ward? Specialty ward ☒ Admissions ward ☐

d) In a hospital receiving emergency patients in *general surgery, vascular surgery, urology and orthopaedics*
How many surgical doctors will be in the hospital to cover these specialties at 3 am? 2 in local hospitals, 3 in regional hospitals, 4-6 in University hospitals
How many surgical doctors will be on duty from home to cover these specialties at 3 am? 1 in local and regional hospitals, 1-2 in University hospitals

Please go back to Question 1 and mark * which levels of doctors (including consultants) would be in the hospital at 3 am? 1 consultant and house officer in local hospital, 1 consultant, 1 registrar and 1 house officer in regional hospital, 2 consultants, 1 registrar and 1 house officer in University hospital at minimum

e) Are non-medical staff used to decrease the workload of trainee doctors in any of the following areas?

| | | | | | |
|---|---|---|---|---|---|
| Clerical Work | Yes ☒ | No ☐ | Admitting patients | Yes ☒ | No ☐ |
| Venepuncture | Yes ☒ | No ☐ | Clinics | Yes ☒ | No ☐ |
| ECGs | Yes ☐ | No ☐ | Endoscopy | Yes ☒ | No ☐ |
| Prescribing drugs | Yes ☐ | No ☒ | Catheters | Yes ☐ | No ☒ |
| First operator | Yes ☐ | No ☒ | Assistant Operator | Yes ☐ | No ☒ |

**7) Further information**

The Board would be very grateful if you could provide further information on the organization of surgical training and the service provided by junior doctors and the way in which this has been affected by the requirements of the working time directive. Please provide details of any measures that have been taken which have helped surgical training to adapt to the shorter working week (e.g. greater use of nurses to reduce junior doctorsí workload).

Thank you very much for your cooperation.

# The European Board of Vascular Surgery
## Surgical Training and Working Time in Europe Questionnaire

| | |
|---|---|
| Name and Title | N. Angelides MD, PhD, FRCS |
| Country | CYPRUS |
| Contact Telephone number | 0035722355230 |

Date working time directive introduced 23 / 06 / 2003

**1) Length of Training**

In the UK surgical training is divided into two blocks following graduation. Years 1-5 (Intern/House Officer and Senior House Officer) include a different specialty every six months; years 6-11 (Registrar) are spent in the single career specialty. Supervised training generally finishes by year 12 (when Consultant/independent practitioner status is achieved).

Please specify the structure of the post-graduate surgical training scheme in your country and please indicate qualifications/achievements that must be made before progressing to the next stage. When do the trainees specialize? *(Please indicate stage next to relevant number of years).*

BLOCK ONE: General Surgery: 3 years

BLOCK TWO: Vascular Surgery: 3 years

BLOCK THREE: Thoracic Surgery: 6 months

Cardiac Surgery: 6 months

| | |
|---|---|
| 2 | 12 |
| 3 | 13 |
| 4 | 14 |
| 5 | 15 |
| 6 | 16 |
| 7 | 17 |
| 8 | 18 |
| 9 | 19 |
| 10 | 20 |

**2) Leave**

In your country, how much time is allowed for

| | |
|---|---|
| a) Vacations and national or religious (e.g. weeks per year) | 15 days |
| b) External training or conferences (e.g. weeks per year) | 4 weeks |
| c) Internal educational meetings (e.g. hours per week) | 7 hours weekly |
| d) Private study time (e.g. hours per week) | Fluctuates |

**3) Assessment**

Please describe how trainees are monitored and assessed during their training in your country.

* Each trainee doctor has a loc book in which he includes all his medical activities

* Each vascular trainee is on call 10 days monthly including a week-end

* One senior doctor is responsible for each trainee

* Each trainee is assessed on an every day basis during the ward's rounds and the other activities in the Unit. He is also directly assessed by the Director of the Department monthly.

**4) Hours of work**

a) When does the normal working day start and finish?
(e.g. 8 am - 6 pm)

7.30 to 15.00 hrs

b) What is the length (in hours) of the longest shift allowed?

24hrs

c) Night working

How often are surgical trainees on duty at 9 pm? 1 night in 4

How often are surgical trainees on duty at 3 am? 1 night in 4

Does the trainee work the day after a night on duty? Yes ☒ No ☐

d) How long are surgical trainees at work for each week?
(please indicate the number of hours per week)

35 hrs + on call

e) Does the time include training and private study? Yes ☐ No ☒

f) What percentage of your country's surgical trainees currently conform to the Working Time Directive, including the 48-hour week?

Approximately 100 %

**5) Team organization**

In UK hospitals a team of doctors consists of one consultant/specialist, one registrar, one senior house officer and maybe a house officer too. That team cares for 10-30 patients. Each patient is cared for only by doctors of that team.

a) How are the teams organized in your country?

*Director of the Unit-Senior Consultant

*Consultant-Registrar-senior house officer

*24 beds

b) How many consultants/specialists are responsible for each patient?

Director of the Unit + One consultant

c) How many consultants/specialists supervise each trainee doctor?

Director of the Unit

**6) Specialty cover at night**

a) At night, do surgeons cover just their own specialty or more than one surgical specialty or subspecialty?

| | | | |
|---|---|---|---|
| Year 1-5 | Own ☐ | Several ☒ | e.g.:Cardiovascular and thoracic |
| Year 6 onwards | Own ☒ | Several ☐ | e.g.: Vascular |
| Consultant/specialist | Own ☒ | Several ☐ | e.g.: |

b) Do surgical trainees cover any non-surgical specialties? Yes ☐ No ☒

c) Are emergency surgical patients admitted straight to the specialty ward or to a general admissions ward? Specialty ward ☒ Admissions ward ☐

d) In a hospital receiving emergency patients in *general surgery, vascular surgery, urology and orthopaedics*

- How many surgical doctors will be in the hospital to cover these specialties at 3 am?

  one

- How many surgical doctors will be on duty from home to cover these specialties at 3 am?

  four

Please go back to Question 1 and mark * which levels of doctors (including consultants) would be in the hospital at 3 am.

e) Are non-medical staff used to decrease the workload of trainee doctors in any of the following areas?

| | | | | | |
|---|---|---|---|---|---|
| Clerical Work | Yes ☒ | No ☐ | Admitting patients | Yes ☒ | No ☐ |
| Venepuncture | Yes ☒ | No ☐ | Clinics | Yes ☐ | No ☒ |
| ECGs | Yes ☒ | No ☐ | Endoscopy | Yes ☐ | No ☒ |
| Prescribing drugs | Yes ☐ | No ☒ | Catheters | Yes ☒ | No ☐ |
| First operator | Yes ☒ | No ☐ | Assistant Operator | Yes ☒ | No ☐ |

* Surgical trainees have the freedom to examine patients, prescribe their medication, plan their investigations but have to report to their supervisor regularly

* Surgical trainees have regular access to operating theatres. As a first stage they assist, as a second stage they perform minor operations and as a third stage they perform more essential operations.

* Concerning the work-load certain measures have been taken so that the trainee doctors are assisted by non-medical personnel

* Some of the vascular trainees are working on a PhD thesis while others are participating in clinical research

**7) Further information**

The Board would be very grateful if you could provide further information on the organization of surgical training and the service provided by junior doctors and the way in which this has been affected by the requirements of the working time directive. Please provide details of any measures that have been taken which have helped surgical training to adapt to the shorter working week (e.g. greater use of nurses to reduce junior doctors' workload).

Thank you very much for your cooperation.

The European Board of Vascular Surgery
Surgical Training and Working Time in Europe Questionnaire

Name and Title MARUSIAK JAN, M.D., PhD.

**Country Czech Republic**

Contact Telephone number
+42048602131295

Date working time directive introduced DD MM YYYY
□□/□□/□□□□

1) Length of Training

In the Czech republic surgical training is divided into two blocks following graduation. Years 1-3 include a different speciality every 3 - 6 months; years 4 - 9 (Registrar) are spent in the single career speciality. Supervised training generally finishes by year 9 - 10 (when Consultant/independent practitioner status is achieved).

After the first period of 3 years, the surgeon has to do 1st degree of confirmation, which is obligatory and during the second period, after 9 years 2nd degree of confirmation, which is obligatory only if the surgeon would like to continue his career in the hospital. Both these exams are from general surgery/common trunk/. Paralelly, but not sooner than after the passing 1st degree, the surgeon can undergo exam from vascular surgery, if he wish to do this speciality as a main speciality. The exam from vascular surgery is done under the Society for Cardiovascular Surgery, because in Czech Republic vascular surgery so far is division of Society for Cardiovascular Surgery.

**Please specify the structure of the post-graduate surgical training scheme in your country and please indicate qualifications/achievements that must be made before progressing to the next stage. When do the trainees specialize? (Please indicate stage next to relevant number of years).**

| | | | |
|---|---|---|---|
| 1 | | 11 | Consultant, Head of the Unit etc. |
| 2 | | 12 | |
| 3 | 1st degree of confirmation in general surgery/obligatory/ | 13 | |
| 4 | | 14 | |
| 5 | Exam from Vascular Surgery /not obligatory/ | 15 | |

| | | | |
|---|---|---|---|
| 6 | | 16 | |
| 7 | | 17 | |
| 8 | | 18 | |
| 9 | 2nd degree of confirmation in GS /not obligatory/ | 19 | |
| 10 | | 20 | |

2) Leave
In your country, how much time is allowed for

a) Vacations and national or religious

(e.g. weeks per year) 4 - 6

not specified

b) External training or conferences

(e.g. weeks per year) /2 – 8/

not specified

c) Internal educational meetings

(e.g. hours per week) /4 – 8/

not specified

d) Private study time

(e.g. hours per week) / 7 – 21 /

**3) Assessment**
**Please describe how trainees are monitored and assessed during their training in your country.**

First 3 years in hospital under the consultant supervision next 4 – 9 years, if they stay in the hospital, they are registrars and have one experienced surgeon as a teacher
if they decide to have private praxis after 3 years and exam from general surgery /1st degree of surgical confirmation/ they are independent with full responsibility
In the hospital they need to undergo 2nd degree of surgical confirmation to become consultant and full responsible surgeon /after 9-10 years after studies in the University/
Vascular Surgery is a speciality which needs qualified vascular surgeons,

In Czech republic is recommended for vascular surgeon to have 2nd degree from general surgery /not obligatory/ and special exam from vascular surgery / obligatory for consultant on vascular surgery unit or department/

4) Hours of work

7 am – 15 pm

a) When does the normal working day start and finish?

(e.g. 8 am - 6 pm)

b) Ask ministry of health
What is the length (in hours) of the longest shift allowed?

c) Night working week
How often are surgical trainees on duty at 9 pm? 1 night in week

How often are surgical trainees on duty at 3 am? 1 night in

Does the trainee work the day after a night on duty? Yes

d) How long are surgical trainees at work for each week?

(please indicate the number of hours per week) 40 - 94

e) Does the time include private study No

f) What percentage of your country's surgical trainees currently conform to the Working Time Directive, including the 48-hour week?
Approximately 15 – 40%

5) Team organization

In Czech republic hospitals a team of doctors consists of one consultant/specialist, two registrar, and trainees. That team cares for 10-30 patients. Only doctors of that team care for each patient.

a) How are the teams organized in your country?

Described above

b) How many consultants/specialists are responsible for each patient?

1 consultant /specialist/ for 15 – 30 patients

c) How many consultants/specialists supervise each trainee doctor?

1 consultant for 2 – 3 trainees

6) Specialty cover at night

a) At night, do surgeons cover just their own specialty or more than one surgical specialty or subspecialty?

| | | |
|---|---|---|
| Year 1-5 | Several | e.g.: |
| Year 6 onwards | Several | e.g.: |
| Consultant/specialist | Several | e.g.: |

b) Do surgical trainees cover any non-surgical specialties? No

c) Are emergency surgical patients admitted straight to the specialty ward or to a general admissions ward? General admissions ward

d) In a hospital receiving emergency patients in general surgery, vascular surgery, urology and orthopaedics

How many surgical doctors will be in the hospital to cover these specialties at 3 am?

§ 2 /20% of hosp./ 3 /80% of hospitals

How many surgical doctors will be on duty from home to cover these specialties at 3 am?

§ 1 - 3

Please go back to Question 1 and mark * which levels of doctors (including consultants) would be in the hospital at 3 am.

In Czech republic, there are 2 – 3 doctors in the hospital all night on the surgery unit with 50 – 100 beds, included consultants and head of department

e) Are non-medical staff used to decrease the workload of trainee doctors in any of the following areas?

| | | | |
|---|---|---|---|
| Clerical Work | No □ | Admitting patients | No □ |
| Venopuncture | No □ | Clinics | No □ |
| ECGs | No □ | Endoscopy | No □ |
| Prescribing drugs | No □ | Catheters | No □ |
| First operator | No □ | Assistant Operator | No □ |

7) Further information

The Board would be very grateful if you could provide further information on the organization of surgical training and the service provided by junior doctors and the way in which this has been affected by the requirements of the working time directive. Please provide details of any measures that have been taken which have helped surgical training to adapt to the shorter working week (e.g. greater use of nurses to reduce junior doctors' workload).

Thank you very much for your cooperation. Our system so far is organized in that way, that the physician serves many many hours per week, included trainees, registrars, consultants and even heads of departments.

## The European Board of Vascular Surgery
## Surgical Training and Working Time in Europe Questionnaire

Name and Title JES SANDERMANN, CONSULTANT

Country DENMARK

Contact Telephone number + 45-8927-2444

Date working time directive introduced DD / MM / YYYY — / / 1981

### 1) Length of Training

In the UK surgical training is divided into two blocks following graduation. Years 1-5 (Intern/House Officer and Senior House Officer) include a different specialty every six months; years 6-11 (Registrar) are spent in the single career specialty. Supervised training generally finishes by year 12 (when Consultant/independent practitioner status is achieved).

Please specify the structure of the post-graduate surgical training scheme in your country and please indicate qualifications/achievements that must be made before progressing to the next stage. When do the trainees specialize? *(Please indicate stage next to relevant number of years).*

| | |
|---|---|
| 1 1 ½ years internship | 11 After the surgical block it will take 2 years In a general surgical unit to |
| 2 2 years basic surgery | 12 become a general surgeon. |
| 3 (1/2 year orthopaedics included) | 13 |
| 4 2 ¼ years in a surgical block, then specialization | 14 None of the last 15 Danish Vascular surgeons are general Surgical specialists. |
| 5 One can go directly into vascular surgical training for 3 years to become a vascular | 15 |
| 6 specialist. | 16 *REF: Sandermann-Panduro Jensen EJVES 2002;23:353-357* |
| 7 After a 4th year, you are qualified to become a consultant | 17 |
| 8 | 18 |
| 9 | 19 |
| 10 | 20 |

**2) Leave**

In your country, how much time is allowed for

| | |
|---|---|
| a) Vacations and national or religious (e.g. weeks per year) | 5 weeks & 3 days |
| b) External training or conferences (e.g. weeks per year) | not defined |
| c) Internal educational meetings (e.g. hours per week) | not defined |
| d) Private study time (e.g. hours per week) | not defined |

**3) Assessment**

Please describe how trainees are monitored and assessed during their training in your country.

Every trainee has a Trainer and there exists a training program baste upon Some tall goals to be achieved. Going through 2 units of which one is a university clinic. The sum of the two training programs fullfill the goals. The trainer is responsible for this and the training is adjusted.

Again please see the ref . *Sandermann-Panduro Jensen EJVES 2002;23:353-357*

**4) Hours of work** in my unit

a) When does the normal working day start and finish? (e.g. 8 am - 6 pm) 08.00 am – 03.00 pm

b) What is the length (in hours) of the longest shift allowed? 17 hrs

c) Night working

How often are surgical trainees on duty at 9 pm? 1 night in 7- 8

How often are surgical trainees on duty at 3 am? 1 night in 7-8

Does the trainee work the day after a night on duty? Yes ☐ No ☒

d) How long are surgical trainees at work for each week? (please indicate the number of hours per week) 37-40 hrs

e) Does the time include training and private study? Yes ☒ No ☒

f) What percentage of your country's surgical trainees currently conform to the Working Time Directive, including the 48-hour week?

Approximately **100** %

**5) Team organization**

In UK hospitals a team of doctors consists of one consultant/specialist, one registrar, one senior house officer and maybe a house officer too. That team cares for 10-30 patients. Each patient is cared for only by doctors of that team.

a) How are the teams organized in your country?

In our general surgical unit we take care of :
surgical patients
urological patients
thoracic patients (no cardiac surgery)
vascular patients

All the 8-9 juniors work in the whole department, but we try to give them a period within each area.
The registrars work in the separate areas as do the consultants (two of the 5 vascular consultants are also thoracic surgeons).
There are 5 registrars (2 train for surgery, one for vascular, one for urology and one for surgical).

b) How many consultants/specialists are responsible for each patient?

All consultants / specialists in the unit

c) How many consultants/specialists supervise each trainee doctor?

The trainer and all the other consultants / specialists supervise the trainee whenever they work together.

**6) Specialty cover at night**

a) At night, do surgeons cover just their own specialty or more than one surgical specialty or subspecialty?

| | | | |
|---|---|---|---|
| Year 1-5 | Own ☐ | Several ☒ | e.g.: the 4 mentioned surgical areas |
| Year 6 onwards | Own ☐ | Several ☒ | e.g.: the 4 mentioned surgical areas |
| Consultant/specialist | Own ☒ | Several ☐ | e.g.: |

b) Do surgical trainees cover any non-surgical specialties? Yes ☐ No ☒

c) Are emergency surgical patients admitted straight to the specialty ward or to a general admissions ward?

Specialty ward ☒ Admissions ward ☐

d) In a hospital receiving emergency patients in *general surgery, vascular surgery, urology and orthopaedics*

- How many surgical doctors will be in the hospital to cover these specialties at 3 am?
  One surgery, orthopaedics 2 } juniors. The registrars (2) one for each area – after a.m. in the hospital, but they are allowed to go home (1/2 hour to arrive!)
- How many surgical doctors will be on duty from home to cover these specialties at 3 am?
  3. : one orthopaedic Consultants, one vascular, one for surgeons or urology

Please go back to Question 1 and mark * which levels of doctors (including consultants) would be in the hospital at 3 am.

e) Are non-medical staff used to decrease the workload of trainee doctors in any of the following areas?

| | | | | | |
|---|---|---|---|---|---|
| Clerical Work | Yes ☒ | No ☐ | Admitting patients | Yes ☐ | No ☒ |
| Venepuncture | Yes ☒ | No ☐ | Clinics | Yes ☐ | No ☒ |
| ECGs | Yes ☒ | No ☐ | Endoscopy | Yes ☐ | No ☒ |
| Prescribing drugs | Yes ☐ | No ☒ | Catheters | Yes ☒ | No ☐ |
| First operator | Yes ☐ | No ☒ | Assistant Operator | Yes ☐ | No ☒ |

**7) Further information**

The Board would be very grateful if you could provide further information on the organization of surgical training and the service provided by junior doctors and the way in which this has been affected by the requirements of the working time directive. Please provide details of any measures that have been taken which have helped surgical training to adapt to the shorter working week (e.g. greater use of nurses to reduce junior doctors' workload).

Thank you very much for your cooperation.

In 1981 in Denmark we went through a period which you are approaching. More young doctors were needed and the training contend was discussed. The work had to be done and I have a good training programs . I - that have been through all this, think we have managed. Accelerating the training period of course might not provide all that sufficient experience for the new specialists compared to the older ones. And so it has been in Sweden even for a longer time.

As you may know, a specialist commission made a report in the year 200 Upon which we are redoing all specialist training programs in Denmark, now focusing on gaining (not loosing on time) – how to teach and how to evaluate. The programs should be ready in Spring and practised for the year 2004.
Within vascular surgery I have been in charge of the community and expressed the important of having the text translated into prepare English.

# The European Board of Vascular Surgery
## Surgical Training and Working Time in Europe Questionnaire

Name and Title Railo Mikael, Deputy head of vascular surgery

Country: Helsinki, Finland

Contact Telephone number

Date working time directive introduced DD MM YYYY

☐☐ / ☐☐ / ☐☐☐☐

**1) Length of Training**

In the UK surgical training is divided into two blocks following graduation. Years 1-5 (Intern/House Officer and Senior House Officer) include a different specialty every six months; years 6-11 (Registrar) are spent in the single career specialty. Supervised training generally finishes by year 12 (when Consultant/independent practitioner status is achieved).

Please specify the structure of the post-graduate surgical training scheme in your country and please indicate qualifications/achievements that must be made before progressing to the next stage. When do the trainees specialize? *(Please indicate stage next to relevant number of years).*

| | | | |
|---|---|---|---|
| 1 | Health care center 3/4 | 11 | |
| 2 | Common trunk surgery 2 1/4 | 12 | |
| 3 | Common trunk surgery 2 1/4 | 13 | |
| 4 | Vascular surgery 3 | 14 | |
| 5 | Vascular surgery 3 | 15 | |
| 6 | Vascular surgery 3 | 16 | |
| 7 | | 17 | |
| 8 | | 18 | |
| 9 | | 19 | |
| 10 | | 20 | |

**2) Leave**

In your country, how much time is allowed for

| | |
|---|---|
| a) Vacations and national or religious (e.g. weeks per year) | **4 weeks** |
| b) External training or conferences (e.g. weeks per year) | **one week** |
| c) Internal educational meetings (e.g. hours per week) | 2.5 hrs / week |
| d) Private study time (e.g. hours per week) | 2 hours a week, other studies beyond the working hours |

**3) Assessment**

Please describe how trainees are monitored and assessed during their training in your country.

**4) Hours of work**

a) When does the normal working day start and finish? (07.30) 8.00-15.30
(e.g. 8 am - 6 pm)

b) What is the length (in hours) of the longest shift allowed? 24 hours

c) Night working

How often are surgical trainees on duty at 9 pm? 1 night in

How often are surgical trainees on duty at 3 am? 1 night in one week

Does the trainee work the day after a night on duty? Yes ☐ No ☒

d) How long are surgical trainees at work for each week? Officially 38.5 hrs
(please indicate the number of hours per week) Practically 48-55 hours

e) Does the time include training and private study? Yes ☐ No ☒ mostly

f) What percentage of your country's surgical trainees currently conform to the Working Time Directive, including the 48-hour week?

Approximately **50** %

**5) Team organization**

In UK hospitals a team of doctors consists of one consultant/specialist, one registrar, one senior house officer and maybe a house officer too. That team cares for 10-30 patients. Each patient is cared for only by doctors of that team.

a) How are the teams organized in your country?

Vasc depts. In university consists of 3-8 consultants + 1-6 registrars + 0-1 house officers (common trunk training).

Each registry (specializing in vascular surgery) has its own tutor. Otherwise separate teams are not available unless there are more than one vascular ward.

b) How many consultants/specialists are responsible for each patient?

1-3

c) How many consultants/specialists supervise each trainee doctor?

1-8

**6) Specialty cover at night**

a) At night, do surgeons cover just their own specialty or more than one surgical specialty or subspecialty?

| | | | | |
|---|---|---|---|---|
| Year 1-5 **1-3 any** surgery | Own ☐ | Several ☒ | e.g.: vascular and soft |
| Year 6 onwards | Own ☐ | Several ☐ | e.g.: |
| Consultant/specialist | Own ☐ | Several ☐ | e.g.: |

b) Do surgical trainees cover any non-surgical specialties? Yes ☐ No ☒

c) Are emergency surgical patients admitted straight to the specialty ward or to a general admissions ward? Specialty ward ☒ Admissions ward ☒
according the local conditions and resources

d) In a hospital receiving emergency patients in *general surgery, vascular surgery, urology and orthopaedics*

- How many surgical doctors will be in the hospital to cover these specialties at 3 am? 1-6 depending on the hospital (2 consultants 4 trainees)

- How many surgical doctors will be on duty from home to cover these specialties at 3 am? 2-4 all consultants

Please go back to Question 1 and mark * which levels of doctors (including consultants) would be in the hospital at 3 am.

e) Are non-medical staff used to decrease the workload of trainee doctors in any of the following areas?

| | | | | | |
|---|---|---|---|---|---|
| Clerical Work | Yes ☒ | No ☐ | Admitting patients | Yes ☒ | No ☐ |
| Venepuncture | Yes ☒ | No ☐ | Clinics | Yes ☐ | No ☒ |
| ECGs | Yes ☒ | No ☐ | Endoscopy | Yes ☐ | No ☒ |
| Prescribing drugs | Yes ☐ | No ☒ | Catheters | Yes ☒ | No ☐ |
| First operator | Yes ☐ | No ☒ | Assistant Operator | Yes ☒ | No ☐ |

**7) Further information**

The Board would be very grateful if you could provide further information on the organization of surgical training and the service provided by junior doctors and the way in which this has been affected by the requirements of the working time directive. Please provide details of any measures that have been taken which have helped surgical training to adapt to the shorter working week (e.g. greater use of nurses to reduce junior doctors' workload).

Thank you very much for your cooperation.

The European Board of Vascular Surgery
Surgical Training and Working Time in Europe Questionnaire

Name and Title PROF. OLIVIER GOËAU-BRISSONNIÈRE

Country FRANCE (French College of Vascular Surgery)

Contact Telephone number + 33 149095585

Date working time directive introduced DD MM YYYY
01 / 01 / 2003

**1) Length of Training**

In the UK surgical training is divided into two blocks following graduation. Years 1-5 (Intern/House Officer and Senior House Officer) include a different specialty every six months; years 6-11 (Registrar) are spent in the single career specialty. Supervised training generally finishes by year 12 (when Consultant/independent practitioner status is achieved).

Please specify the structure of the post-graduate surgical training scheme in your country and please indicate qualifications/achievements that must be made before progressing to the next stage. When do the trainees specialize? *(Please indicate stage next to relevant number of years).*

In France, surgical training is divided into two blocks. Years 1-5 (Intern) include a different area every 6 months. During the first 2 years, the intern should work for 6 months in the specialty that he will then choose. During these 5 years he must spend a total of 2 years in the chosen surgical specialty. Years 6-9 are spent in the single career specialty. However, only years 6 and 7 are always performed and the surgeon can work as an independent specialist from year 7. Nevertheless more than 50% spend 3 to 4 years in a supervised training faculty in vascular surgery.

**2) Leave**

In your country, how much time is allowed for

| | |
|---|---|
| a) Vacations and national or religious (e.g. weeks per year) | about 6 weeks |
| b) External training or conferences (e.g. weeks per year) | variable, about 1 week |
| c) Internal educational meetings (e.g. hours per week) | 4 to 6 |
| d) Private study time (e.g. hours per week) | 5 |

**3) Assessment**

Please describe how trainees are monitored and assessed during their training in your country.

--------------------------------

In each French academic region (7 in total) training is organized and supervised by a Professor Director (for each surgical specialty, and in particular for vascular surgery). Every 6 months, the work of the house officers has to be validated by the chairman of the unit where they work. A final oral examination, with a presentation of a clinical research work has to be done at the end of the first year of work as a senior officer; the Jury is composed of 4 vascular surgery professors After success in the examination the surgeon can work independently (however, he often still serves as a senior officer for a farther 1-3 years more).

During training, evaluation is also preformed daily in the unit (science and technique, clinical presentation,) and a surgical logbook will implemented soon.

**4) Hours of work**

a) When does the normal working day start and finish? (e.g. 8 am - 6 pm) — 7.30 am-6 pm

b) What is the length (in hours) of the longest shift allowed? — 24 hrs

c) Night working

How often are surgical trainees on duty at 9 pm? — 1 night in 8 (about)

How often are surgical trainees on duty at 3 am? — 1 night in 8 (about)

Does the trainee work the day after a night on duty? — Yes ☐ No ☒

d) How long are surgical trainees at work for each week? (please indicate the number of hours per week) — 48 hrs

e) Does the time include training and private study? — Yes ☐ No ☒ **training=yes**

f) What percentage of your country's surgical trainees currently conform to the Working Time Directive, including the 48-hour week?

Approximately **100** %

### 5) Team organization

In UK hospitals a team of doctors consists of one consultant/specialist, one registrar, one senior house officer and maybe a house officer too. That team cares for 10-30 patients. Only doctors of that team care for each patient.

a) How are the teams organized in your country?

In France, a team usually consists of one or two consultants, one registrar, 1-3 (often 2) senior house officers in university hospitals and 2-3 house officers in university hospitals. Surgical house officers are often pooled for the emergency duties in general surgery. A team cares for 25-40 patients. Only doctors of that team care for each patient.

b) How many consultants/specialists are responsible for each patient?

1 consultant for each patient

c) How many consultants/specialists supervise each trainee doctor?

In general two, sometimes three, but due to reconstruction and consultation, sometimes more (with more beds and more trainers)

**6) Specialty cover at night**

a) At night, do surgeons cover just their own specialty or more than one surgical specialty or subspecialty?

| | | | |
|---|---|---|---|
| Year 1-5 | Own ☒ | Several ☐ | e.g.: |
| Year 6 onwards | Own ☒ | Several ☐ | e.g.: |
| Consultant/specialist | Own ☒ | Several ☐ | e.g.: |

b) Do surgical trainees cover any non-surgical specialties? Yes ☐ No ☒

c) Are emergency surgical patients admitted straight to the specialty ward or to a general admissions ward? Specialty ward ☒ Admissions ward ☐

d) In a hospital receiving emergency patients in *general surgery, vascular surgery, urology and orthopaedics*

- How many surgical doctors will be in the hospital to cover these specialties at 3 am? Usually one orthopaedics house officer, one orthopaedics senior house officer and the same (2 people) for general surgery → 4 doctors
- How many surgical doctors will be on duty from home to cover these specialties at 3 am?
  One urology senior house officer
  One vascular surgery senior house officer } on duty of the home

**Please go back to Question 1 and mark * which levels of doctors (including consultants) would be in the hospital at 3 am.**

e) Are non-medical staff used to decrease the workload of trainee doctors in any of the following areas?

| | | | | | |
|---|---|---|---|---|---|
| Clerical Work | Yes ☒ | No ☐ | Admitting patients | Yes ☐ | No ☒ |
| Venepuncture | Yes ☒ | No ☐ | Clinics | Yes ☐ | No ☒ |
| ECGs * | Yes ☒ | No ☐ | Endoscopy | Yes ☐ | No ☒ |
| Prescribing drugs | Yes ☐ | No ☒ | + Catheters | Yes ☒ | No ☐ |
| First operator | Yes ☐ | No ☒ | Assistant Operator | Yes ☐ | No ☒ |

* recording not interpreting + urinary

**7) Further information**

The Board would be very grateful if you could provide further information on the organization of surgical training and the service provided by junior doctors and the way in which this has been affected by the requirements of the working time directive. Please provide details of any measures that have been taken which have helped surgical training to adapt to the shorter working week (e.g. greater use of nurses to reduce junior doctors' workload).

Thank you very much for your cooperation.

Before the directive, house officers worked in academic and non-academic hospitals. Due to the Directive and also a decrease in the number of trainees in surgical specialties, house officers are progressively removed from non-university hospitals. These factors will probably contribute to a series reconstruction of the surgical network. Due the numerous implications of that reconstruction, few measures have yet being taken, but discussions are on going.

## The European Board of Vascular Surgery
## Surgical Training and Working Time in Europe Questionnaire

| | |
|---|---|
| Name and Title | DR KLAUS BALTER |
| Country | GERMANY |
| Contact Telephone number | +492083092440 |
| Date working time directive introduced | DD / MM / YYYY<br>12 / 04 / 2003 |

**1) Length of Training**

In the UK surgical training is divided into two blocks following graduation. Years 1-5 (Intern/House Officer and Senior House Officer) include a different specialty every six months; years 6-11 (Registrar) are spent in the single career specialty. Supervised training generally finishes by year 12 (when Consultant/independent practitioner status is achieved).

Please specify the structure of the post-graduate surgical training scheme in your country and please indicate qualifications/achievements that must be made before progressing to the next stage. When do the trainees specialize? *(Please indicate stage next to relevant number of years).*

| Year | Stage | Year | Stage |
|---|---|---|---|
| 1–5 | General surgery | 11 | } |
| 6–8 | vascular surgery including all kinds of diagnostic, open surgery and endovascular examination in vascular surgery | 12 | possibility of teaching vascular surgery (1.2.3 years depending on the facilities and the number of operation) |
| 9–10 | clinical practice in hospital or as a practitioner | 13 | |
| | | 14 | |
| | | 15 | |
| | | 16 | |
| | | 17 | |
| | | 18 | |
| | | 19 | |
| | | 20 | |

**2) Leave**

In your country, how much time is allowed for

a) Vacations and national or religious (e.g. weeks per year) **7**

b) External training or conferences (e.g. weeks per year) **1**

c) Internal educational meetings (e.g. hours per week) **4**

d) Private study time (e.g. hours per week) Ø

**3) Assessment**

Please describe how trainees are monitored and assessed during their training in your country.

Only for assistance of a fully trained Vascular Surgeon a trainee is allowed to perform diagnostic or therapeutic procedures. He has to perform a certain number of procedures in the different fields of Vascular surgery and all the diagnostic procedure. The number he has to do is fixed by a special national catalogue.

**4) Hours of work**

a) When does the normal working day start and finish? 7.30-16.30
(e.g. 8 am - 6 pm)

b) What is the length (in hours) of the longest shift allowed? 12 hours

c) Night working

How often are surgical trainees on duty at 9 pm? 1 night in 10

How often are surgical trainees on duty at 3 am? 1 night in 10

Does the trainee work the day after a night on duty? Yes ☐ No ☒

d) How long are surgical trainees at work for each week? ~ 60
(please indicate the number of hours per week)

e) Does the time include training and private study? Yes ☒ No ☐

f) What percentage of your country's surgical trainees currently conform to the Working Time Directive, including the 48-hour week?

Approximately **20** %

**5) Team organization**

In UK hospitals a team of doctors consists of one consultant/specialist, one registrar, one senior house officer and maybe a house officer too. That team cares for 10-30 patients. Each patient is cared for only by doctors of that team.

a) How are the teams organized in your country?

| |
|---|
| Head of Vascular Surgical Department 1-3 substitutes (employed in the hospital).<br>Depending on the number of beds, assistance surgeons<br><br>1 doctor (surgeon) in total for 8-10 patients |

b) How many consultants/specialists are responsible for each patient?

| |
|---|
| 1 |

c) How many consultants/specialists supervise each trainee doctor?

| |
|---|
| 1-3 |

**6) Specialty cover at night**

a) At night, do surgeons cover just their own specialty or more than one surgical specialty or subspecialty?

| | | | |
|---|---|---|---|
| Year 1-5 | Own ☐ | Several ☒ | e.g.: |
| Year 6 onwards | Own ☒ | Several ☐ | e.g.: |
| Consultant/specialist | Own ☒ | Several ☐ | e.g.: |

b) Do surgical trainees cover any non-surgical specialties? Yes ☐ No ☒

c) Are emergency surgical patients admitted straight to the specialty ward or to a general admissions ward? Specialty ward ☒ Admissions ward ☐

d) In a hospital receiving emergency patients in *general surgery, vascular surgery, urology and orthopaedics*

- How many surgical doctors will be in the hospital to cover these specialties at 3 am? 2
- How many surgical doctors will be on duty from home to cover these specialties at 3 am? 3

Please go back to Question 1 and mark * which levels of doctors (including consultants) would be in the hospital at 3 am.

e) Are non-medical staff used to decrease the workload of trainee doctors in any of the following areas?

| | | | | | |
|---|---|---|---|---|---|
| Clerical work | Yes ☐ | No ☒ | Admitting patients | Yes ☐ | No ☒ |
| Venepuncture | Yes ☐ | No ☒ | Clinics | Yes ☐ | No ☒ |
| ECGs | Yes ☒ | No ☐ | Endoscopy | Yes ☒ | No ☐ |
| Prescribing drugs | Yes ☐ | No ☒ | Catheters | Yes ☒ | No ☐ |
| First operator | Yes ☐ | No ☒ | Assistant Operator | Yes ☐ | No ☒ |

**7) Further information**

The Board would be very grateful if you could provide further information on the organization of surgical training and the service provided by junior doctors and the way in which this has been affected by the requirements of the working time directive. Please provide details of any measures that have been taken which have helped surgical training to adapt to the shorter working week (e.g. greater use of nurses to reduce junior doctors' workload).

Thank you very much for your cooperation.

The European Board of Vascular Surgery
Surgical Training and Working Time in Europe Questionnaire

| | |
|---|---|
| Name and Title | ALEX CH. NIKOLAOU M.D. |
| Country | GREECE |
| Contact Telephone number | 030 210 7456347 |
| Date working time directive introduced | DD MM YYYY<br>☐☐/☐☐/☐☐☐☐ |

**1) Length of Training**

In the UK surgical training is divided into two blocks following graduation. Years 1-5 (Intern/House Officer and Senior House Officer) include a different specialty every six months; years 6-11 (Registrar) are spent in the single career specialty. Supervised training generally finishes by year 12 (when Consultant/independent practitioner status is achieved).

Please specify the structure of the post-graduate surgical training scheme in your country and please indicate qualifications/achievements that must be made before progressing to the next stage. When do the trainees specialize? *(Please indicate stage next to relevant number of years).*

| | |
|---|---|
| 1 | 11 |
| 2 | 12 |
| 3 | 13 |
| 4 | 14 |
| 5 | 15 |
| 6 | 16 |
| 7 vascular surgery specialty | 17 |
| 8 | 18 |
| 9 | 19 |
| 10 | 20 |

**2) Leave**

In your country, how much time is allowed for

| | |
|---|---|
| a) Vacations and national or religious (e.g. weeks per year) | 23 days |
| b) External training or conferences (e.g. weeks per year) | After request and acceptance |
| c) Internal educational meetings (e.g. hours per week) | After request and acceptance |
| d) Private study time (e.g. hours per week) | 0 |

**3) Assessment**

Please describe how trainees are monitored and assessed during their training in your country.

Trainees are supervised by specialized doctors throughout their specialty training, involving all the activities of the department (outpatients clinics, ward, surgery, vascular laboratory etc.). There are no obligatory examinations during the years of specialty training.
After completion of training years ( 7years for vascular surgery), trainees give oral and written examinations to become specialized doctors.

**4) Hours of work**

a) When does the normal working day start and finish? (e.g. 8 am - 6 pm) — 7.30am – 3.30pm

b) What is the length (in hours) of the longest shift allowed? — 32 hours

c) Night working

How often are surgical trainees on duty at 9 pm? 1 night in — 4 days

How often are surgical trainees on duty at 3 am? 1 night in — 4 days

Does the trainee work the day after a night on duty? Yes ⊞ No ☐

d) How long are surgical trainees at work for each week? (please indicate the number of hours per week) — 72 hours

e) Does the time include training and private study? Yes ☐ No ⊞

f) What percentage of your country's surgical trainees currently conform to the Working Time Directive, including the 48-hour week?

Approximately 0 %

**5) Team organization**

In UK hospitals a team of doctors consists of one consultant/specialist, one registrar, one senior house officer and maybe a house officer too. That team cares for 10-30 patients. Each patient is cared for only by doctors of that team.

a) How are the teams organized in your country?

| |
|---|
| |

b) How many consultants/specialists are responsible for each patient?

| |
|---|
| One (1) |

c) How many consultants/specialists supervise each trainee doctor?

| |
|---|
| 1-3 |

**6) Specialty cover at night**

a) At night, do surgeons cover just their own specialty or more than one surgical specialty or subspecialty?

| | | | |
|---|---|---|---|
| Year 1-5 | Own ⊞ | Several ☐ | e.g.: |
| Year 6 onwards | Own ⊞ | Several ☐ | e.g.: |
| Consultant/specialist | Own ⊞ | Several ☐ | e.g.: |

b) Do surgical trainees cover any non-surgical specialties? Yes ☐ No ⊞

c) Are emergency surgical patients admitted straight to the specialty ward or to a general admissions ward? Specialty ward ⊞ Admissions ward ☐

d) In a hospital receiving emergency patients in *general surgery, vascular surgery, urology and orthopaedics*

- How many surgical doctors will be in the hospital to cover these specialties at 3 am? 15
- How many surgical doctors will be on duty from home to cover these specialties at 3 am? 6

Please go back to Question 1 and mark * which levels of doctors (including consultants) would be in the hospital at 3 am.

e) Are non-medical staff used to decrease the workload of trainee doctors in any of the following areas?

| | | | | | |
|---|---|---|---|---|---|
| Clerical Work | Yes ☐ | No ⊞ | Admitting patients | Yes ⊞ | No ☐ |
| Venopuncture | Yes ⊞ | No ☐ | Clinics | Yes ⊞ | No ☐ |
| ECGs | Yes ⊞ | No ☐ | Endoscopy | Yes ☐ | No ⊞ |
| Prescribing drugs | Yes ☐ | No ⊞ | Catheters | Yes ☐ | No ⊞ |
| First operator | Yes ☐ | No ⊞ | Assistant Operator | Yes ☐ | No ⊞ |

**7) Further information**

The Board would be very grateful if you could provide further information on the organization of surgical training and the service provided by junior doctors and the way in which this has been affected by the requirements of the working time directive. Please provide details of any measures that have been taken which have helped surgical training to adapt to the shorter working week (e.g. greater use of nurses to reduce junior doctors' workload).

Thank you very much for your cooperation.

The European Board of Vascular Surgery
Surgical Training and Working Time in Europe Questionnaire

| | |
|---|---|
| Name and Title | Prof. Attila Nemes MD, PhD, DSc<br>Zsolt Antal Varga MD, PhD |
| Country | Hungary |
| Contact Telephone number | +36 1 4586789<br>+36 30 9 476 614 |
| Date working time directive introduced | DD / MM / YYYY<br>☐☐ / ☐☐ / ☐☐☐☐ |

**1) Length of Training**

In the UK surgical training is divided into two blocks following graduation. Years 1-5 (Intern/House Officer and Senior House Officer) include a different specialty every six months; years 6-11 (Registrar) are spent in the single career specialty. Supervised training generally finishes by year 12 (when Consultant/independent practitioner status is achieved).

Please specify the structure of the post-graduate surgical training scheme in your country and please indicate qualifications/achievements that must be made before progressing to the next stage. When do the trainees specialize? *(Please indicate stage next to relevant number of years).*

| | | |
|---|---|---|
| 1 resident centrally financed | * | 11 |
| 2 resident centrally financed | * | 12 |
| 3 resident hospital financed | * | 13 |
| 4 resident hospital financed | * | 14 |
| 5 assistant surgeon | * | 15 |
| 6 assistant surgeon<br>fellowship exam | * | 16 |
| 7 specialist in surgery<br>higher surgical training | * | 17 |
| 8 specialist in surgery<br>fellowship exam in sub-specialty | * | 18 |
| 9 specialist in surgery | * | 19 |
| 10 specialist in surgery<br>can be appointed | * | 20 |

**2) Leave**

In your country, how much time is allowed for

| | |
|---|---|
| a) Vacations and national or religious (e.g. weeks per year) | 16-20 days |
| b) External training or conferences (e.g. weeks per year) | not specified |
| c) Internal educational meetings (e.g. hours per week) | not specified |
| d) Private study time (e.g. hours per week) | not specified |

**3) Assessment**

Please describe how trainees are monitored and assessed during their training in your country.

No official interim assessment during training.

**4) Hours of work**

a) When does the normal working day start and finish? (e.g. 8 am - 6 pm) — 7 30 – 15 30

b) What is the length (in hours) of the longest shift allowed? — 30 hours

c) Night working

How often are surgical trainees on duty at 9 pm? 1 night in 4-6

How often are surgical trainees on duty at 3 am? 1 night in 4-6

Does the trainee work the day after a night on duty? Yes ☒ No ☐

d) How long are surgical trainees at work for each week? (please indicate the number of hours per week) — 60?

e) Does the time include training and private study? Yes ☐ No ☐

f) What percentage of your country's surgical trainees currently conform to the Working Time Directive, including the 48-hour week?

Approximately n.a. %

**5) Team organization**

In UK hospitals a team of doctors consists of one consultant/specialist, one registrar, one senior house officer and maybe a house officer too. That team cares for 10-30 patients. Each patient is cared for only by doctors of that team.

a) How are the teams organized in your country?

A chief of services or chief of department is responsible for running the service. According to the number of beds, sub-specialties involved some of the responsibilities are given to senior consultants. Trainees are subordinates of chief of services.

b) How many consultants/specialists are responsible for each patient?

Chief of services is responsible for the professional quality of the service. Specialist however have their own responsibility. It is all the matter of mutual cooperation.

c) How many consultants/specialists supervise each trainee doctor?

Usually one. In the first two years of residency there is a tutor appointed by the regional university.

**6) Specialty cover at night**

a) At night, do surgeons cover just their own specialty or more than one surgical specialty or subspecialty?

| | | | |
|---|---|---|---|
| Year 1-5 | Own ☒ | Several ☐ | e.g.: |
| Year 6 onwards | Own ☒ | Several ☐ | e.g.: |
| Consultant/specialist | Own ☒ | Several ☐ | e.g.: |

b) Do surgical trainees cover any non-surgical specialties? Yes ☐ No ☒

c) Are emergency surgical patients admitted straight to the specialty ward or to a general admissions ward? Specialty ward ☒ Admissions ward ☐

d) In a hospital receiving emergency patients in *general surgery, vascular surgery, urology and orthopaedics*

- How many surgical doctors will be in the hospital to cover these specialties at 3 am? 3
- How many surgical doctors will be on duty from home to cover these specialties at 3 am? 2

Please go back to Question 1 and mark * which levels of doctors (including consultants) would be in the hospital at 3 am.

e) Are non-medical staff used to decrease the workload of trainee doctors in any of the following areas?

| | | | | | |
|---|---|---|---|---|---|
| Clerical Work | Yes ☒ | No ☐ | Admitting patients | Yes ☐ | No ☒ |
| Venopuncture | Yes ☒ | No ☐ | Clinics | Yes ☐ | No ☒ |
| ECGs | Yes ☒ | No ☐ | Endoscopy | Yes ☐ | No ☒ |
| Prescribing drugs | Yes ☐ | No ☒ | Catheters | Yes ☒ | No ☐ |
| First operator | Yes ☐ | No ☒ | Assistant Operator | Yes ☐ | No ☒ |

**7) Further information**

The Board would be very grateful if you could provide further information on the organization of surgical training and the service provided by junior doctors and the way in which this has been affected by the requirements of the working time directive. Please provide details of any measures that have been taken which have helped surgical training to adapt to the shorter working week (e.g. greater use of nurses to reduce junior doctors' workload).

Thank you very much for your cooperation.

The European Board of Vascular Surgery
Surgical Training and Working Time in Europe Questionnaire

| | |
|---|---|
| Name and Title | Dermot Moore |
| Country | IRELAND |
| Contact Telephone number | 00 353 1 4742410 |
| Date working time directive introduced | DD MM YYYY<br>1 / 08 / 2004 |

**1) Length of Training**

In the UK surgical training is divided into two blocks following graduation. Years 1-5 (Intern/House Officer and Senior House Officer) include a different specialty every six months; years 6-11 (Registrar) are spent in the single career specialty. Supervised training generally finishes by year 12 (when Consultant/independent practitioner status is achieved).

Please specify the structure of the post-graduate surgical training scheme in your country and please indicate qualifications/achievements that must be made before progressing to the next stage. When do the trainees specialize? *(Please indicate stage next to relevant number of years).*

| | |
|---|---|
| *1 Intern | 11 SpR Vascular |
| 2 Junior House Officer BST | 12 |
| *3 Senior House Officer BST AFRCSI = Three part exam | 13 |
| 4 Junior Registrar Clinical gap years | 14 |
| *5 Registrar Clinical gap years | 15 |
| 6 HST SpR training six years training, four clinical, last two sub speciality. Exit exam at year 12. | 16 |
| 7 SpR | 17 |
| 8 SpR | 18 |
| 9 SpR | 19 |
| 10 SpR Vascular | 20 |

**2) Leave**

In your country, how much time is allowed for

| | |
|---|---|
| a) Vacations and national or religious (e.g. weeks per year) | 6 weeks |
| b) External training or conferences (e.g. weeks per year) | 2 weeks |
| c) Internal educational meetings (e.g. hours per week) | 4 hours |
| d) Private study time (e.g. hours per week) | 2 x ½ days per week |

**3) Assessment**

Please describe how trainees are monitored and assessed during their training in your country.

Annual counseling
Trainee/Trainer forum
Individual trainers monitor trainees progress and report to the SPR training committee
Three trainers per unit

**4) Hours of work**

a) When does the normal working day start and finish? (e.g. 8 am - 6 pm) — 7.30am – 6.00pm

b) What is the length (in hours) of the longest shift allowed? — No shifts

c) Night working

How often are surgical trainees on duty at 9 pm? 1 night in 4

How often are surgical trainees on duty at 3 am? 1 night in 4

Does the trainee work the day after a night on duty? Yes ☒ No ☐

d) How long are surgical trainees at work for each week? (please indicate the number of hours per week) — 50-100 hours

e) Does the time include training and private study? Yes ☒ No ☐

f) What percentage of your country's surgical trainees currently conform to the Working Time Directive, including the 48-hour week?

Approximately 5 %

**5) Team organization**

In UK hospitals a team of doctors consists of one consultant/specialist, one registrar, one senior house officer and maybe a house officer too. That team cares for 10-30 patients. Each patient is cared for only by doctors of that team.

a) How are the teams organized in your country?

| |
|---|
| Generally the same as the U.K. |

b) How many consultants/specialists are responsible for each patient?

| |
|---|
| 1-3 |

c) How many consultants/specialists supervise each trainee doctor?

| |
|---|
| 3 |

**6) Specialty cover at night**

a) At night, do surgeons cover just their own specially or more than one surgical specialty or subspecialty?

| | | | | | | |
|---|---|---|---|---|---|---|
| Year 1-5 | Own | ☐ | Several | ☒ | e.g.:gen+vasc |
| Year 6 onwards | Own | ☐ | Several | ☒ | e.g.:gen+vasc |
| Consultant/specialist | Own | ☐ | Several | ☒ | e.g.:gen+vasc: |

b) Do surgical trainees cover any non-surgical specialties? Yes ☐ No ☒

c) Are emergency surgical patients admitted straight to the specialty ward or to a general admissions ward? Specialty ward ☒ Admissions ward ☒

d) In a hospital receiving emergency patients in *general surgery, vascular surgery, urology and orthopaedics*

- How many surgical doctors will be in the hospital to cover these specialties at 3 am? 4
- How many surgical doctors will be on duty from home to cover these specialties at 3 am? One each

Please go back to Question 1 and mark * which levels of doctors (including consultants) would be in the hospital at 3 am:LIVING IN

e) Are non-medical staff used to decrease the workload of trainee doctors in any of the following areas?

| | | | | | |
|---|---|---|---|---|---|
| Clerical Work | Yes ☐ | No ☒ | Admitting patients | Yes ☐ | No ☒ |
| Venepuncture | Yes ☒ | No ☐ | Clinics | Yes ☐ | No ☒ |
| ECGs | Yes ☒ | No ☐ | Endoscopy | Yes ☐ | No ☒ |
| Prescribing drugs | Yes ☐ | No ☒ | Catheters | Yes ☐ | No ☒ |
| First operator | Yes ☐ | No ☒ | Assistant operator | Yes ☐ | No ☒ |

**7) Further information**

The board would be very grateful if you could provide further information on the organization of surgical training and the service provided by junior doctors and the way in which this has been affected by the requirements of the working time directive. Please provide details of any measures that have been taken which have helped surgical training to adapt to the shorter working week (e.g. greater use of nurses to reduce junior doctors' workload).

Thank you very much for your cooperation.

As yet very few changes have been made and all hospital are being asked to review their current practice.

The European Board of Vascular Surgery
Surgical Training and Working Time in Europe Questionnaire

Name and Title PROF. FABRIZIO BENEDETTI-VALENTINI

Country ROME - ITALY

Contact Telephone number + 39 – 06 - 490255

Date working time directive introduced DD MM YYYY
08 / 08 / 1991

See comments numbered as circled (1)

**1) Length of Training**

In the UK surgical training is divided into two blocks following graduation. Years 1-5 (Intern/House Officer and Senior House Officer) include a different specialty every six months; years 6-11 (Registrar) are spent in the single career specialty. Supervised training generally finishes by year 12 (when Consultant/independent practitioner status is achieved).

Please specify the structure of the post-graduate surgical training scheme in your country and please indicate qualifications/achievements that must be made before progressing to the next stage. When do the trainees specialize? *(Please indicate stage next to relevant number of years).*

| | | | | |
|---|---|---|---|---|
| 1 | | 11 | | |
| 2 | | 12 | | |
| 3 | | 13 | | |
| 4 | | 14 | | |
| 5 | C C S T obtained after final exam | 15 | | (2) |
| 6 | | 16 | | |
| 7 | | 17 | | |
| 8 | | 18 | | |
| 9 | | 19 | | |
| 10 | | 20 | | |

**2) Leave**

In your country, how much time is allowed for

| | |
|---|---|
| a) Vacations and national or religious (e.g. weeks per year) | 30 days / year |
| b) External training or conferences (e.g. weeks per year) | if certified are included in working time |
| c) Internal educational meetings (e.g. hours per week) | included in working time |
| d) Private study time (e.g. hours per week) | not included<br>up to the trainee |

**3) Assessment**

Please describe how trainees are monitored and assessed during their training in your country.

They work every day with staff surgeons. Main trainer is the Chief of the Service or Division.
They are monitored and assessed by those same persons and have a final assessment each year by the Faculty of the School of Specialty.
They must pass the final assessment in order to be allowed into the following year of training and to maintain their grant (+- Euro 930 / month).

**4) Hours of work**

a) When does the normal working day start and finish? 8 – 2.30 pm (3)
(e.g. 8 am - 6 pm)

b) What is the length (in hours) of the longest shift allowed? 12 hrs

c) Night working

How often are surgical trainees on duty at 9 pm? 1 night in 7d 8 pm – 8 am

How often are surgical trainees on duty at 3 am? 1 night in 7d (4)

Does the trainee work the day after a night on duty? Yes ☒ No ☐ (5)

d) How long are surgical trainees at work for each week? 90 hrs
(please indicate the number of hours per week)

e) Does the time include training and private study? Yes ☒ No ☒

f) What percentage of your country's surgical trainees currently conform to the Working Time Directive, including the 48-hour week?

Approximately %

**Nil at least in Surgery and certainly not in Vascular Surgery**

**5) Team organization**

In UK hospitals a team of doctors consists of one consultant/specialist, one registrar, one senior house officer and maybe a house officer too. That team cares for 10-30 patients. Each patient is cared for only by doctors of that team.

a) How are the teams organized in your country?

Each service or Division (10-30 beds) has a regular staff of 4-7 (1 chief, 1-2 senior assistants, 3-4 assistants) surgeons all with CCST and experience according to ..... seniorship. The patients are cared for only by the doctors of that team.

Additionally, from 1- 6-8 trainees are working in the Service/Division according to the size of the Service/Division and the relevance of the Training Centre.

b) How many consultants/specialists are responsible for each patient?

The entire staff is responsible for all the patients. The final responsibility lies with the chief of the service and "flows downwards"

c) How many consultants/specialists supervise each trainee doctor?

At least 3: Chief of the service ; Senior Assistant, assistant

**6) Specialty cover at night**

a) At night, do surgeons cover just their own specialty or more than one surgical specialty or subspecialty?

| | | | |
|---|---|---|---|
| Year 1-5 | Own ☐ | Several ☒ | e.g.: general surgery<br>thoracic surgery<br>emergencies |
| Year 6 onwards | Own ☒ | Several ☐ | e.g.: |
| Consultant/specialist | Own ☒ | Several ☐ | e.g.: |

b) Do surgical trainees cover any non-surgical specialties? Yes ☒ No ☐
in vascular field

c) Are emergency surgical patients admitted straight to the specialty ward or to a general admissions ward?

Specialty ward ☐ Admissions ward ☒

d) In a hospital receiving emergency patients in *general surgery, vascular surgery, urology and orthopaedics*

- How many surgical doctors will be in the hospital to cover these specialties at 3 am? 6
- How many surgical doctors will be on duty from home to cover these specialties at 3 am?

Please go back to Question 1 and mark * which levels of doctors (including consultants) would be in the hospital at 3 am.

e) Are non-medical staff used to decrease the workload of trainee doctors in any of the following areas?

| | | | | | |
|---|---|---|---|---|---|
| Clerical Work | Yes ☒ | No ☐ | Admitting patients | Yes ☐ | No ☒ |
| Venepuncture | Yes ☒ | No ☐ | Clinics | Yes ☐ | No ☒ |
| ECGs * | Yes ☒ | No ☐ | Endoscopy | Yes ☐ | No ☒ |
| Prescribing drugs | Yes ☐ | No ☒ | + Catheters | Yes ☒ | No ☐ |
| First operator | Yes ☐ | No ☒ | Assistant Operator | Yes ☐ | No ☒ |

* recording not interpreting + urinary

**7) Further information**

The Board would be very grateful if you could provide further information on the organization of surgical training and the service provided by junior doctors and the way in which this has been affected by the requirements of the working time directive. Please provide details of any measures that have been taken which have helped surgical training to adapt to the shorter working week (e.g. greater use of nurses to reduce junior doctorsí workload).

Thank you very much for your cooperation.

The 48 hours directive is not yet a law in our Country.
There is a much stricter regulation (38 h/week) which has been ignored so far.
But there is a particular facet of our regulations that should be taken into account.

There trainees do not receive a salary, they receive a grant. It means that they do not have worker status, but through an admission examination they gain a scholarship granted by they Ministry of Education. Recently (1998) a Degree granted the trainees worker status; however due to financial reasons, despite walkouts and all sorts of quarrelling, it is not yet in effect so far.

**COMMENTS**

1) The European Directive 93/104/EC Nov. 23rd 1993 has not become a law in Italy as yet.
However there is a Decree (n.257 Aug. 8th 1991) of the Ministers of Education and Public Health stating that working hours for trainees are the same as for Staff Medical Personnel in Public Hospitals: 38 hours!

2) Training is focused on Vascular Surgery. There are 12 months, which can and actually are divided in two 6 months periods, of common trunk including general surgery/emergencies, thoracic and cardiac surgery.
The trainee has to sit an assessment (oral and practical, though not surgical) each year and cannot proceed to the following year if failed. The trainers do Surgical/technical assessment during the year.
Participation to scientific work and research is considered but, practically, nobody is failed this ground.

3) Theoretically at least in the surgical field

4) On duty at 9 pm is the same as 3 am since when they are on call they start at 8 pm and finish at 8 am.

5) They are not supposed to, but they do.

6) It depends on the hospital (if dealing with Training Centers they are University or Regional Hospitals).
General surgeons are on call in the hospital anywhere: 1 consultant, 1 senior assistant, 1 assistant + some trainees from general surgery or other specialities connected by a common trunk.
At least one orthopaedist is on call: an entire team is specialized hospitals or tauma centers. Urologist is usually on duty from home.
Vascular sergeons are on call inside the hospital (usually 1 senior assistant, 1 assistant, 1-2 Trainees) in some hospitals. In others they are on duty from home (more or less the same number and levels).

## The European Board of Vascular Surgery
## Surgical Training and Working Time in Europe Questionnaire

| | |
|---|---|
| Name and Title | J.H. van Bockel |
| Country | The Netherlands |
| Contact Telephone number | + 31 71 5263968 |
| Date working time directive introduced | DD MM YYYY<br>01 / 07 / 1997 |

**1) Length of Training**

In the UK surgical training is divided into two blocks following graduation. Years 1-5 (Intern/House Officer and Senior House Officer) include a different specialty every six months; years 6-11 (Registrar) are spent in the single career specialty. Supervised training generally finishes by year 12 (when Consultant/independent practitioner status is achieved).

Please specify the structure of the post-graduate surgical training scheme in your country and please indicate qualifications/achievements that must be made before progressing to the next stage. When do the trainees specialize? *(Please indicate stage next to relevant number of years).*

| | |
|---|---|
| 1 6 years of general surgery training (= consultant | |
| 2 Thereafter (postgraduate) voluntary 2 years if vascular surgery | |
| 3 (last surgical year may also be devoted to vascular or other specialty training) | |
| 4 | 14 |
| 5 | 15 |
| 6 | 16 |
| 7 | 17 |
| 8 | 18 |
| 9 | 19 |
| 10 | 20 |

**2) Leave**

In your country, how much time is allowed for

| | |
|---|---|
| a) Vacations and national or religious (e.g. weeks per year) | app. 6 weeks |
| b) External training or conferences (e.g. weeks per year) | app. 2 weeks |
| c) Internal educational meetings (e.g. hours per week) | app. 3-4 hours |
| d) Private study time (e.g. hours per week) | not included in working hours |

**3) Assessment**

Please describe how trainees are monitored and assessed during their training in your country.

Varies between hospitals

- daily meetings
- weekly meetings
- personal monitoring
- assessment of performance
- no examination except for examination (basic) within the first 2 years of training

**4) Hours of work**

a) When does the normal working day start and finish? (e.g. 8 am - 6 pm) — 7.45 am-5.30 pm

b) What is the length (in hours) of the longest shift allowed? — 13

c) Night working

How often are surgical trainees on duty at 9 pm? 1 night in 8

How often are surgical trainees on duty at 3 am? 1 night in 8

Does the trainee work the day after a night on duty? Yes ☐ No ☒

d) How long are surgical trainees at work for each week? (please indicate the number of hours per week) — 48

In practice: 53 hours (incl. on call hours)

e) Does the time include training and <u>private study</u>? Yes ☐ No ☒

f) What percentage of your countryís surgical trainees currently conform to the Working Time Directive, including the 48-hour week?

unknown: expect guess 25% Approximately 25 %

**5) Team organization**

In UK hospitals a team of doctors consists of one consultant/specialist, one registrar, one senior house officer and maybe a house officer too. That team cares for 10-30 patients. Each patient is cared for only by doctors of that team.

a) How are the teams organized in your country?

b) How many consultants/specialists are responsible for each patient?

c) How many consultants/specialists supervise each trainee doctor?

**6) Specialty cover at night**

a) At night, do surgeons cover just their own specialty or more than one surgical specialty or subspecialty?

| | | | |
|---|---|---|---|
| Year 1-5 | Own ☒ | Several ☐ | e.g.: |
| Year 6 onwards | Own ☒ | Several ☐ | e.g.: |
| Consultant/specialist | Own ☒ | Several ☐ | e.g.: |

b) Do surgical trainees cover any non-surgical specialties? Yes ☒ No sometimes

c) Are emergency surgical patients admitted straight to the specialty ward or to a general admissions ward? Specialty ward ☐ Admissions ward ☒

d) In a hospital receiving emergency patients in *general surgery, vascular surgery, urology and orthopaedics*

- How many surgical doctors will be in the hospital to cover these specialties at 3 am? 1-2
- How many surgical doctors will be on duty from home to cover these specialties at 3 am? 3-4

Please go back to Question 1 and mark * which levels of doctors (including consultants) would be in the hospital at 3 am.

e) Are non-medical staff used to decrease the workload of trainee doctors in any of the following areas?

| | | | | | |
|---|---|---|---|---|---|
| Clerical Work | Yes ☒ | No ☐ | Admitting patients | Yes ☒ | No ☐ |
| Venepuncture | Yes ☐ | No ☒ | Clinics | Yes ☐ | No ☒ |
| ECGs | Yes ☒ | No ☐ | Endoscopy | Yes ☐ | No ☒ |
| Prescribing drugs | Yes ☐ | No ☒ | Catheters | Yes ☐ | No ☒ |
| First operator | Yes ☐ | No ☒ | Assistant Operator | Yes ☐ | No ☒ |

**7) Further information**

The Board would be very grateful if you could provide further information on the organization of surgical training and the service provided by junior doctors and the way in which this has been affected by the requirements of the working time directive. Please provide details of any measures that have been taken which have helped surgical training to adapt to the shorter working week (e.g. greater use of nurses to reduce junior doctors' workload).

Thank you very much for your cooperation.

The European Board of Vascular Surgery

**Surgical Training and Working Time in Europe Questionnaire**

| | |
|---|---|
| Name and Title | Anne Karin Lindahl, MD, PhD |
| Country | Norway |
| Contact Telephone number | 47-67809693 |

Date working time directive introduced DD MM YYYY

Norway is not a member of the EU, and thus the working time directive is not applicable, We have however, had a general law against long working hours, but doctors are excempt from it on a general basis. The regular working week in Norway is 37,4 hours for daytime workers and 35 for people working shifts. □□/□□/□□□□

**1) Length of Training**

In the UK surgical training is divided into two blocks following graduation. Years 1-5 (Intern/House Officer and Senior House Officer) include a different specialty every six months; years 6-11 (Registrar) are spent in the single career specialty. Supervised training generally finishes by year 12 (when Consultant/independent practitioner status is achieved).

Please specify the structure of the post-graduate surgical training scheme in your country and please indicate qualifications/achievements that must be made before progressing to the next stage. When do the trainees specialize? *(Please indicate stage next to relevant number of years).*

1 *1,5 year of internship (6 months surgery, 6 months internal medicine, 6 months general practice). Needs a certification to pass to next level.
11
2 *General surgical practice: 5 years plus one year relevant practice from other specialty areas or research. The practice needs to be at different departments, and at least 1, 5 years at a larger hospital (University hospital or other larger hospital with approval for such training). 12
To obtain a specialty certificate as a general surgeon, a specified number of procedures needs to be performed, as well attending a certain number of theoretical courses.
3 *Vascular surgery as a branch specialty: After (or partly during) qualifying as a general surgeon, 3 years of practice in vascular surgery, of which 2 years must be in a hospital of large volume of vascular procedures. A specified list of procedures needs to be performed, as well as participation in a certain number of theoretical courses. No exams, but a committee evaluates the merits before qualification as a Vascular Surgeon is approved. 13
4 14
5 15
6 16
7 17
8 18
9 19
10 20

**2) Leave**

In your country, how much time is allowed for

| | |
|---|---|
| a) Vacations and national or religious (e.g. weeks per year) | Approx 7 (5 weeks holiday + religious days |
| b) External training or conferences (e.g. weeks per year) | Minimum of two |
| c) Internal educational meetings (e.g. hours per week) | Minimum of two hours |
| d) Private study time (e.g. hours per week) | 2-4 hours |

**3) Assessment**

Please describe how trainees are monitored and assessed during their training in your country.

Assessment is done in each individual department, where the trainee is appointed a special councillor to guide and monitor progress. A logbook of procedures is required, with type of procedure only listed (not outcome). Before final approval, this list must be confirmed and signed by the department head.

After the training is finished, the candidate sends an application to a national committee to seek his or her Specialty of Vascular Surgery Certificate.

**4) Hours of work**

a) When does the normal working day start and finish? (e.g. 8 am - 6 pm) — 7.30am – 4 pm

b) What is the length (in hours) of the longest shift allowed? — 19 hours (often violated)

c) Night working

How often are surgical trainees on duty at 9 pm? 1 night in 6-10

How often are surgical trainees on duty at 3 am? 1 night in 6-10

Does the trainee work the day after a night on duty? Yes ☐ No ☒

d) How long are surgical trainees at work for each week? (please indicate the number of hours per week) — Average 45 (paid)

e) Does the time include training and private study? Yes ☒ No ☐

f) What percentage of your country's surgical trainees currently conform to the Working Time Directive, including the 48-hour week?

Approximately 85 %

**5) Team organization**

In UK hospitals a team of doctors consists of one consultant/specialist, one registrar, one senior house officer and maybe a house officer too. That team cares for 10-30 patients. Each patient is cared for only by doctors of that team.

a) How are the teams organized in your country?

In the University hospitals and the larger training centres, the vascular surgery wards are 10-20 patients, cared for by a team of 3-7 consultants, 1-2 registrars (training for vascular surgery only) and 1-2 house officers (training for general surgery).

b) How many consultants/specialists are responsible for each patient?

Varies, but should in theory be only one main contact for the patient.

c) How many consultants/specialists supervise each trainee doctor?

On a day to day basis, all consultants supervise each trainee, depending on the different work schedules. Each candidate gets one appointed councillor who is not responsible for the practical surgical training, but for guiding the candidate in areas to develop and how to cope with surgical and relational work problems.

**6) Specialty cover at night**

a) At night, do surgeons cover just their own specialty or more than one surgical specialty or subspecialty?

| | | | |
|---|---|---|---|
| Year 1-5 | Own ☐ | Several ☒ | e.g.: gastroenterlogly, vascular surgery, urology, sometimes orthopaedics |
| Year 6 onwards | Own ☐ | Several ☒ | e.g.: |
| Consultant/specialist | Own ☒ | Several ☐ | e.g.: (most of the times, but there are exceptions) |

b) Do surgical trainees cover any non-surgical specialties? Yes ☐ No ☒

c) Are emergency surgical patients admitted straight to the specialty ward or to a general admissions ward? Specialty ward ☐ Admissions ward ☒

d) In a hospital receiving emergency patients in *general surgery, vascular surgery, urology and orthopaedics*

How many surgical doctors will be in the hospital to cover these specialties at 3 am?

1-2

How many surgical doctors will be on duty from home to cover these specialties at 3 am?

1

Please go back to Question 1 and mark * which levels of doctors (including consultants) would be in the hospital at 3 am.

e) Are non-medical staff used to decrease the workload of trainee doctors in any of the following areas? ( * indicates help from nurses or other medically trained personel)

| | | | | | |
|---|---|---|---|---|---|
| Clerical Work | Yes ☒ | No ☐ | Admitting patients | Yes ☐ | No ☒ |
| Venepuncture | Yes * | No ☐ | Clinics | Yes ☐ | No ☐ |
| ECGs | Yes * | No ☐ | Endoscopy | Yes ☐ | No ☐ |
| Prescribing drugs | Yes ☐ | No ☒ | Catheters | Yes * | No ☐ |
| First operator | Yes ☐ | No ☒ | Assistant Operator | Yes * | No ☐ |

## 7) Further information

The Board would be very grateful if you could provide further information on the organization of surgical training and the service provided by junior doctors and the way in which this has been affected by the requirements of the working time directive. Please provide details of any measures that have been taken which have helped surgical training to adapt to the shorter working week (e.g. greater use of nurses to reduce junior doctors' workload).

Thank you very much for your cooperation

In Norway we have practiced less than 48 hours a week for surgical specialty training for many years. Some feel the lack of continuity in the follow up of the patients due to the need to practice comp. time to decrease the numbers of hours worked is harmful to the training. However, it is commonly accepted that a surgeon who has been on duty all night cannot stay at work the day after, due to the quality of the work and of the training while sleep deprivated. The consultants must do more routine work, I think, than in many other countries. It also emphasizes the need for intense training with good planning of repetitive procedures during a short period of time for the candidate, to obtain a good enough surgical training qualitatively.

The European Board of Vascular Surgery
Surgical Training and Working Time in Europe Questionnaire

| | |
|---|---|
| Name and Title | J.D. Menezes M.D. |
| Country | Portugal |
| Contact Telephone number | 00351214104211 |
| Date working time directive introduced | DD MM YYYY<br>09 04 2003 |

**1) Length of Training**

In the UK surgical training is divided into two blocks following graduation. Years 1-5 (Intern/House Officer and Senior House Officer) include a different specialty every six months; years 6-11 (Registrar) are spent in the single career specialty. Supervised training generally finishes by year 12 (when Consultant/independent practitioner status is achieved).

Please specify the structure of the post-graduate surgical training scheme in your country and please indicate qualifications/achievements that must be made before progressing to the next stage. When do the trainees specialize? *(Please indicate stage next to relevant number of years).*

| | | | |
|---|---|---|---|
| 1 | Intern | 11 | |
| 2 | Examination /access to specialty | 12 | |
| 3 | | 13 | |
| 4 | Resident (years 4–9) | 14 | Examination /Consultant |
| 5 | | 15 | |
| 6 | | 16 | |
| 7 | | 17 | |
| 8 | | 18 | Examination / Chief of service (few places ) |
| 9 | | 19 | Examination / Specialist |
| 10 | | 20 | |

**2) Leave**

In your country, how much time is allowed for

| | |
|---|---|
| a) Vacations and national or religious (e.g. weeks per year) | 4 to 6 weeks |
| b) External training or conferences (e.g. weeks per year) | 2 weeks |
| c) Internal educational meetings (e.g. hours per week) | Depends on programs |
| d) Private study time (e.g. hours per week) | Not schedule |

**3) Assessment**

Please describe how trainees are monitored and assessed during their training in your country.

Continuous monitoring, plus in each year discussion of the annual report, and a theoretical and practical (clinical) examination, following the instructions of College of Angiology and Vascular Surgery (Organ of the Portuguese Medical Association.
Each year trainees have a classification (0 to 20).
After the 6 years of training there is a National Examination, (with discussion of the "logbook", theoretical and practical examination) getting another classification (0 to 20).
The final result / classification is the average of those obtained during the training plus that of the final examination.

**4) Hours of work**

a) When does the normal working day start and finish? (e.g. 8 am - 6 pm) | 8 to 17

b) What is the length (in hours) of the longest shift allowed? | 24

c) Night working

How often are surgical trainees on duty at 9 pm? 1 night in | 7

How often are surgical trainees on duty at 3 am? 1 night in | 7

Does the trainee work the day after a night on duty? Yes ☒ No ☐

d) How long are surgical trainees at work for each week? (please indicate the number of hours per week) | 42 plus extras

e) Does the time include training and private study? Yes No ☒

f) What percentage of your country's surgical trainees currently conform to the Working Time Directive, including the 48-hour week?

Approximately | 10 | %

**5) Team organization**

In UK hospitals a team of doctors consists of one consultant/specialist, one registrar, one senior house officer and maybe a house officer too. That team cares for 10-30 patients. Each patient is cared for only by doctors of that team.

a) How are the teams organized in your country?

| |
|---|
| Depends on the Unit.<br>1 to 3 Consultants, 2 to 8 senior house officers (or equivalent), 2 to 5 residents.<br>Portuguese medical staff on Public Hospitals (Head of the Unit ,with the degree of Chief of Service, Chief of Service, Consultant, Assistant (specialist-first five years ) and Residents. |

b) How many consultants/specialists are responsible for each patient?

| |
|---|
| 1 |

c) How many consultants/specialists supervise each trainee doctor?

| |
|---|
| 1 (the supervisor of the resident ) |

**6) Specialty cover at night**

a) At night, do surgeons cover just their own specialty or more than one surgical specialty or subspecialty?

| | | | | | |
|---|---|---|---|---|---|
| Year 1-4 | Own | ☐ | Several | ☒ | e.g.☹General Surgery |
| Year 6 onwards | Own | ☒ | Several | ☐ | e.g.: |
| Consultant/specialist | Own | ☒ | Several | ☐ | e.g.: |

b) Do surgical trainees cover any non-surgical specialties? Yes ☐ No ☒

c) Are emergency surgical patients admitted straight to the specialty ward or to a general admissions ward? Specialty ward ☐ Admissions ward ☒

d) In a hospital receiving emergency patients in *general surgery, vascular surgery, urology and orthopaedics*

- How many surgical doctors will be in the hospital to cover these specialties at 3 am? > 6
- How many surgical doctors will be on duty from home to cover these specialties at 3 am? 2 /3

Please go back to Question 1 and mark * which levels of doctors (including consultants) would be in the hospital at 3 am.

e) Are non-medical staff used to decrease the workload of trainee doctors in any of the following areas?

| | | | | | |
|---|---|---|---|---|---|
| Clerical Work | Yes ☐ | No ☐ | Admitting patients | **Yes** ☒ | No ☐ |
| Venepuncture | Yes ☒ | No ☐ | Clinics | Yes ☐ | **No** ☒ |
| ECGs | **Yes** ☒ | No ☐ | Endoscopy | Yes ☐ | **No** ☒ |
| Prescribing drugs | Yes ☐ | **No** ☒ | Catheters | Yes ☐ | **No** ☒ |
| First operator | Yes ☐ | No ☐ | Assistant Operator | Yes ☐ | No ☐ |

**7) Further information**

The problem of paying extra-hours in public Hospitals is actually a major concern of the administrations.
So, it is necessary to find solutions to solve it, perhaps with reorganization of the Urgencies.
The "48 hours-week" does not seemed to be a major concern in this coutrry where Vascular Surgery is a recognized monospeciality.

The European Board of Vascular Surgery
Surgical Training and Working Time in Europe Questionnaire

| | |
|---|---|
| Name and Title | Vladimir SEFRANEK, MD, |
| Country | Slovak Republic |
| Contact Telephone number | +421259320650 |
| Date working time directive introduced | DD MM YYYY<br>01 / 03 / 2003 |

**1) Length of Training**

In the UK surgical training is divided into two blocks following graduation. Years 1-5 (Intern/House Officer and Senior House Officer) include a different specialty every six months; years 6-11 (Registrar) are spent in the single career specialty. Supervised training generally finishes by year 12 (when Consultant/independent practitioner status is achieved).

Please specify the structure of the post-graduate surgical training scheme in your country and please indicate qualifications/achievements that must be made before progressing to the next stage. When do the trainees specialize? *(Please indicate stage next to relevant number of years).*

| | | | |
|---|---|---|---|
| 1 | house officer | 11 | |
| 2 | main trunk | 12 | |
| 3 | main trunk | 13 | |
| 4 | main trunk | 14 | |
| 5 | vascular surg. | 15 | |
| 6 | vascular surg. | 16 | |
| 7 | vascular surg. | 17 | |
| 8 | vascular surg. | 18 | |
| 9 | | 19 | |
| 10 | | 20 | |

**2) Leave**

In your country, how much time is allowed for

| | |
|---|---|
| a) Vacations and national or religious (e.g. weeks per year) | 7 weeks |
| b) External training or conferences (e.g. weeks per year) | 1 week |
| c) Internal educational meetings (e.g. hours per week) | 3 hours |
| d) Private study time (e.g. hours per week) | not allowed |

**3) Assessment**

Please describe how trainees are monitored and assessed during their training in your country.

Specialization in vascular surgery in Slovakia has been implemented in a centralized institution „Slovak Healthcare University" and its Department for Vasculars Surgery. Every applicant of the specialization and trainee process has to fulfill some basic requirements: specialization in surgery, opportunity to perform active vascular surgery in the home department and sufficient numbers of major vascular reconstructions personally operated on by the applicant. All trainees have to stay minimally one year in accredited departments of vascular surgery in Slovakia/abroad before accepting him/her to the exam. During this time they have to take part in consultations and seminars. Every trainee has got his personal tutor. Tutors have to monitor and check the individual training level of each trainee.

**4) Hours of work**

a) When does the normal working day start and finish? (e.g. 8 am - 6 pm) — 7 a.m. - 3 p.m.

b) What is the length (in hours) of the longest shift allowed? — 24 hours

c) Night working

How often are surgical trainees on duty at 9 pm? 1 night in week

How often are surgical trainees on duty at 3 am? 1 night in week

Does the trainee work the day after a night on duty? Yes ☒

d) How long are surgical trainees at work for each week? (please indicate the number of hours per week) — 58

e) Does the time include training and private study? No ☒

f) What percentage of your country's surgical trainees currently conform to the Working Time Directive, including the 48-hour week?

Approximately 100 %

**5) Team organization**

In UK hospitals a team of doctors consists of one consultant/specialist, one registrar, one senior house officer and maybe a house officer too. That team cares for 10-30 patients. Each patient is cared for only by doctors of that team.

a) How are the teams organized in your country?

In Slovakia we do not have any special type of team organization – there are fixed working places in each institution without exact determining of the level of training or specialization. It is the role of the chief to monitor the training process of his doctors.

b) How many consultants/specialists are responsible for each patient?

2

c) How many consultants/specialists supervise each trainee doctor?

1

**6) Specialty cover at night**

a) At night, do surgeons cover just their own specialty or more than one surgical specialty or subspecialty?

| | | | |
|---|---|---|---|
| Year 1-5 | Own ☐ | Several ☒ | e.g.: main trunk |
| Year 6 onwards | Own ☒ | Several ☐ | e.g.: |
| Consultant/specialist | Own ☒ | Several ☐ | e.g.: |

b) Do surgical trainees cover any non-surgical specialties? Yes ☐ No ☒

c) Are emergency surgical patients admitted straight to the specialty ward or to a general admissions ward? Specialty ward ☒ Admissions ward ☐

d) In a hospital receiving emergency patients in *general surgery, vascular surgery, urology and orthopaedics*

- How many surgical doctors will be in the hospital to cover these specialties at 3 am? 1 (surgeons/consultants)
- How many surgical doctors will be on duty from home to cover these specialties at 3 am? 3

Please go back to Question 1 and mark * which levels of doctors (including consultants) would be in the hospital at 3 am.

e) Are non-medical staff used to decrease the workload of trainee doctors in any of the following areas?

| | | | | | |
|---|---|---|---|---|---|
| Clerical Work | Yes ☐ | No ☒ | Admitting patients | Yes ☐ | No ☒ |
| Venepuncture | Yes ☒ | No ☐ | Clinics | Yes ☐ | No ☒ |
| ECGs | Yes ☒ | No ☐ | Endoscopy | Yes ☐ | No ☒ |
| Prescribing drugs | Yes ☐ | No ☒ | Catheters | Yes ☐ | No ☒ |
| First operator | Yes ☐ | No ☒ | Assistant Operator | Yes ☐ | No ☒ |

**7) Further information**

The Board would be very grateful if you could provide further information on the organization of surgical training and the service provided by junior doctors and the way in which this has been affected by the requirements of the working time directive. Please provide details of any measures that have been taken which have helped surgical training to adapt to the shorter working week (e.g. greater use of nurses to reduce junior doctors' workload).

Thank you very much for your cooperation.

| The European Board of Vascular Surgery<br>Surgical Training and Working Time in Europe Questionnaire | |
|---|---|
| Name and Title | Marc Cairols & Jordi Maeso Lebrún |
| Country | Spain |
| Contact Telephone number | +34 93 260 76 65 (M Cairols) |
| Date working time directive introduced | Not fully introduced yet |

**1) Length of Training**

In the UK surgical training is divided into two blocks following graduation. Years 1-5 (Intern/House Officer and Senior House Officer) include a different specialty every six months; years 6-11 (Registrar) are spent in the single career specialty. Supervised training generally finishes by year 12 (when Consultant/independent practitioner status is achieved).

Please specify the structure of the post-graduate surgical training scheme in your country and please indicate qualifications/achievements that must be made before progressing to the next stage. When do the trainees specialize? *(Please indicate stage next to relevant number of years).*

**TRAINING PROGRAMME (5 years)**

1 General Surgery

2 Intensive Care Unit for 2 months and Vascular Surgery for 9 months

3 Cardiothoracic Surgery (4 m) and Different Specialties (3 m)
vascular Surgery for the rest of the year

4 Interventional radiology (5 m) and Vascular Surgery

5 Vascular Surgery

After this period of time the Residents have the National Diploma that allows them to opt for a job in a Hospital. The Diploma in Angiologia y Cirugia Vascular is mandatory to act as a Vascular Surgeon.
During a period of few years is considered as Junior Staff (Medico Adjunto)
The access to a top post depends on the possibilities different hospital have to offer.

**2) Leave**

In your country, how much time is allowed for

| | |
|---|---|
| a) Vacations and national or religious (e.g. weeks per year) | 4 weeks per year |
| b) External training or conferences (e.g. weeks per year) | According to needs. No limits |
| c) Internal educational meetings (e.g. hours per week) | Not regulated |
| d) Private study time (e.g. hours per week) | Not regulated |

**3) Assessment**

Please describe how trainees are monitored and assessed during their training in your country.

The Teaching Committee is in charge of monitoring the progress for all residents. Each department of Vascular Surgery has its own tutor who control the number of procedures the resident is allowed to carry out according to his merits and capabilities.
Every year there a final evaluation made by the Hospital Teaching Committee.
Only accredited services are allowed to have resident in training and only through this period of training is possible to obtain the Diploma in Angiology and Vascular Surgery.
There is no final examination but a global evaluation. The chief of the service has to back up the Committee's decision.

**4) Hours of work**

a) When does the normal working day start and finish? (e.g. 8 am - 6 pm) — 8am-5pm

b) What is the length (in hours) of the longest shift allowed? — 24 h

c) Night working

How often are surgical trainees on duty at 9 pm? 1 night in — 4

How often are surgical trainees on duty at 3 am? 1 night in — 

Does the trainee work the day after a night on duty? Yes ☒ No ☐

d) How long are surgical trainees at work for each week? (please indicate the number of hours per week) — 52 h

e) Does the time include training and private study? Yes No ☒

f) What percentage of your country's surgical trainees currently conform to the Working Time Directive, including the 48-hour week?

Approximately ? %

**5) Team organization**

In UK hospitals a team of doctors consists of one consultant/specialist, one registrar, one senior house officer and maybe a house officer too. That team cares for 10-30 patients. Each patient is cared for only by doctors of that team.

a) How are the teams organized in your country?

The teaching services consist by and large (minimum):

1. Chief of Section (Consultant)
2. 1 Chief of Section (bigger departments 2)
3. 4 staff (medico Adjunto) bigger departments 6
4. There is a vascular lab under the direction of the Chief of Service

We take care exclusively of vascular patients (20-40 patients).
On duty calls are limited to younger staff (under 50 years) therefore most services have to ask for external ex-trainees for fulfilling all emergencies.
My department is divided into two team (4 each) with assigned patients and on duty rota.

b) How many consultants/specialists are responsible for each patient?

The Chief of Service is responsible for all patients.
However each patient is under the care of a team

c) How many consultants/specialists supervise each trainee doctor?

There is one resident per year therefore each chief of service has 5 residents to supervise.

**6) Specialty cover at night**

a) At night, do surgeons cover just their own specialty or more than one surgical specialty or subspecialty?

| | | | |
|---|---|---|---|
| Year 1-5 | Own ☒ | Several ☒ | e.g.: General Surgery |
| Year 6 onwards | Own ☒ | Several ☐ | e.g.: |
| Consultant/specialist | Own ☒ | Several ☐ | e.g.: |

b) Do surgical trainees cover any non-surgical specialties? Yes ☐ No ☒

c) Are emergency surgical patients admitted straight to the speciality ward or to a general admissions ward? Speciality ward ☒ Admissions ward ☐

d) In a hospital receiving emergency patients in *general surgery, vascular surgery, urology and orthopaedics*.

- How many surgical doctors will be in the hospital to cover these specialties at 3 am? I cannot see the interest in
- How many surgical doctors will be on duty from home to cover these specialties at 3 am? I do not know

Please go back to Question 1 and mark * which levels of doctors (including consultants) would be in the hospital at 3 am.

There is one doctor on duty at the hospital (the resident) and another doctor (staff) at home just for vascular emergencies.

e) Are non-medical staff used to decrease the workload of trainee doctors in any of the following areas?

| | | | | | |
|---|---|---|---|---|---|
| Clerical Work | Yes ☐ | No ☒ | Admitting patients | Yes ☐ | No ☒ |
| Venepuncture | Yes ☐ | No ☒ | Clinics | Yes ☐ | No ☒ |
| ECGs | Yes ☒ | No ☐ | Endoscopy | Yes ☐ | No ☒ |
| Prescribing drugs | Yes ☐ | No ☒ | Catheters | Yes ☐ | No ☒ |
| First operator | Yes ☐ | No ☒ | Assistant Operator | Yes ☒ | No ☐ |

**7) Further information**

The Board would be very grateful if you could provide further information on the organization of surgical training and the service provided by junior doctors and the way in which this has been affected by the requirements of the working time directive. Please provide details of any measures that have been taken which have helped surgical training to adapt to the shorter working week (e.g. greater use of nurses to reduce junior doctors' workload).

Thank you very much for your cooperation.

-----------------------------

*As stated, the directive is not fully implemented therefore no special measures have been taken. Just reducing the number of on call duties by allowing external people to help and the duty begins rather than at 8 am at 5 pm Nevertheless as the resident is in the hospital the measure is more legal than practical.*
*As a matter of fact this is still a problem unresolved in my hospital (M Cairols).*

The European Board of Vascular Surgery
Surgical Training and Working Time in Europe Questionnaire

| | |
|---|---|
| Name and Title | Professor Lars Norgren |
| Country | Sweden |
| Contact Telephone number | +46 70 5473259 |
| Date working time directive introduced | DD MM YYYY<br>☐☐ / ☐☐ / ☐☐☐☐ |

**1) Length of Training**

In the UK surgical training is divided into two blocks following graduation. Years 1-5 (Intern/House Officer and Senior House Officer) include a different specialty every six months; years 6-11 (Registrar) are spent in the single career specialty. Supervised training generally finishes by year 12 (when Consultant/independent practitioner status is achieved).

Please specify the structure of the post-graduate surgical training scheme in your country and please indicate qualifications/achievements that must be made before progressing to the next stage. When do the trainees specialize? *(Please indicate stage next to relevant number of years).*

| | |
|---|---|
| 1 Basically 5 y General Surgery | 11 |
| 2 e.g. 2 y General Surgery | 12 |
| 3 e.g. 3 y Vascular Surgery (combined with General Surgery) | |
| 4 Further 4-6 m in e.g. Urology, Anesthesiology etc. | |
| 5 No definite time point to become "Consultant" "Specialist" at 5,5 years | |
| 6 | 16 |
| 7 | 17 |
| 8 | 18 |
| 9 | 19 |
| 10 | 20 |

**2) Leave**

In your country, how much time is allowed for

| | |
|---|---|
| a) Vacations and national or religious (e.g. weeks per year) | About 6 weeks |
| b) External training or conferences (e.g. weeks per year) | 2-4 weeks |
| c) Internal educational meetings (e.g. hours per week) | 2-4 h/week |
| d) Private study time (e.g. hours per week) | Usually not in schedule |

**3) Assessment**

Please describe how trainees are monitored and assessed during their training in your country.

One responsible tutor
"All" consultants have the responsibility to guide trainees
Trainee first operator, assisted by consultant
Scientific discussions
M&M conferences by the trainee
Head of department assesses the full specialisation

**4) Hours of work**

a) When does the normal working day start and finish? (e.g. 8 am - 6 pm) — 7.30 – 17.00

b) What is the length (in hours) of the longest shift allowed? — 7.30 – 7.30 (when on duty)

c) Night working

How often are surgical trainees on duty at 9 pm? 1 night in ~ week

How often are surgical trainees on duty at 3 am? 1 night in ~ week

Does the trainee work the day after a night on duty? Yes ☐ No ☒

d) How long are surgical trainees at work for each week? (please indicate the number of hours per week) — 40+ duties

e) Does the time include training (and private study)? Yes ☒ No ☐

f) What percentage of your country's surgical trainees currently conform to the Working Time Directive, including the 48-hour week?

Approximately nobody %

**5) Team organization**

In UK hospitals a team of doctors consists of one consultant/specialist, one registrar, one senior house officer and maybe a house officer too. That team cares for 10-30 patients. Each patient is cared for only by doctors of that team.

a) How are the teams organized in your country?

| |
|---|
| Consultant – head of Section (eg. Vascular)<br>Consultants, senior registrars 2-4<br>House officer ( trainee) 1-2 |

b) How many consultants/specialists are responsible for each patient?

| |
|---|
| One |

c) How many consultants/specialists supervise each trainee doctor?

| |
|---|
| One or more |

**6) Specialty cover at night**

a) At night, do surgeons cover just their own specialty or more than one surgical specialty or subspecialty? Great variation!

| | | | |
|---|---|---|---|
| Year 1-5 | Own ☒ | Several ☐ | e.g.: Some hospitals + |
| Year 6 onwards | Own ☒ | Several ☐ | e.g.: orthopedics etc |
| Consultant/specialist | Own ☒ | Several ☐ | e.g.: -“- only as above |

b) Do surgical trainees cover any non-surgical specialties? Yes ☒ No ☐

c) Are emergency surgical patients admitted straight to the specialty ward or to a general admissions ward? Specialty ward ☐ Admissions ward ☒

Variations!

d) In a hospital receiving emergency patients in *general surgery, vascular surgery, urology and orthopaedics*

- How many surgical doctors will be in the hospital to cover these specialties at 3 am? 1-4 (great variation due to hospital type
- How many surgical doctors will be on duty from home to cover these specialtics at 3 am? 4 (3)

Please go back to Question 1 and mark * which levels of doctors (including consultants) would be in the hospital at 3 am.
? Done by nurses and aids

e) Are <u>non-medical</u> staff used to decrease the workload of trainee doctors in any of the following areas?

| | | | | | |
|---|---|---|---|---|---|
| Clerical Work | Yes ☒ | No ☐ | Admitting patients | Yes ☒ | No ☐ |
| Venepuncture | Yes ☒ | No ☐ | Clinics | Yes ☐ | No ☒ |
| ECGs | Yes ☒ | No ☐ | Endoscopy | Yes ☐ | No ☒ |
| Prescribing drugs | Yes ☐ | No ☒ | Catheters | Yes ☒ | No ☐ |
| First operator | Yes ☐ | No ☒ | Assistant Operator | Yes ☐ | No ☒ |

**7) Further information**

The Board would be very grateful if you could provide further information on the organization of surgical training and the service provided by junior doctors and the way in which this has been affected by the requirements of the working time directive. Please provide details of any measures that have been taken which have helped surgical training to adapt to the shorter working week (e.g. greater use of nurses to reduce junior doctors' workload).

Thank you very much for your cooperation.

So far no attempts

**Annexes**

# Guidelines for CME Activities Accredited by the EBVS

J.H. van Bockel, D. Bergqvist, C.D. Liapis, D. Palombo, J.H.N. Wolfe

The Committee for Continuing Medical Education of the European Board of Vascular Surgery (EBVS) of the Union Européenne des Médecins Spécialistes (UEMS), The Netherlands

Eur J Vasc Endovasc Surg 27, 534–536 (2004)

Author Keywords: Guidelines; CME; Accredited; EBVS; UEMS

Corresponding author:

J. Hajo van Bockel, M.D.
Department of Vascular Surgery
Leiden University Medical Center
PO Box 9600, 2300 RC Leiden
The Netherlands

## Introduction

Continuing medical education (CME) can be defined as "educational activities that serve to maintain, develop, or increase the knowledge, skills and professional performance (and) relationships used by a physician to provide services for patients, the public, or the profession" [1]. It is a professional responsibility for all practicing physicians, and it has become increasingly important in a fast-moving medical world.

Many CME activities are organized on a national level. For CME organized on a European level, the European Board of Vascular Surgery of the Union Européenne des Médecins Spécialistes (UEMS) has accepted a responsibility concerning the quality of CME activities. It is important to realize that the EBVS is not a provider of Continuing Medical Education (CME), but must be seen as an independent authority that by its activities may assist as a clearinghouse for CME credits from a European to a national level. The EBVS has proposed accreditation for European Vascular CME activities since 1999 [2]. The CME Committee has been very active and accredits many quality European vascular meetings each year according to simple published criteria. Criteria for CME initially focused on major meetings in order to ensure that our criteria were reliable. CME activities have now been extended to technical skills workshops, again with specific and transparent criteria.

Why are guidelines necessary? Traditionally, the pharmaceutical and medical device manufacturers have generously supported CME for physicians. Without industrial support, the quality of many activities would have been reduced and some activities would have been cancelled. During the last decade, physicians, editorial boards of scientific journals and authorities have increasingly scrutinised the role of industry supporting these activities [3,4,5]. The basis for the concern that scientific activities may be used for promotional activities without clearly identifying these activities. In 1993, Mannick reported on the 'scientific symposium' grafted onto the national meetings. For many of these, both the program and the speakers are both picked and sponsored by a company. Under these circumstances, an unbiased presentation is difficult to attain [6]. It is clear that a conflict of interest may easily occur if organizers of CME activities need the support of the industry. In fact, travel funds, honoraria for nominal consultancies, free lunches, elegant dinners accompanied by product demonstrations and guest lectures with favourable views of the sponsors' products all threaten our integrity [7]. Fortunately, both CME providers and the industry have recognized this issue and both are keen to resolve the problem.

The CME Committee of the European Board of Vascular Surgery has discussed this issue at length and believes that for both CME providers and industry, as well as for participants of CME activities, it would be helpful to provide clear and objective guidelines describing the relationship between the various parties. These guidelines are meant to stimulate a healthy and clear relationship between organizers of CME activities and the industry. The EBVS of the UEMS approved these guidelines on 3rd September 2003 in Dublin. The guidelines are published on the Web site of the EBVS and will be handed to both CME providers and the industry. For practical purposes, the guidelines have been subdivided in those for providers of CME activities, speakers and faculty and industrial sponsors. The guidelines will be evaluated regularly and comments are encouraged.

# 1. Guidelines for CME Activities accredited by the European Board of Vascular Surgery

## 1.1. Introduction

Continual Medical Education (CME) consists of educational activities that serve to maintain, develop or increase the knowledge, skills and/or professional performance of a physician. CME is provided by CME providers by means of organizing conferences, workshops, etc., and is an important element of Continuing Physician Professional Development (CCPD). Providers of CME are responsible for the provision of objective, balanced and scientifically rigorous information. CME should not be biased.

The relationship between the provision of educational activities and industrial support is essential and acknowledged with gratitude. Subsidies to underwrite the costs of CME activities can contribute to the improvement of those activities and help reduce the costs of the activity for the participants. However, financial support should never influence the content and quality of the scientific programme. Therefore, financial support from the industry should come in the form of an educational grant with grateful acknowledgement. The need for financial (industrial) support may generate a conflict of interest for the provider of CME or the faculty. To prevent such a conflict of interest, the European Board of Vascular Surgery has established the following guidelines to assist both parties.

# 2. Guidelines

## 2.1. For Organizers of CME Activities

- Physicians involved in providing CME activities should ensure that the program is balanced.
- Physicians who serve as presenters, moderators or other faculty at CME conferences should ensure that research findings and therapeutic recommendations are based upon scientifically accurate, up-to-date information and are presented in a balanced, objective manner.
- All conflicts of interest or biases, such as a financial connection to a particular commercial company or product, should be disclosed by faculty members to the audience in the programme and/or at the beginning of a presentation.
- A direct financial relationship between speakers and industry should be discouraged. Speakers and faculty should not accept direct subsidies from industry to pay for the costs of travel, lodging or other personal expenses. Costs should be reimbursed by the organizer/provider of the CME activities.
- The scientific programme committee is responsible for moderators, presenters and other faculty and welcomes suggestions from those companies that have been generous enough to support the programme. Clearly, the responsibility for the moderators, presenters and other faculty lies with the scientific committee.
- Non-CME activities, i.e. primarily promotional seminars, should be clearly identified as such in the programme.

### 2.2. For Speakers and other Faculty

- Speakers and other faculty involved in providing CME activities should present a broad range of scientifically supportable viewpoints related to the topics.
- Speakers and other faculty who present, chair or moderate at CME conferences should ensure that research findings and therapeutic recommendations are based on scientifically accurate, up-to-date information and are presented in a balanced, objective manner.
- All conflicts of interest should be disclosed by faculty members to the audience in the programme and/or at the beginning of a presentation.
- A direct financial relationship between speakers or other faculty and industry should be discouraged. Speakers and faculty should not accept direct subsidies from industry to pay for the costs of travel, lodging or other personal expenses. Costs should be reimbursed by the organizer/provider of the CME activities.
- Non-CME activities, i.e. primarily promotional seminars, should be clearly identified as such in the programme.

### 2.3. For Industrial Sponsors

- Financial support of CME activities is greatly appreciated by the organizers of CME activities and it is gratefully recognized that these activities would not be viable without industrial sponsorship. The support should be provided by educational grants to the organizers of the CME activities.
- A direct financial relationship between speakers or other faculty and industry should be discouraged. Speakers and faculty should not offer direct subsidies from industry to pay for the costs of travel, lodging or other personal expenses. Costs should be reimbursed by the organizer/provider of the CME activities.
- The scientific programme committee is responsible for moderators, presenters and other faculty. Suggestions from those companies that have been generous enough to support the programme are welcome. Clearly, the responsibility for the moderators, presenters and other faculty lies with the scientific committee.
- CME symposia supported by a sponsor should be fully acknowledged in the appropriate section of the programme. However, a company name in the title of the symposium unintentionally suggests a promotional relationship. For this reason, sponsor names should not be included in the title of the CME symposium.
- Non-CME activities, i.e. primarily promotional seminars, should be clearly identified in the programme.

## References

[1] AMA PRA Information Booklet for Physicians V3.0. (http://www.ama-assn.org/ama/pub/category/2923.html).
[2] J.H. Wolfe, European CME. Eur. J. Vasc. Endovasc. Surg. 18 (4) (1999) 277–279.
[3] L. Tritsmans, P. Briscoe, P. Lemmens, G.V. Bussche, Pharmaceutical company trials and the integrity of medical research. Lancet 347 (9015) (1996) 1628–1629.
[4] E. Wager, How to dance with porcupines: rules and guidelines on doctors' relations with drug companies. BMJ 326 (7400) (2003) 1196–1198.
[5] K. Abbasi, R. Smith, No more free lunches. BMJ 326 (7400) (2003) 1155–1156.
[6] J.A. Mannick, Vascular surgeons—are they for sale? J. Vasc. Surg. 17 (2) (1993) 245–248.
[7] J.W. Jones, L.B. McCullough, Surgeon–industry relationships: ethically responsible management of conflicts of interest. J. Vasc. Surg. 35 (4) (2002) 825–826.

# EVCME APPROVED CONGRESSES IN 2002

| Application # | Congress title | Country | Date of Congress | Submission date | CME Points Requested | CME Points Awarded | Approval date | Evaluations received on |
|---|---|---|---|---|---|---|---|---|
| 1 | Ajaccio Meeting | France | 16–19 Jun 02 | 15.01.02 | 20h45 | 16 | 26.04.02 | 28.06.02 |
| 2 | Charing Cross Symposium London | UK | 08–09 Apr 02 | 15.01.02 | 17 | 17 | 17.01.02 | 04.07.02 |
| 3 | Pontresina Workshop | Switzerland | 02–05 Feb 02 | 04.01.02 | – | 18 | 21.01.02 | 04.03.02 |
| 4 | Paphos Summit Conference | Cyprus | 22–26 May 02 | 04.03.02 | 21 | 17 | 28.03.02 | 20.06.02 |
| 5 | ESCVS Congress Helsinki | Finland | 28 Jun–1 Jul 02 | 23.04.02 | 20 | 19 | 21.05.02 | 10.08.02 |
| 6 | Femoro-Distal Course London | UK | 29–30 May 02 | 17.04.02 | 13 | 13 | 10.05.02 | 09.07.02 |
| 7 | SAVS Course Trondheim | Norway | 06–07 Jun 02 | 06.05.02 | 7.5 | 8 | 23.05.02 | |
| 8 | Endovascular Treatment Course Milan | Italy | 16–17 Oct 02 | 16.05.02 | 15 | 15 | 12.07.02 | 20.11.03 |
| 9 | ESVS 2002 Meeting Istanbul | Turkey | 26–29 Sep 2002 | 19.06.02 | 26 | 26 | 28.06.02 | 16.12.02 |
| 10 | Bringing Basic Science into Clinical Practice Stockholm | Sweden | 30 Jan–1 Feb 03 | 19.06.02 | 12 | 12 | 07.08.02 | |
| 11 | SICVE 2nd Nat Congress (European Session Cagliari | Italy | 26 Oct–02 | 31.07.02 | 3 | 3 | 28.08.02 | 10.12.02 |
| 12 | Controversies and Update in Vasc and Cardiovasc Surg Paris | France | 24–25 Jan 03 | 27.08.02 | 11,5 | 12 | 30.09.02 | 06.06.03 |
| 13 | XI Int Meeting in Ang and Vasc Surgery Lisbon | Portugal | 13–14 Dec 02 | 05.11.02 | 10 | 10 | 11.11.02 | |
| 14 | Selected Topics in Aortic Surgery Rome | Italy | 16–18 Jan 03 | 27.11.02 | 18 | 10 | 10.12.02 | 17.04.03 |

# EVCME APPROVED CONGRESSES IN 2003

| Application # | Congress title | Country | Date of Congress | Submission date | CME Points Requested | CME Points Awarded | Approval date | Evaluations received on |
|---|---|---|---|---|---|---|---|---|
| 1 | IV Int Symp on Endovasc Therapeutics, Barcelona | Spain | 7–8 Mar 03 | 02.01.03 | 15 | 14 | 10.01.03 | 02.07.03 |
| 2 | Pontresina Workshop | Switzerland | 24–26 Jan 03 | 03.01.03 | 13 | 13 | 15.01.03 | 21.07.03 |
| 3 | Charing Cross | UK | 12–15 Apr 03 | 09.01.03 | 24,5 | 19 | 17.02.03 | 21.03.03 |
| 4 | Aorto-Iliac Course Strasbourg | France | 13–15 Feb 03 | 15.01.03 | 21 | 12 | 10.02.03 | 22.04.03 |
| 5 | Aorto-Iliac Course Strasbourg | France | 25–27 Sep 03 | 15.01.03 | 21 | 21 | 07.05.03 | 20.11.03 |
| 6 | EVC 2003 Marseilles | France | 13–15 Mar 03 | 30.01.03 | 21 | 12 | 07.03.03 | 30.06.03 |
| 7 | MEET 2003 Marseilles | France | 26–28 Jun 03 | 31.01.03 | 17 | 17 | 10.04.03 | 16.02.04 |
| 8 | IVEC Milan | Italy | 2–3 Oct 2003 | 11.04.03 | 16h40m | 17 | 12.05.03 | 24.02.04 |
| 9 | Ajaccio Corsica | France | 22–25 Jun 03 | 10.05.03 | 16h45m | 16 | 13.06.03 | 21.07.03 |
| 10 | ESVS Dublin | Ireland | 5–7 Sept 03 | 10.06.03 | 24 | 24 | 24.06.03 | 04.04.04 |
| 11 | Baltic Vascular 2003 Tallin | Estonia | 25–28 Sep 03 | 15.07.03 | 10 | 11 | 27.08.03 | 06.11.03 |
| 12 | AAA Screening Viborg | Denmark | 24 Oct 2003 | 10.07.03 | 5h30m | 6 | 02.10.03 | 15.11.03 |
| 13 | Technovasc Andorra | Spain | 11–13 Dec 03 | 02.08.03 | 12 hrs | 8.40 hrs | 14.11.03 | 20.01.04 |
| 14 | Controversies and Updates Paris | France | 23–24 Jan 04 | 10.11.03 | 12 hrs | 11 hrs | 05.12.03 | Pending completed forms |

Union Européenne de Médecins Spécialistes

**Division of Vascular Surgery**

Associated with the Specialist Section Surgery

&

**European Board of Vascular Surgery**

Associated with the European Board of Surgery

## EVCME COMMITTEE:

(European Vascular Continuing Medical Education)

Chairman: J Hajo van Bockel

Members: D Bergqvist, C D Liapis, D Palombo, J H N Wolfe

## CONGRESS:

## PROGRAMME EVALUATION FORM

Please take a few minutes to give us your opinion of this conference. Your comments will be useful in planning future meetings.

***Note:** apart from the title and names of the congress organizers which should be entered above (top righthand corner), the format of this form should not be altered.*

1. Please indicate your primary reason for attending the conference (one √ only).

| | |
|---|---|
| a) | First-time introduction to main topic |
| b) | Update overall knowledge about vascular surgery |
| c) | Learn more about one particular technique - which one? |
| d) | Obtain CME credits |
| e) | Other |

2. How well did the Congress programme do in fulfilling this goal?

| a) Excellent | b) Good | c) Fair | d) Poor |
|---|---|---|---|
| | | | |

3. Evaluate then rate the following elements of this meeting in fulfilling your goal.

| | Excellent | Good | Fair | Poor |
|---|---|---|---|---|
| a) Abstracts | | | | |
| b) Meeting with faculty | | | | |
| c) Demonstrations | | | | |
| d) Discussion periods | | | | |
| e) Exhibits | | | | |
| f) Lectures by faculty | | | | |
| g) Presentations by non faculty | | | | |
| h) Programme book | | | | |
| i) Satellite symposia | | | | |

4. Please rate how relevant each of these educational needs are to you.

| | Extremely Important | Important | Somewhat Important | Not Relevant |
|---|---|---|---|---|
| a) Examine new diagnostic modes | | | | |
| b) Examine new therapeutic potential | | | | |
| c) Learn about new devices | | | | |
| d) Learn about endoluminal grafts | | | | |
| e) Receive hands-on training | | | | |
| f) Classical Surgical techniques | | | | |
| g) Other | | | | |

5. How important are the following topics to your practice.

| | Extremely Important | Important | Somewhat Important | Not Relevant |
|---|---|---|---|---|
| a) Diagnostic investigation | | | | |
| b) Risk factor management | | | | |
| c) Evidence-based practice | | | | |
| d) Experimental studies | | | | |
| e) Drug therapy | | | | |
| f) Classical Surgical treatment | | | | |
| g) Endovascular treatment | | | | |

6. Please rate the following items.

| | Excellent | Good | Fair | Poor |
|---|---|---|---|---|
| a) Organization of the programme | | | | |
| b) Overall rating of Congress | | | | |
| c) Hotel accommodation/facilities | | | | |
| d) Prices | | | | |
| e) Meeting facilities | | | | |
| f) Congress staff | | | | |

7. Please rate:

| | Excellent | Acceptable | Poor |
|---|---|---|---|
| a) Information about potential conflicts of interest by chairman / presenter / programme | | | |
| b) Balanced views presented during the Congress | | | |
| c) Information free of commercial bias during the scientific sessions | | | |

8. Please give a summary of the information you received which will be useful in your practice.
Please continue overleaf if necessary

9. Further comments (please continue overleaf if necessary)

EVCME COMMITTEE

**Participants should leave this form with the organizers on collection of their certificate of attendance before leaving the auditorium.**

C D Liapis, MD FACS FRCS, Secretary General
U E M S Division and Board of Vascular Surgery, Secretariat: c/o Athens University School of Medicine
"Laiko" General Hospital - 2nd Dept of Propedeutic Surgery, Vascular Laboratory - 16, Sevastoupoleos St, 11526 Athens, Greece
Tel: +30-210 7456 128, Fax: +30-210 7456 130 E-mail: liapivas@panafonet.gr Website: www.uems-vasc.org

**Acknowledgements**

The following evaluation report, kindly submitted to the EVCME Committee for completion of the accreditation cycle, has been prepared by the working group under Professor Michael Horrocks, ESVS Secretary.

## CONGRESS ESVS 2002—QUESTIONNAIRE FEEDBACK

## INTRODUCTION

The feedback received in 2002, in units, rose from 418 in 2001 to 436. However, this margin can only be significant when compared to the attendance recorded at both conferences. In 2001, the attendance at Lucerne was approx. 1500. This rose by 10% to approx. 1650 at Istanbul. Therefore, feedback rose at less than half the attendance rate. Despite this fact, feedback is the necessary tool with which to make improvements for Dublin 2003.

The results from Dublin will be most useful in creating a trio of feedback. As you will see in the report, comparisons can only be made with the previous year. Acting upon the evidence in this year's feedback will make Dublin responses all the more accurate. Additions to the current questionnaire framework next year may show a number of variables more useful when planning the conference for 2004.

This feedback is in two parts. The first is based upon 'closed questioning', using tick boxes. The second is an annotated representation of the 'open questions'—Numbers. 1.c), 1.e), 7. and 8. The former compares feedback in percent to Lucerne. 'Trace' refers to the fact that the feedback given was not near 1%, while 'Even' suggests little or no change whatsoever. Finally '% Swing' shows an upward or downward trend when compared to Lucerne. The downward figure is in red, but is not necessarily always a 'bad' indication: If 'Poor' equals − 7%, then the news is good. The latter part will be described later in the report.

## PART ONE—RESPONSES TO CLOSED QUESTIONS

*Based on the standard evaluation form created by the European Vascular CME Committee of the UEMS Division and Board of Vascular Surgery*

### 1. Please indicate your primary reason for attending the conference (one ✓ only)

| Answer categories | 2001 % | 2002 Response | 2002 % | % Swing |
|---|---|---|---|---|
| a) First-time introduction to main topic | 2% | 22 | 6% | +4% |
| b) Update overall knowledge about vascular surgery | 82% | 326 | 75% | − 7% |
| c) Learn more about one particular technique —which one? | 5% | 35 | 8% | +3% |
| d) Obtain CME credits | 4% | 22 | 5% | +1% |
| e) Other | 5% | 26 | 6% | +1% |
| No answer | Trace | 5 | 1% | +1% |

## 2. How well did the Congress programme do in fulfilling this goal?

| Answer categories | 2001 % | 2002 Response | 2002 % | % Swing |
|---|---|---|---|---|
| a) Excellent | 17% | 68 | 16% | − 1% |
| b) Good | 69% | 284 | 65% | − 4% |
| c) Fair | 12% | 68 | 16% | + 4% |
| d) Poor | Trace | 15 | 3% | + 3% |
| No answer | Trace | 1 | Trace | Even |

## 3. Evaluate then rate the following elements of this meeting in fulfilling your goal

| Answer categories | 2001 % | 2002 Response | 2002 % | % Swing |
|---|---|---|---|---|
| *a) Abstracts* | | | | |
| a) Excellent | 13% | 61 | 14% | + 1% |
| b) Good | 69% | 301 | 69% | Even |
| c) Fair | 15% | 51 | 12% | − 3% |
| d) Poor | Trace | 9 | 2% | + 2% |
| No answer | 2% | 14 | 3% | + 1% |
| *b) Meeting with faculty* | | | | |
| a) Excellent | 13% | 49 | 11% | − 2% |
| b) Good | 60% | 269 | 62% | + 2% |
| c) Fair | 14% | 74 | 17% | + 3% |
| d) Poor | 1% | 8 | 2% | + 1% |
| No answer | 10% | 36 | 8% | − 2% |
| *c) Demonstrations* | | | | |
| a) Excellent | 15% | 66 | 15% | Even |
| b) Good | 52% | 257 | 59% | + 7% |
| c) Fair | 17% | 71 | 16% | − 1% |
| d) Poor | 4% | 7 | 2% | − 2% |
| No answer | 10% | 35 | 8% | − 2% |
| *d) Discussion periods* | | | | |
| a) Excellent | 16% | 93 | 21% | + 5% |
| b) Good | 56% | 257 | 59% | + 3% |
| c) Fair | 19% | 66 | 15% | − 4% |
| d) Poor | 4% | 3 | 1% | − 3% |
| No answer | 4% | 17 | 4% | Even |
| *e) Exhibits* | | | | |
| a) Excellent | 4% | 70 | 16% | + 12% |
| b) Good | 56% | 257 | 59% | + 3% |
| c) Fair | 19% | 75 | 17% | − 2% |
| d) Poor | 1% | 6 | 1% | Even |
| No answer | 7% | 28 | 7% | Even |

*(continued on next page)*

| Answer categories | 2001 % | 2002 Response | 2002 % | % Swing |
|---|---|---|---|---|
| *f) Lectures by faculty* | | | | |
| a) Excellent | 18% | 52 | 12% | – 6% |
| b) Good | 58% | 265 | 60% | + 2% |
| c) Fair | 11% | 60 | 14% | + 3% |
| d) Poor | 1% | 13 | 3% | + 2% |
| No answer | 9% | 46 | 11% | + 2% |
| *g) Presentations by non-faculty* | | | | |
| a) Excellent | 6% | 26 | 6% | Even |
| b) Good | 56% | 254 | 58% | + 2% |
| c) Fair | 20% | 86 | 20% | Even |
| d) Poor | 1% | 11 | 3% | + 2% |
| No answer | 14% | 59 | 13% | – 1% |
| *h) Programme book* | | | | |
| a) Excellent | 26% | 97 | 22% | – 4% |
| b) Good | 52% | 246 | 57% | + 5% |
| c) Fair | 12% | 63 | 14% | + 2% |
| d) Poor | 1% | 10 | 2% | + 1% |
| No answer | 5% | 20 | 5% | Even |
| *i) Satellite symposia* | | | | |
| a) Excellent | 26% | 82 | 19% | – 7% |
| b) Good | 58% | 236 | 54% | – 4% |
| c) Fair | 7% | 63 | 14% | + 7% |
| d) Poor | 1% | 13 | 3% | + 2% |
| No answer | 6% | 42 | 10% | + 4% |

## 4. Please rate how relevant each of these educational needs are to you

| Answer categories | 2001 % | 2002 Response | 2002 % | % Swing |
|---|---|---|---|---|
| *a) Examine new diagnostic modes* | | | | |
| a) Extremely important | 23% | 102 | 23% | Even |
| b) Important | 61% | 264 | 61% | Even |
| c) Somewhat important | 11% | 45 | 10% | – 1% |
| d) Not relevant | Trace | 3 | 1% | + 1% |
| No answer | 2% | 22 | 5% | + 3% |
| *b) Examine new therapeutic potential* | | | | |
| a) Extremely important | 37% | 157 | 36% | – 1% |
| b) Important | 47% | 225 | 52% | + 5% |
| c) Somewhat important | 9% | 35 | 8% | – 1% |
| d) Not relevant | Zero | 2 | Trace | Trace |
| No answer | 4% | 17 | 4% | Even |
| *c) Learn about new devices* | | | | |
| a) Extremely important | 28% | 133 | 31% | + 3% |
| b) Important | 51% | 223 | 51% | Even |
| c) Somewhat important | 14% | 54 | 12% | – 2% |
| d) Not relevant | Trace | 2 | Trace | Even |
| No answer | 4% | 24 | 6% | + 2% |

| Answer categories | 2001 % | 2002 Response | 2002 % | % Swing |
|---|---|---|---|---|
| *d) Learn about endoluminal grafts* | | | | |
| a) Extremely important | 25% | 126 | 29% | + 4% |
| b) Important | 46% | 189 | 43% | − 3% |
| c) Somewhat important | 22% | 90 | 21% | − 1% |
| d) Not relevant | 1% | 6 | 1% | Even |
| No answer | 4% | 25 | 6% | + 2% |
| *e) Receive hands-on training* | | | | |
| a) Extremely important | 18% | 112 | 26% | + 8% |
| b) Important | 33% | 152 | 35% | + 2% |
| c) Somewhat important | 26% | 100 | 23% | − 3% |
| d) Not relevant | 12% | 34 | 8% | − 4% |
| No answer | 8% | 38 | 8% | Even |
| *f) Classical surgical techniques* | | | | |
| a) Extremely important | 16% | 98 | 22% | + 6% |
| b) Important | 49% | 192 | 44% | − 5% |
| c) Somewhat important | 20% | 97 | 22% | + 2% |
| d) Not relevant | 8% | 24 | 6% | − 2% |
| No answer | 4% | 25 | 6% | + 2% |
| *g) Other* | | | | |
| a) Extremely important | Trace | 19 | 4% | + 4% |
| b) Important | 9% | 74 | 17% | + 8% |
| c) Somewhat important | 9% | 41 | 9% | Even |
| d) Not relevant | 7% | 21 | 5% | − 2% |
| No answer | 73% | 281 | 65% | − 8% |

## 5. How important are the following topics to your practice

| Answer categories | 2001 % | 2002 Response | 2002 % | % Swing |
|---|---|---|---|---|
| *a) Diagnostic investigation* | | | | |
| a) Extremely important | 28% | 125 | 29% | + 1% |
| b) Important | 55% | 243 | 56% | + 1% |
| c) Somewhat important | 11% | 45 | 10% | − 1% |
| d) Not relevant | 1% | 1 | Trace | − 1% |
| No answer | 2% | 22 | 5% | + 3% |
| *b) Risk factor management* | | | | |
| a) Extremely important | 31% | 132 | 30% | − 1% |
| b) Important | 48% | 222 | 51% | + 3% |
| c) Somewhat important | 15% | 59 | 14% | − 1% |
| d) Not relevant | 1% | 1 | Trace | − 1% |
| No answer | 3% | 22 | 5% | + 2% |
| *c) Evidence-based practice* | | | | |
| a) Extremely important | 39% | 165 | 38% | − 1% |
| b) Important | 45% | 203 | 46% | + 1% |
| c) Somewhat important | 10% | 36 | 8% | − 2% |
| d) Not relevant | Trace | 4 | 1% | + 1% |
| No answer | 3% | 28 | 7% | + 4% |

*(continued on next page)*

| Answer categories | 2001 % | 2002 Response | 2002 % | % Swing |
|---|---|---|---|---|
| *d) Experimental studies* | | | | |
| a) Extremely important | 12% | 72 | 17% | + 5% |
| b) Important | 41% | 182 | 42% | + 1% |
| c) Somewhat important | 36% | 132 | 30% | − 6% |
| d) Not relevant | 4% | 26 | 6% | + 2% |
| No answer | 5% | 24 | 5% | Even |
| *e) Drug therapy* | | | | |
| a) Extremely important | 11% | 55 | 13% | + 2% |
| b) Important | 54% | 228 | 52% | − 2% |
| c) Somewhat important | 26% | 119 | 27% | + 1% |
| d) Not relevant | 1% | 8 | 2% | + 1% |
| No answer | 5% | 26 | 6% | + 1% |
| *f) Classical surgical treatment* | | | | |
| a) Extremely important | 36% | 155 | 35% | − 1% |
| b) Important | 50% | 225 | 52% | + 2% |
| c) Somewhat important | 8% | 31 | 7% | − 1% |
| d) Not relevant | 1% | 3 | 1% | Even |
| No answer | 2% | 22 | 5% | + 3% |
| *g) Endovascular treatment* | | | | |
| a) Extremely important | 34% | 158 | 36% | + 2% |
| b) Important | 47% | 196 | 45% | − 2% |
| c) Somewhat important | 12% | 53 | 12% | Even |
| d) Not relevant | 2% | 7 | 2% | Even |
| No answer | 2% | 22 | 5% | + 3% |

## 6. Please rate the following items

| Answer categories | 2001 % | 2002 Response | 2002 % | % Swing |
|---|---|---|---|---|
| *a) Organization of the programme* | | | | |
| a) Excellent | 47% | 182 | 42% | − 5% |
| b) Good | 44% | 215 | 49% | + 5% |
| c) Fair | 3% | 18 | 4% | + 1% |
| d) Poor | Trace | 4 | 1% | + 1% |
| No answer | 3% | 17 | 4% | + 1% |
| *b) Overall rating of Congress* | | | | |
| a) Excellent | 32% | 110 | 25% | − 7% |
| b) Good | 53% | 256 | 59% | + 6% |
| c) Fair | 8% | 38 | 9% | + 1% |
| d) Poor | Trace | 9 | 2% | + 2% |
| No answer | 3% | 23 | 5% | + 2% |
| *c) Hotel accommodation/facilities* | | | | |
| a) Excellent | 22% | 164 | 37% | + 15% |
| b) Good | 52% | 204 | 47% | − 5% |

| Answer categories | 2001 % | 2002 Response | 2002 % | % Swing |
|---|---|---|---|---|
| *c) Hotel accommodation/facilities* | | | | |
| c) Fair | 16% | 38 | 9% | − 7% |
| d) Poor | 1% | 4 | 1% | Even |
| No answer | 6% | 26 | 6% | Even |
| *d) Prices* | | | | |
| a) Excellent | 4% | 48 | 11% | + 7% |
| b) Good | 37% | 233 | 53% | + 16% |
| c) Fair | 38% | 106 | 24% | − 14% |
| d) Poor | 14% | 21 | 5% | − 9% |
| No answer | 5% | 28 | 7% | + 2% |
| *e) Meeting facilities* | | | | |
| a) Excellent | 34% | 115 | 26% | − 8% |
| b) Good | 51% | 252 | 58% | + 7% |
| c) Fair | 9% | 36 | 8% | − 1% |
| d) Poor | Trace | 4 | 1% | + 1% |
| No answer | 4% | 29 | 7% | + 3% |
| *f) Congress staff* | | | | |
| a) Excellent | 45% | 166 | 38% | − 7% |
| b) Good | 46% | 233 | 53% | + 7% |
| c) Fair | 3% | 16 | 4% | + 1% |
| d) Poor | Trace | 3 | 1% | + 1% |
| No answer | 3% | 18 | 4% | + 1% |

## PART TWO—RESPONSES TO OPEN QUESTIONS

This, the latter of the two parts of the 2002 Congress Questionnaire Feedback, attempts to highlight the positives and negatives voiced by the 163 members (37% of those who filled out questionnaires) who took part in a combination of one, some, or all of the following four questions: 1.c); 1.e); 7. and 8. Questions 7. and 8. will be annotated, but firstly, we refer to the two open answers from categories c) and e) in question number 1.

### 1. Please indicate your primary reason for attending the conference (one ✓ only)

| Answer categories | 2001 % | 2002 Response | 2002 % | % Swing |
|---|---|---|---|---|
| c) Learn more about one particular technique—which one? | 5% | 35 | 8% | + 3% |

From the 35 responses (ticks) to the question, only 12 answered ‘which one?’—(34%):

| | |
|---|---|
| MIAS | 1 |
| Endovascular surgery | 1 |
| AAA | 3 |
| EVAR | 7 |

**1. Please indicate your primary reason for attending the conference (one ✓ only)**

| Answer categories | 2001 % | 2002 Response | 2002 % | % Swing |
|---|---|---|---|---|
| e) Other | 5% | 26 | 6% | +1% |

From the 26 responses (ticks) to this part of question 1, only 4 described the 'other' primary reason for attending the conference—(15%):

| | |
|---|---|
| Social | 3 |
| Tutoring | 1 |

**NB—It is worth noting that 1 of the 'Social' 3 later commented that the Congress had: *"no scientific value"***

**7. Please give a summary of the information you received which will be useful in your practice**

The results from 'question' 7 were varied, but we were able to categorise them into 5 key areas: (i) Updating Devices and Techniques; (ii) Treatment; (iii) Surgery; (iv) Discussion Groups; and (v) Research. Out of the 163 total responses for part two of the questionnaire, 119 were answering this 'question'. The best way to annotate these responses is to table them under the 5 key areas, listing them in order of strength of response within each category. The percentage marked to the side represents the percent of the response to this question only, i.e. a percentage of the 119 people who commented, or 'answered' the question.

| | |
|---|---|
| *Devices and Techniques* | |
| Update and learning latest advances in new techniques, inc. diagnosis and therapies | **33** (27%) |
| *Treatment* | |
| Endovascular treatment | **8** (6%) |
| Long-term evaluation of endoluminal grafts, inc. treatment of infected grafts | **5** (4%) |
| Carotid endovascular treatment | **4** (3%) |
| Post surgery treatment, inc. drug therapy | **3** (2.5%) |
| Carotid angioplasty | **1** (0.8%) |
| EBP | **1** (0.8%) |
| Endoprosthesis | **1** (0.8%) |
| *Surgery* | |
| EVAR | **14** (11%) |
| AAA inc. risk factors | **12** (10%) |
| Carotid stenting, inc. stent grafts | **12** (10%) |
| Classical surgical treatment | **5** (4%) |

| | |
|---|---|
| *Surgery* | |
| Endo treatment of ruptured aneurysms | **3** (2.5%) |
| Vein/vessel surgery | **2** (1.5%) |
| Dorsa lateral | **1** (0.8%) |
| Endovascular surgery complications | **1** (0.8%) |
| Endovascular based practice | **1** (0.8%) |
| Open surgery | **1** (0.8%) |
| Robotic repair | **1** (0.8%) |
| *Discussion Groups* | |
| Discussion on 48 hr Working Wk for Trainees | **1** (0.8%) |
| Hands-on Workshops | **1** (0.8%) |
| Management concepts | **1** (0.8%) |
| Risk management in CEA | **1** (0.8%) |
| Successful vascular surgery = learning endovascular techniques | **1** (0.8%) |
| Video conferencing | **1** (0.8%) |
| *Research* | |
| Vascular surgery research | **1** (0.8%) |
| Vascular disease | **1** (0.8%) |
| Randomised trials and evidence-based medicines | **1** (0.8%) |

## 8. Further Comments

Like question 7, question 8 is separated into 3 definable topics: (i) Positive Comments, (ii) Negative Comments, and (iii) Future Suggestions. There were 50 responses out of the 163 to this 'question', and, they are accompanied by their respective percentage terms.

| | |
|---|---|
| *Positive comments* | |
| Excellent opportunity to update | **2** (4%) |
| Good auditorium | **1** (2%) |
| Good to be reassured of treatment methods | **1** (2%) |
| *Negative comments* | |
| Food | **3** (6%) |
| Discriminative use of English language | **2** (4%) |
| Congress is of "no scientific value" | **2** (4%) |
| Congress failed to update from last year | **1** (2%) |
| Inconsistent level of quality of contributors (speakers) | **1** (2%) |
| Too young and inexperienced speakers | **1** (2%) |
| Symposia by sponsored companies is not right—should be independent | **1** (2%) |
| There were no "'unsponsored' roundtables" | **1** (2%) |
| There were no lectures | **1** (2%) |
| No focus on some important topics (the topics were not listed) | **1** (2%) |
| Too little discussion | **1** (2%) |
| Congress did not "reflect the best Vascular Surgery of Europe" | **1** (2%) |
| No interesting topics | **1** (2%) |
| "Miserable abstracts" | **1** (2%) |
| Difficulty in understanding discussions (did not state reason why) | **1** (2%) |

*(continued on next page)*

| | |
|---|---|
| *Negative comments* | |
| Registration difficulties | **1** (2%) |
| Bad shuttle bus service | **1** (2%) |
| Social programme different to that advertised | **1** (2%) |
| No internet, post office, currency exchange | **1** (2%) |
| Problems of EVAR and carotid stenting class—"not acceptable" | **1** (2%) |
| No class on angioplasty surgery | **1** (2%) |
| Poor acoustics | **1** (2%) |
| Large meetings have less valuable discussions | **1** (2%) |
| *Future suggestions* | |
| Use ID badges—(speakers and senior Congress members) | **1** (2%) |
| Better info on Eurostar services/connections | **1** (2%) |
| Need more emphasis on "clinical importance" | **1** (2%) |
| Need more workshops | **1** (2%) |
| Need genetic map incorporated into vascular diseases | **1** (2%) |
| Better symposia topics (did not suggest any) | **1** (2%) |
| More support needed for experimental and diagnostic research | **1** (2%) |
| More info needed on techniques, treatment and drug therapy | **1** (2%) |
| Meet big names (invite high(er) profile guests) | **1** (2%) |
| More practical info needed (did not state what sort of practical info) | **1** (2%) |
| Congress should be longer | **1** (2%) |
| Bring own interpreter if you cannot speak enough English | **1** (2%) |
| More evidence-based medicine | **1** (2%) |
| More EVAR treatment | **1** (2%) |
| More emphasis on clinical trials | **1** (2%) |
| Live demos (did not suggest what sort of topics) | **1** (2%) |
| Videos needed showing different techniques | **1** (2%) |
| Live video demo for future symposium | **1** (2%) |
| Make CD-ROM of talks | **1** (2%) |

## CONCLUSIONS AND SUGGESTIONS

The statistics relating to Part One speak for themselves. There are big gains in popularity for some workshops and Hotel/Accommodation. Conversely, the Satellite Symposia took some criticism. Anything that a 'Tick Box' could not show is reflected in Part Two.

There were 173 different written responses on 163 forms. This can be seen as positive, in that few people felt 'bothered' enough to comment. However, along with the proportionate decrease in responses (– 5% in real terms), there could be signs of Member 'apathy'.

Thankfully, the members who see Congress as a non-scientific social are well into the minority. However, the comments to 'question' 8 do ask for more science overall, as well as better communications facilities and the incorporation of multimedia.

The latter idea, if incorporated, would ease the fear that Congress is too short. Creating CD-ROMs and demo videos would also please the socialites and could be included into a long-term budget, cutting costs. Of course, members have to be encouraged to attend Congress.

The 'Negative comments' should work hand-in-hand with 'Future suggestions', although there are contradictory anomalies claiming that certain classes did not exist. What could be a valuable inclusion into the questionnaire would be the introduction of

Equal Opps Monitoring, or something that, via the Data Protection Act, would give a picture of who is saying what. For example, it is a Norwegian surgeon who suggests interpreting for those with a low command of English, not those who are typically accused of discriminating with the language.

It would be also good to confirm that the newer members are very enthusiastic and full of praise, while the more experienced are becoming bored and even disillusioned. This could explain why the Satellite Symposia plummeted in popularity. Interest has to be retained as well as attained, and this could perhaps be encouraged by the introduction of 'take-home' multimedia.

**Acknowledgements**

The following evaluation report, kindly submitted to the EVCME Committee for the completion of the accreditation cycle, has been prepared by the working group under Professor Roger Greenhalgh, Programme Chairman, President of the European Board of Surgery.

## Charing Cross Symposium Evaluation 2004

This summarises the major sponsor meeting that took place on April 3–6 2004. The summary includes data from 268 delegates who completed the official UEMS evaluation form of the 1282-delegate total:

### 1. Overall 2003

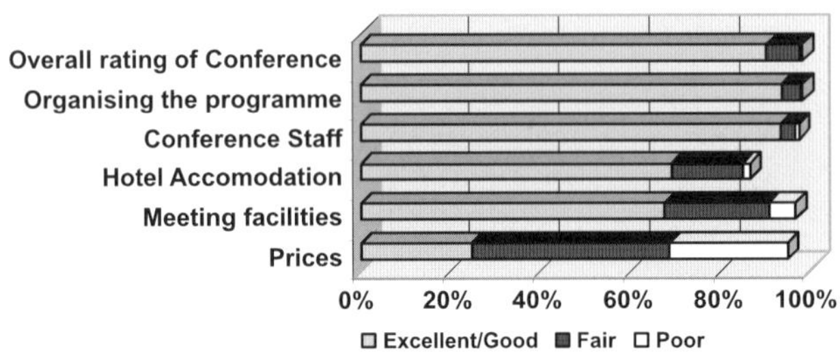


### Overall 2004

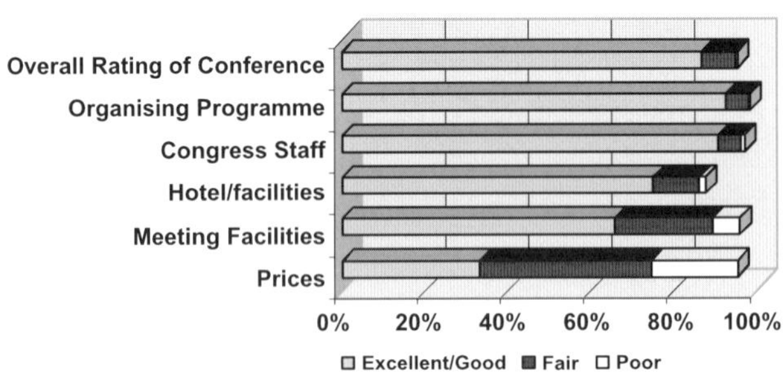


### 2. Attendance

This year, Charing Cross had a record attendance of over 1282 delegates, an increase of 28.1% on the previous year

| 1999 | 2000 | 2001 | 2002 | 2003 | 2004 | % Difference on previous year |
|---|---|---|---|---|---|---|
| 502 | 515 | 630 | 882 | 1001 | 1282 | 28.1% |

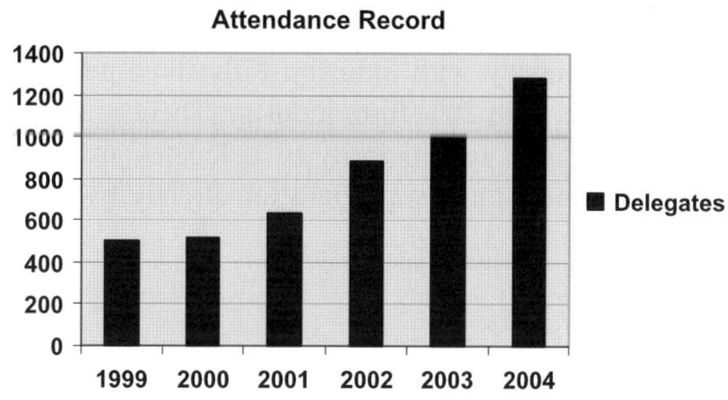


## The Charing Cross has become more international than ever

There was an overall growth of 28.1% year on year, with Rest of World rising by 72.9%, Western Europe rising by 18.9% and the UK rising by 26.2%

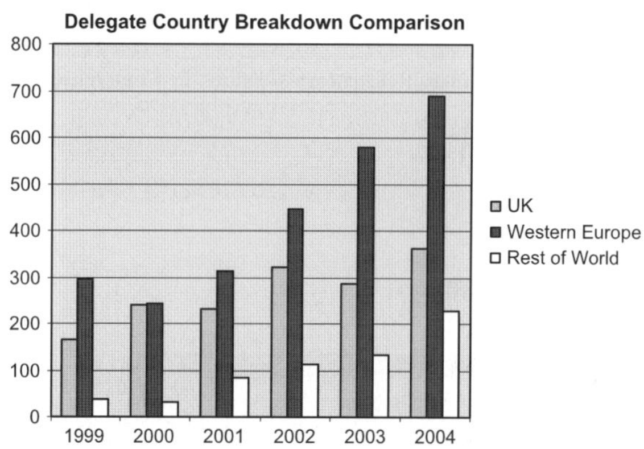


For the fourth year, the number of countries represented rose and reached 55 this year (from 48 in 2003).

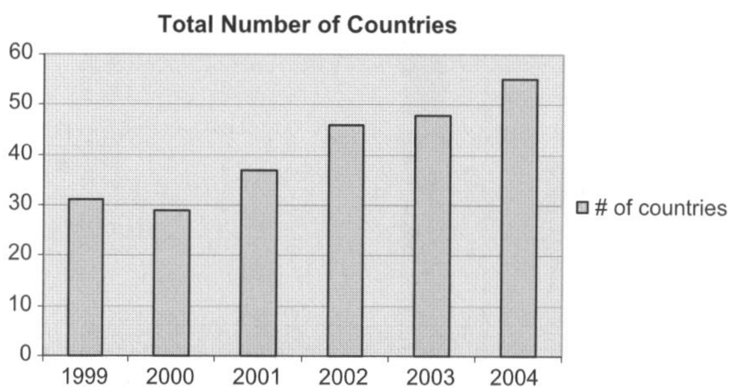

Charing Cross currently attracts around a large number of vascular specialists with opportunities for greater partnership with industry. Fifty-three percent of those attending were senior vascular specialists with 20% from industry. There is an opportunity to partner more closely with industry as the vast majority of delegates are not directly funded by industry. One hundred and ninety-three were paid for directly by exhibiting companies.

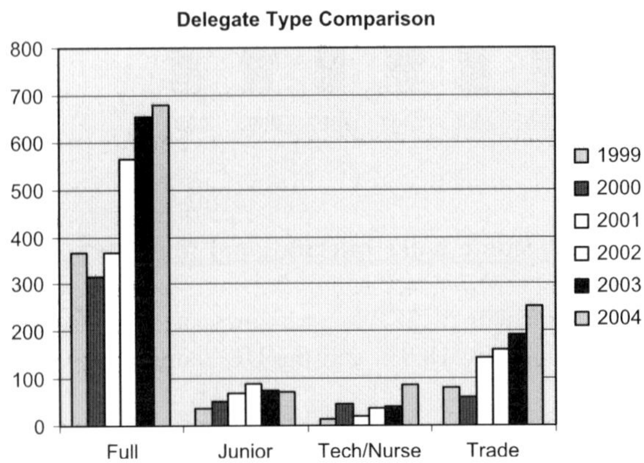


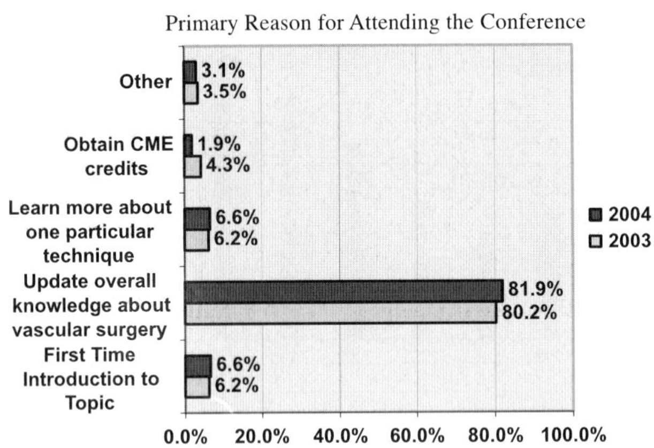


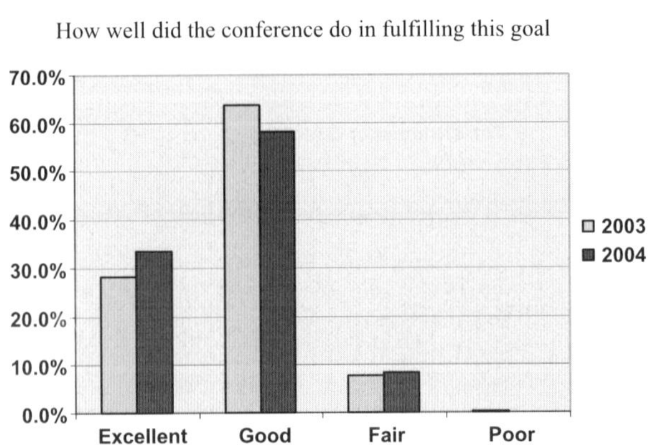

How relevant each of these educational needs to you 2004

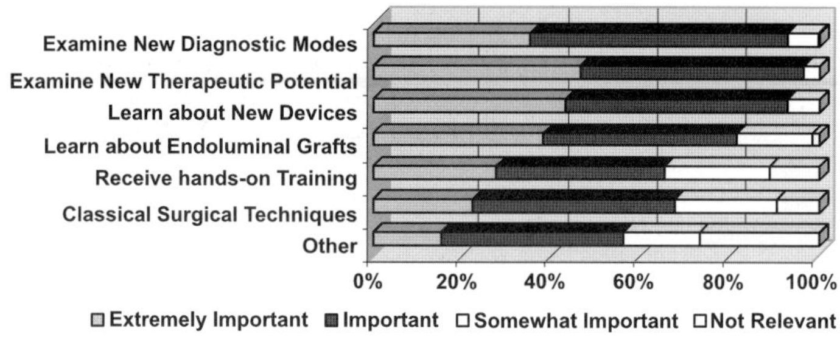


Importance of the following topics to your practice 2003

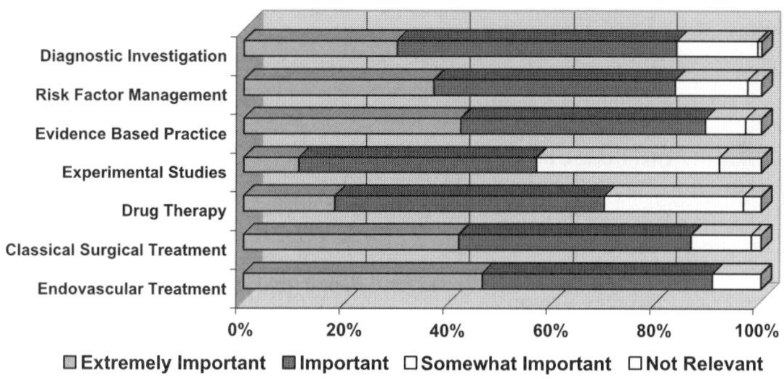


Importance of the following topics to your practice 2004

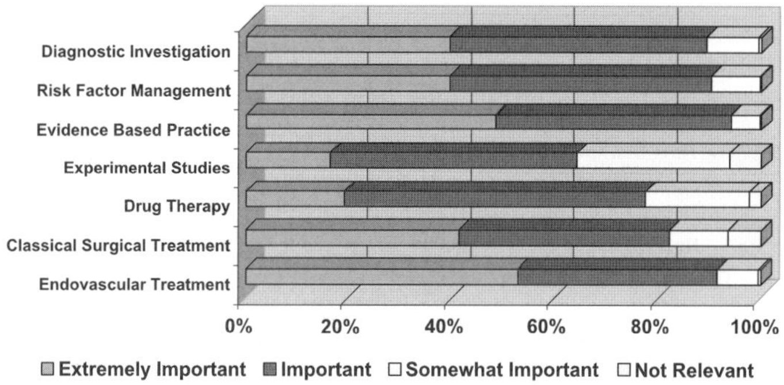

Evaluation of Elements of the meeting fulfilling Goals 2003

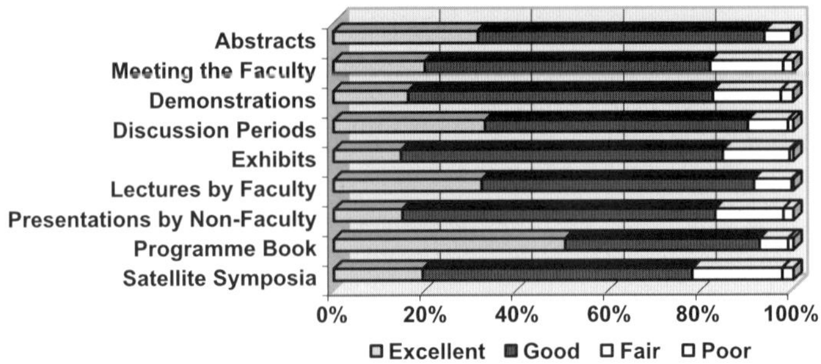


Evaluation of Elements of the meeting fulfilling Goals 2004

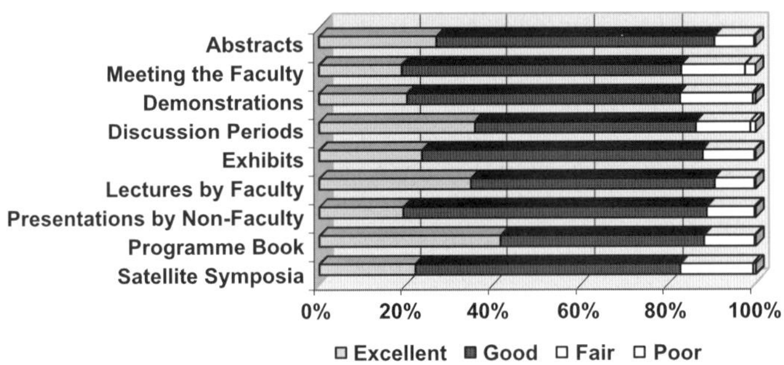


How relevant each of these educational needs are to you 2003

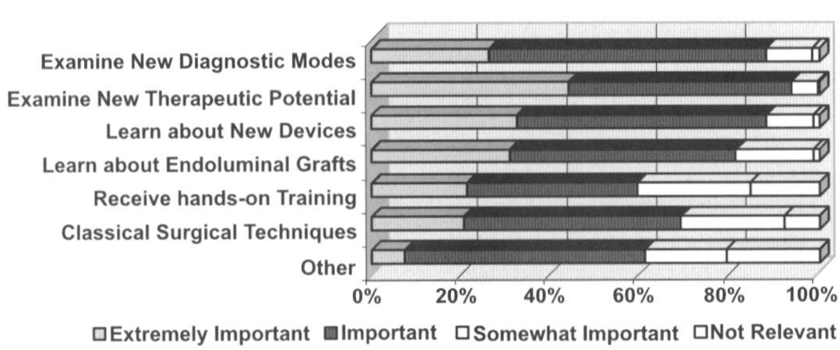

## Acknowledgements

The following evaluation report, kindly submitted to the EVCME Committee for the completion of the accreditation cycle, has been prepared by the working group under Professors Alain Branchereau and Michael Jacobs, Directors of the European Vascular Course.

## EUROPEAN VASCULAR COURSE

## Amsterdam 2004

## CME Accreditation—Short Report

This report (copy enclosed) is based on the UEMS questionnaires returned by participants of the EVC congress in March 2004.

The primary reason for vascular surgeons to attend the course appears to be to *update overall knowledge* in their field.

The congress program was highly appreciated by well over half of the attendees.

The textbook was rated between good and excellent by almost all participants.

When it came to rating the possibilities of *meeting with the faculty*, *lectures*, *discussions*, *exhibits* and *satellite symposia* held by the industry, most of the attendees ticked the *good* box.

The participants graded their educational needs as follows: extremely important was *new therapeutic potential*, important was *new diagnostic modes* and *learning about open surgical techniques*. Then followed *learning about new devices* and *endoluminal techniques* just before *receive hands-on training*.

Concerning the question: *How important are the following topics for your practice?*, over half of the attendees thought important diagnostic investigation, risk factor management, classical surgical treatment as well as endovascular treatment, whereas drug therapy seemed to be extremely important to two-thirds of the participants.

Furthermore, almost everyone was satisfied with the *balanced views presented during the course*. And, all in all, *information free of commercial bias during the scientific sessions* was perceived as excellent and acceptable with very few exceptions.

Finally, fees, meeting facilities, accommodations, organization of the program and congress staff were graded as good or excellent by the majority of the participants.

## SURVEY ANALYSIS EVC 2004 Amsterdam

### Question 1: Primary reasons for attending

| 1st Intro to main topic | Update overall knowledge | One particular technique | CME credits | Other |
|---|---|---|---|---|
| 13% | **79%** | 7% | / | / |

## Question 2: Rate the congress program

| Excellent | Good | Fair | Poor |
|---|---|---|---|
| **31%** | **61%** | 7% | / |

## Question 3: Rate the following elements of the meeting with regard to your expectations

| | Excellent | Good | Fair | Poor | No comment |
|---|---|---|---|---|---|
| Textbook | 38% | **56%** | 4% | / | / |
| Meeting faculty | / | **76%** | 21% | 1.5% | 1.5% |
| Demonstrations | 16% | **56%** | 16% | 4% | 6% |
| Discussions | 18% | **67%** | 13% | 1.5% | 0% |
| Exhibits | 19% | **67%** | 13% | / | / |
| Lectures by faculty | 21% | **67%** | 6% | / | 4% |
| Presentations by non-faculty | 13% | **72%** | 12% | 1.5% | 2% |
| Satellite symposia | 24% | **63%** | 9% | 1.5% | 3% |

## Question 4: Please rate these educational needs

| | Extremely important | Important | Somewhat important | Not relevant | No comment |
|---|---|---|---|---|---|
| New diagnostic modes | 33% | **58%** | 6% | 3% | 0% |
| New therapeutic potential | **48%** | 46% | 6% | / | / |
| Learning about new devices | 39% | **55%** | 6% | / | / |
| Learning about endoluminal techniques | 31% | **52%** | 13% | 1,5% | 2% |
| Learning about open surgical techniques | **18%** | **58%** | 19% | 4% | / |
| Receive hands-on training | 25% | **36%** | 34% | 4% | / |
| Other | Harmonized training in Europe | | | | |

## Question 5: How important are the following topics for your practice

| | Extremely important | Important | Somewhat important | Not relevant | No comment |
|---|---|---|---|---|---|
| Diagnostic investigation | 28% | **58%** | 12% | / | / |
| Risk factor management | 30% | **58%** | 12% | / | / |
| Evidence-based practice | 39% | **43%** | 15% | 3% | / |
| Experimental studies | 15% | **48%** | 36% | 1.5% | / |
| Drug therapy | 7% | **63%** | 27% | 3% | / |
| Classical surgical treatment | 31% | **58%** | 10% | / | / |
| Endovascular treatment | 46% | **52%** | 2% | / | / |

## Question 6: Please rate the following items

| | Excellent | Good | Fair | Poor | No comment |
|---|---|---|---|---|---|
| Organization of the program | 43% | **54%** | 3% | / | / |
| Overall congress | 33% | **60%** | 7% | / | / |
| Accommodations/facilities | 37% | **55%** | 3% | / | 4% |
| Prices | 6% | **49%** | 39% | 3% | 3% |
| Meeting facilities | 24% | **69%** | 6% | 1.5% | / |
| Congress staff | 37% | **55%** | 6% | / | / |

## Question 7: Please grade the following items

| | Excellent | Acceptable | Poor | No comment |
|---|---|---|---|---|
| Information about potential conflicts of interest by chairman/presenter/program | 28% | **51%** | 12% | 9% |
| Balanced views presented during the congress | 30% | **63%** | 1.5% | 6% |
| Information free of commercial bias during the scientific sessions | 28% | **60%** | 6% | 6% |

International Congress Series 1272 (2004) 285–286

www.ics-elsevier.com

# The status of vascular surgery in Austria in 2004

Josef Klocker*

*Klinische Abteilung für Gefässchirurgie, Universitätsklinik für Chirurgie, Innsbruck 6020, Austria*

*Keywords:* Vascular surgery

In Austria, the organisation and delivery of general medical services and vascular medicine and surgery is considerably variable within this country of approximately 8 million people, predominantly as a result of the country's geography. Departments of Vascular Surgery are restricted to the four medical universities (Vienna, Graz, Salzburg and Innsbruck) and a small number of multi-specialty hospitals in administrative centers. Primary diagnosis and treatment of vascular disease, however, is frequently performed by physicians trained in internal medicine or general surgery in local hospitals, especially in the remote countryside. As a consequence, it is estimated that only 50% of vascular surgical procedures are performed in the 23 Austrian vascular surgery (sub-) units (departments of vascular surgery: $n=6$; cardiothoracic and vascular surgery: $n=3$; general surgery plus vascular subunit: $n=14$), whereas the other 50% is carried out by surgeons without longstanding experience and/or without a primary interest in vascular surgery. This situation has several implications.

## 1. In terms of the training of surgeons performing vascular surgery

At present, there are 35 training positions for vascular surgeons in Austria, all which are allocated to the vascular surgery (sub-) units. In order to obtain certification as a "vascular surgeon" by the Austrian Medical Board, 6 years of training in general surgery (including two years of related subjects like anaesthesiology, pathology and internal medicine) is a mandatory requirement with an additional 3 years of training in vascular surgery. Compared with other countries, this long training period of 9 years seems unreasonable, although it may be of benefit in the local setting, keeping in mind that half of all vascular surgical procedures are performed there. Many regional hospitals nowadays employ at least one surgeon with additional vascular training to perform vascular procedures, mostly emergency cases.

* Tel.: +43-512-504-80787; fax: +43-512-504-2559.
*E-mail address:* josef.klocker@uibk.ac.at (J. Klocker).


doi:10.1016/j.ics.2004.04.090

## 2. In terms of qualification and certification of surgeons performing vascular surgery

Up until now, following a minimum of 9 years of training, vascular surgeons received a certificate from the Austrian Medical Board proclaiming sufficient knowledge and proficiency to treat patients with arterial, venous and/or lymphatic disease, either conservatively or operatively (including endovascular therapy). At the end of the 6-year period in general surgery, a board exam in general surgery has become mandatory since 1996. Presently, however, there is no such vascular surgery exam, which tests knowledge and skills, following the additional 3 years of training. In future, as intended by the Austrian Society of Vascular Surgery, vascular surgeons will have to be examined at the end of their training period, and a system similar to the one used by the European Society of Vascular Surgery is proposed.

At present, the number of vascular procedures performed during training is not monitored with adequate quality control. Essential subjects like interventional radiology and angiology are also not yet included in the basic training requirements of vascular surgeons in Austria, as also seen in many other countries.

## 3. In terms of controlling the efficacy and cost of vascular surgery

Since vascular procedures are performed by surgeons trained without the need to meet specific quality and cost requirements, monitoring of efficacy, volume and costs of treatment is difficult but essential. Several steps have been initiated to improve the patient outcome by the Austrian Society of Vascular Surgery. In the late 1990s, the society started to collect and analyse nationwide data concerning the results of carotid surgery (approximately 3900 patients up until March 2003) and of aortic aneurysm repair (more than 500 patients up until March 2003), allowing for outcome analysis and comparison of results achieved at different institutions. Second, the society recently published consensus statements on the treatment of vascular diseases, such as the endovascular treatment of carotid stenosis or stent-grafting of aortic aneurysms. It also facilitates and organises exchange programs during training to allow for a broadened individual experience in vascular medicine.

International Congress Series 1272 (2004) 287–288

www.ics-elsevier.com

# Status of vascular surgery in Belgium

André Nevelsteen

*Department of Vascular Surgery, U.Z. Gasthuisberg, Herestraat 49, Leuven 300, Belgium*

In 1997, Raphael Suy presented a review on vascular surgery in Belgium in the European Journal of Vascular and Endovascular Surgery [1]. The most important findings were:

1. Belgium is a small, but politically complex, country. Overall, six ministers are involved in public health.
2. Belgium is confronted with a plethora of physicians (one physician for every 300 inhabitants).
3. Vascular surgery is not recognized as a monospecialty, but remains under the umbrella of "general surgery." Nevertheless, 83% of the 160 hospitals with surgical beds have at least one surgeon exclusively involved with vascular surgery.
4. Belgium is the European leader for all types of vascular surgery, with a total number of 15,000 arterial operations, 18,500 venous operations, 6600 endovascular procedures and 900 thrombolytic procedures for 10 million inhabitants in 1995. Surgeons in the operating room do the majority of endovascular procedures.

In the meantime, the federal government started with an entrance examination for medical studies. The number of medical students has reduced significantly, but until now this has not influenced the number of surgical residents nor the plethora of physicians (medical studies take at least 7 years in Belgium). It can, however, be foreseen that in the near future the number of surgical residents will also reduce significantly. The Belgian Society for Vascular Surgery, founded in 1992, now has over 150 surgical members, the overwhelming majority exclusively involved with vascular surgery.

Vascular surgery remains under the umbrella of general surgery and is still not officially recognized as a subspecialty. In order to stimulate official certification, the Belgian Society for Vascular Surgery has created guidelines for training centers and education in vascular surgery. At this moment, 17 centers are certified for training in vascular surgery by the Belgian Society. In 1997, the Belgian Society also initiated a certificate of "competence in vascular surgery." The conditions to obtain this certificate are:

1. The candidate should be a citizen of an EU country. He/she should have a CCST for general surgery, recognized by the Belgian government.

*E-mail address:* Andre.Nevelsteen@us.kuleuven.ac.be (A. Nevelsteen).


doi:10.1016/j.ics.2004.04.074

2. The candidate should have done 2 years of training in vascular surgery in a recognized center. The first year might be combined with the previous year.
3. The candidate should present a logbook showing that he performed at least
   (a) 200 major arterial operations (aortic, carotid, infra-inguinal) with a good balance between open and endovascular reconstruction
   (b) 50 venous operations
   (c) 100 diagnostic procedures (preferably duplex).
4. The candidate must prove that he/she has at least one publication or presentation at a national or international congress.

This certificate is not a legal requirement to perform vascular surgery in Belgium, and it does not mean that a certified surgeon will perform better than a non-certified one. It is, however, a guarantee that the holder has had adequate training in a dedicated training center. In the meantime, young Belgian vascular surgeons are also encouraged towards the EBSQ-VASC examination. It is hoped that these programs will create a stimulus for the federal government to officially recognize vascular surgery as a surgical subspecialty in Belgium.

## Reference

[1] R. Suy, Vascular surgery in Belgium, Eur. J. Vasc. Endovasc. Surg. 14 (1997) 233–234.

International Congress Series 1272 (2004) 289–291

ELSEVIER

www.ics-elsevier.com

# The status of vascular surgery in Croatia

Tomislav Šoša*, Lidija Erdelez

*Department of Surgery and Vascular Surgery, University Hospital Merkur, Zajceva 19, Zagreb X, Croatia*

*Keywords:* Vascular surgery

## 1. Introduction

In Croatia, one can find 19 vascular departments with 43 surgeons situated in six University centers and in 13 Regional hospitals. Out of these, 24 vascular surgeons working in the University centers are monospecialists, each with >150 arterial procedures/year, while other 19 are general surgeons who deal with vascular surgery in their Regional hospitals (each with <50 arterial procedures/year). Vascular departments are geographically equally distributed in the long and narrow country. Monospecialists are trained throughout Europe, in the USA and Australia.

## 2. Vascular epidemiology

In Croatia, 52.3% of population die from cardiac and vascular diseases. Of these, 31.2% are cardiac, 33% cerebrovascular and 35.8% peripheral vascular patients. Thirty thousand patients suffer from PAOD. There are 2700 amputations per year, and 1900 patients with critical limb ischaemia. According to the current epidemiological data, about 14,000 patients with AA live in Croatia. Out of these, 1800 aneurysms/year need surgery. Incidence of stroke is in competition with MI incidence. Real need for CEA/CAS is 2700 per year. In the working population, the incidence of varicose veins is up to 39%. In the population, 11.3% males and 23.7% females with varicose veins can be found. CVI with ulcer bear 90,000 patients.

## 3. Brief history

First published aneurysmal operations were performed in Zagreb by D. Schwartz in 1904 (Liječ. Vjesn. 27 (2) (1905) 53–54). F. Jurisic published his results in the vascular paper "Kirurgija zilja-Angiosurgery" (Liječ. Vjesn. 40 (8) (1918) 263–269). From 1921–1943, more than 1000 vascular procedures were done. The first department for vascular surgery was founded in 1964 by V. Luetic. From 1964–1975, three University

* Corresponding author. Tel.: +385-1-2431-390/394; fax: +385-1-2332-270.
*E-mail address:* klinicka-bolnica-merkur1@zg.hinet.hr (T. Šoša).


doi:10.1016/j.ics.2004.04.072

centers seeded vascular surgeons throughout the country. CME from vascular surgery and angiology started in 1972. In the past 20 years, 1043 papers in national and international journals, and nine national books with chapters from vascular surgery were published.

In 1994, Croatia became a full member of ESVS and, in 1995, of EAVST. The Croatian Phlebological Society (CPS) founded in 1993, became a member of UIP in 1995. The same year Croatian Academy of Sciences and Arts founded Committee for detecting, studying, preventing and treating atherosclerosis. Finally, in 1996, the Croatian Society for Vascular Surgery (CSVS) was founded during the International Symposium of Vascular Surgery in Zagreb.

## 4. State of the art

In the past 30 years, the number of arterial procedures rose from <100/million to >900 operations/million. The experience from the University centers in the past 10 years showed comparable results to the European and the US vascular centers data. University centers deal with complex vascular problems, i.e., re-do procedures, surgery of the aortic arch, supraaortic surgery, thoracoscopic sympathectomies, carotid body tumours, aortorenal and visceral procedures, thoracic and thoracoabdominal aneurysms, congenital malformations, etc. During the war (1991–1993), Croatian vascular surgeons gained experience in resolving various types of military vascular injuries.

At the present time, informational link between vascular centers is still missing. Due to the lack of equipment, EVAR is done in only two University centers with <20 procedures/year. However, PTA/stent peripheral and carotid procedures have been done routinely since 1996 (starting in 1992); they make up >10% of the total volume of the arterial surgery.

**Education in croatian vascular surgery**

Education can be summarized by program of specialization in vascular surgery which was issued 10 years ago and is listed as follows. As the adjunct to this program, each candidate should provide at least 30 CME points each year as it is requested from the Croatian Chamber of Physicians in order to prolong his licence.

## 5. Program of specialisation in vascular surgery issued by the Ministry of Health, Republic of Croatia, 1994

During subspecialization in vascular surgery, the specialist in general surgery will spend: (a) at the vascular ward of the Department of Internal Medicine: 2 months; (b) at the vascular radiology ward with invasive diagnostics: 1 month; (c) at the transfusion ward: 1 month; (d) at the cardiosurgery ward: 1 month; (e) at the intensive care ward: 1 month; (f) at the Division (Department) of Vascular Surgery: 16 months.

Ad (a) At the vascular ward of the Department of Internal Medicine, the specialist is supposed to learn the pathophysiologic changes in blood vessel diseases, symptomatology and diagnosis, differential diagnosis and methods of conservative treatment.

Ad (b) At the vascular radiology ward, radiological diagnosis of blood vessels, as well as invasive diagnostic procedures, are supposed to be mastered.

Ad (c) At the transfusion ward, the specialist has to acquire the skills of basic transfusion diagnosis (blood grouping, cross-matching, Rh factors, etc.), autologous transfusion, storing blood for cardiovascular patients and intraoperative blood saving.

Ad (d) At the cardiovascular ward, the specialist is supposed to master the extracorporal circulation technique, haemodilution technique, hemoseparation and autotransfusion, the heart electrostimulation technique, and circulation supporting the guidelines for organ transplantation.

Ad (e) At the intensive care ward for vascular patients, endotracheal intubation, monitoring, instituting mechanical ventilation, basic recovery characteristics for anaesthesia, and resuscitation procedures are supposed to be mastered.

Ad (f) At the Division (Department) of Vascular Surgery, the specialist is supposed to master the following.

## 6. Theoretical aspects

### *6.1. General*

Armamentarium, the basic operative technique, vascular prosthesis, medical records, experimental vascular surgery.

### *6.2. Specialised*

Particular issues and assessment of vascular patients, arterial occlusive disease, aneurysms, cerebrovascular diseases, vascular diseases of the upper extremities, visceral arterial diseases, blood vessel injuries, venous diseases, arteriovenous fistulae, amputations, transplantation, and vascular surgery for sexual difficulties.

## 7. Practical aspects

(A) Prior to performing surgical procedures independently, the specialist has to assist vascular operations (25), independently prepare the operative field (from preparations to perivascular dissection (25), and administer sutures and arterial anastomoses (5).

(B) List and number of obligatory surgical procedures: carotid artery (3), thoracic outlet syndrome (3), abdominal aorta (aneurysm) (5), aortoiliacal region (12), femoropopliteal region (20), femorocrural region (10), visceral arteries (3), pulmonary thromboembolism (10), sympathectomies (10), injuries of the arteries and large veins (10), fasciotomies and amputations (10), extraanatomical bypass (5), varicose veins (20), prevention of pulmonary thromboembolism (2), and portal hypertension (2).

Total: 125 operations.

From a total of 125 surgical procedures, the candidate is supposed to perform 60% of them independently.

International Congress Series 1272 (2004) 292–293

www.ics-elsevier.com

# The status of vascular surgery in Cyprus

Nicos S. Angelides

*Department of Cardiovascular Surgery, Nicosia General Hospital, 6 Evangelistrias Street, 2057 Strovolos-Nicosia, Cyprus*

*Keywords:* Vascular surgery; Cyprus; Atherosclerosis

Atherosclerosis is a common disease in Cyprus. People eat well, smoke a lot and always use a car, even for very short distances! In other words, all factors predisposing to atherosclerosis are very high among the Cypriot population. Statistical analysis for coronary artery disease demonstrated that Cyprus has a significant problem with a need for more than 650 coronary bypass operations per million per year. Similarly, carotid artery disease, either symptomatic or asymptomatic, is very common and carotid endarterectomy shows a mean hospital value of 13 individuals per 100,000 population per year. Finally, it is estimated that 1050 patients per million per year suffer from critical limb ischaemia and are in need of urgent treatment.

As with any other specialization, vascular surgery in Cyprus is carried out either in the hospitals or in the private sector. The greatest majority of vascular examinations and operations are performed in the hospitals, which are governmental. All hospitals have the facility for non-invasive assessment, and this allows the patients to be scrutinised and to be referred mainly to the Nicosia General Hospital, which is the referral hospital in the capital of Cyprus. In this hospital, a well-developed and well-equipped vascular laboratory has been functioning since 1984. Cyprus, being a small island with a population of less than a million inhabitants, means that it is very difficult to "loose" patients in this environment. Patients come at regular intervals for a follow-up examination, which is carried out by the same personnel, allowing the ongoing observation of the natural history of the disease. Since 1984, 28,970 patients are on record in the Vascular Laboratory of the Nicosia General Hospital, with follow-up investigations going on up to 20 years. Smaller laboratories exist in the private sector and serve to scrutinise patients needing some form of further intervention and treatment.

Conventional angiography is carried out at the Nicosia General Hospital, while MR or spiral CT angiography is performed both in the hospitals and in the private sector. Since multifocal atherosclerosis is very common in Cyprus, there is always a tendency to

*E-mail address:* n_angelides@hotmail.com (N.S. Angelides).


doi:10.1016/j.ics.2004.04.073

investigate by non-invasive and invasive means the three most popular focuses of the disease, i.e. the carotids, the coronary arteries and the peripheral arteries.

Endovascular treatment has been performed since 1984. It includes the peripheral arteries, the coronary arteries, the thoracic and abdominal aorta, the subclavian arteries, the renal arteries and, more recently, the carotids. A team of doctors, including vascular surgeons, cardiologists, radiologists, nephrologists and specialized nurses, carries out these procedures. The results are within the standards, taking into consideration that there is always a reasonable selection of patients.

Surgery is carried out principally in the Nicosia General Hospital and in some private clinics. At Nicosia General, the first Vascular Department started functioning in 1978, and in 1989 this department was upgraded to a cardiovascular unit. Carotid surgery, coronary bypass surgery, peripheral vascular surgery and aortic surgery, above and below the diaphragm, are carried out with a referral of patients from all parts of Cyprus. In parallel, there are some specialized clinics in various towns of the island where cardiac surgery and limited vascular surgery are performed.

Training in vascular surgery has recently been undertaken at the Cardiovascular Unit of the Nicosia General Hospital. This training includes 3 years in General Surgery, 3 years in Vascular Surgery, 6 months in Thoracic Surgery and 6 months in Cardiac Surgery, ending with examinations for specialization. Throughout the whole of the training, the trainee has to keep a logbook of his/her experience, indicating whether he is the main operator or the assistant at a particular operation. Also, he has to keep a record of whether he was assisted with any particular operation by a more senior surgeon. He also has the opportunity to spend at least 1 year in research and can use the outcome of his research for an MD thesis.

Research in vascular surgery is carried out both in the hospitals and in the private sector. The vascular laboratory is a good source of material for research purposes and the Statistical Service of the Republic of Cyprus always ensures that the final results are produced in a scientific manner.

I would like to end this short analysis of the vascular background of Cyprus by using the words of Hippocrates that are very appropriate to the theme. "Life is short, the art long, opportunity fleeting, experience uncertain, and judgement difficult. The physician must be ready not only to do his duty but also to secure the cooperation of the patient, of the attendants and of externals."

International Congress Series 1272 (2004) 294–295

www.ics-elsevier.com

# Status of vascular surgery in the Czech Republic

Jan Marusiak*

*Department of Vascular and Reconstructive Surgery, Liberec General Teaching Hospital, Czech Republic*

**Abstract.** In the Czech Republic, there has been Czech Society for Cardiovascular Surgery, which has about 250 members. Vascular Surgery is the division/section and has its representatives in the Council of the Czech Society for Cardiovascular Surgery. Every surgeon after finishing studies has to have 2.5 years praxis in the hospital, after which he is allowed to pass exams and will get "1st degree of general surgery confirmation" which is obligatory. Then, if he wish to continue in the hospital, he needs to past the next exam—"2nd degree of general surgery confirmation", usually during next 5 years. It means when in hospital, after 7–8 years after the studies we have fully qualified and skilled general surgeons in the hospitals /common trunk/. 

*Keywords:* Vascular surgery

The Czech Society for Cardiovascular Surgery in the Czech Republic has about 250 members. Vascular Surgery is the division/section and has its Representatives in the Council of the Czech Society for Cardiovascular Surgery.

Every surgeon, after finishing studies, has to have 2.5 years praxis in the hospital, after which he is allowed to pass exams and will get a 1st degree of general surgery confirmation, which is obligatory. Then, if he wishes to continue in the hospital, he needs to pass the next exam, the 2nd degree of general surgery confirmation, usually during the next 5 years. This means, while working in hospital and after 7–8 years of study, we have fully qualified and skilled general surgeons in the hospitals /common trunk/.

In a parallel manner, after the first degree exam, if the general surgeon wishes only to do a vascular or cardiac speciality, he is allowed to do exams from vascular surgery or cardiac surgery directly. He needs to have practical and theoretical knowledge, and the exams are separated in two parts—theoretical and practical—during 2 days. The responsible authority is the Board for Cardiovascular Surgery and its examiners from university hospitals.

The number of skilled, graduated vascular surgeons is about 100 in 2003 in the Czech Republic.

* Tel.: +420-485-31-2243.
*E-mail address:* jan.marusiak@nemlib.cz (J. Marusiak).

0531-5131/ 
doi:10.1016/j.ics.2004.04.102

This is, in fact, acceptable only in very specialized departments in the country, meaning departments of Cardiovascular or Vascular Surgery, university or teaching hospitals. If a general surgeon wishes to do vascular cases in the Department of General Surgery, he needs first to pass the 2nd degree exam of general surgery confirmation and only then do exams from vascular surgery. Likewise, in university hospitals it is possible to do a PhD in the general or vascular surgery trunk and after scientific work, become a professor.

The main problem, generally speaking, is that surgeons spend many hours in the hospitals. For example, in departments with 135 beds—60 general surgery, 40 traumatology, 20 vascular surgery, 15 intensive care—every afternoon and all night there are three surgeons in the hospital, plus the other specialists on call.

Altogether, if we have 40 h per week as a normal working time, we serve from 15 to 55 h every week at night, in addition to specialists who are permanently on call. So, at present, it is hard to keep and respect the European directive of 48 h per week.

We need more surgeons and more specialists, many of whom are coming mainly from Eastern Europe, Slovakia, etc. On the other hand, our specialists try to be employed in Germany, Austria, the United Kingdom or Ireland, where hospitals also need more doctors to keep the 48 h directive.

According to our Vascular Surgery Register, there are about 8000 major vascular cases out of 10,000,000 inhabitants operated on per year.

Endovascular cases are dealt with mainly by interventional radiologists, but during the last several years the number of young vascular surgeons skilled in endovascular techniques has been increasing.

## 1. Summary

Czech Republic: 10,000,000 inhabitants
Common trunk: general surgery exams/
1. exam 2–3 years after finishing medical studies
2. exam 4–5 years after the 1st exam

Number of senior registrars in vascular surgery: 100
Specialization:
Vascular Surgery—3 years after 1st exam in general surgery
Cardiac Surgery—3 years after 1st exam in general surgery
The responsible authority for exams from vascular or cardiac surgery—Czech Society for Cardiovascular Surgery Scientific Board
The number of major vascular cases per year: 8000–10,000
The number of peripheral endovascular cases treated via interventional radiology: 6000.

International Congress Series 1272 (2004) 296–297

www.ics-elsevier.com

# Status of vascular surgery in Denmark

Jes Sandermann[a,*], Henrik Sillesen[b,1]

[a] *Vascular Surgery Unit, Viborg Hospital, 8800 Viborg, Denmark*
[b] *University Hospital Gentofte, DK 2900 Hellerup, Denmark*

*Keywords:* Vascular surgery

## 1. Aspects of vascular surgery in Denmark in 2003

Since 1983 vascular surgery has been a recognised subspecialty and from 1st of January 2004 it is a mono-speciality parallel to thoracic surgery, plastic and reconstructive surgery, urology and surgery. (Surgery covers what is not included under the first four mentioned surgical specialities and with surgical gastroenterology as a main part).

The basic structure of vascular surgery in Denmark is almost settled with nine major vascular units covering a population of more or less 500,000 inhabitants each, and the staff includes at least four to five vascular consultants/specialists. Five of the units have university status. All units can offer endovascular treatment during daytime and in many occasions also during call hours.

All vascular surgery is related to the vascular units and all vascular operations are performed by vascular surgeons. There are no angiologists in Denmark.

The main vascular task is evaluating patients with peripheral arterial disease and arterial reconstructions of which around 5500 primary procedures are performed annually—20% are endovascular.

A few years ago, venous surgery became related to vascular surgery in the sense that vascular specialists in general are responsible for making recommendations for treatment and performing the re-operations and complex cases. The vascular surgery units today do not have the capacity to perform all primary venous operations or the re-operations. Venous reconstruction is very rarely performed while venous thrombectomy has been replaced by thrombolyses (followed by endovascular treatment in two thirds of the cases), performed in one unit only with less than 25 cases a year.

The vascular surgeon is more and more recognised as a vascular specialist. Evaluating patients with peripheral arterial disease includes advice on lifestyle changes and pharmacological secondary prevention. In many cases of intermittent claudication, the effect of

* Corresponding author. Fax: +45-8927-3580
*E-mail addresses:* vskarjs@vibamt.dk (J. Sandermann), hens@gentoftehosp.kbhamt.dk (H. Sillesen).
[1] Fax: +45-3977-7674.


doi:10.1016/j.ics.2004.04.067

non-interventional measures has to be evaluated before surgical or endovascular intervention is considered. Thus, the vascular specialist has a central role in the total management of these patients. This leads to discussions on the infrastructure of the vascular units including training of doctors and involvement of specially trained nurses. In this setup, it is important to have a close relationship with medical areas such as cardiology, diabetology and nephrology together with dermatology, wound centres, orthopaedic surgeons, foot therapists, etc.

The new role of the vascular specialist demands more manpower. At the moment, serious lacks of applicants for surgical specialist training blocks are seen within all surgical areas. Our manpower prognosis goes towards qualification of five specialists in vascular surgery per year and aiming for 70–80 vascular specialists in Denmark.

This year all specialist training programmes in Denmark are being revised, and all the needed minimum competencies for specialist recognition have been defined thoroughly including learning strategies and evaluation methods. Besides the role of the medical expert in vascular surgery also areas such as communication, collaboration, health advocating, management, professionalism, academic attitude, etc. have been defined in the same way. Vascular surgical trainees in Denmark will, following the new training programme, also be educated in endovascular techniques. All this is based upon the conclusion of a Danish Specialist Commission report from May 2000, and many ideas seem to have come from Canada. The implementation is running 2003/2004 including coordination of the relationship to the other surgical specialities.

Whether this will have an impact on recruitment of new surgical candidates only the future can tell. Today, 60–70% of medical candidates from University are women. Having the five mentioned surgical mono-specialities, it might be an advantage for Vascular Surgery, as the on-call workload is low and most of the surgery is very delicate.

International Congress Series 1272 (2004) 298

www.ics-elsevier.com

# The status of vascular surgery in Finland

Mikael Railo

*HUCH, Department of Vascular Surgery, Meilahti Hospital, P.O. Box 340 (Haartmaninkatu 4), FIN-00029 HUS, Helsinki, Finland*

*Keywords:* Vascular surgery

Surgical training in vascular surgery in Finland is based on a 3-year period of common trunk training succeeded by a 3-year training in pure vascular surgery.

The training period also includes vascular physiology, 1–3 months; interventional radiology, 1–3 months; thorax-surgery, 6 months (either in the common trunk period or vascular period); optional plastic and reconstructive surgery, 1–3 months.

Weekly scientific meeting and teaching activity is 2–5 h/week.

Theory and teaching, 60 h (during the common trunk) and 80 h in vascular training period.

A logbook with at least 200 vascular surgical procedures partly as first assistant and partly as main surgeon. (A list of the procedures is available if needed.)

A national board examination is taken at the end of the vascular surgery training.

Literature required for the examination:

Rutherford R.B : Vascular surgery (Saunders)
Bernstein E.R.F: Noninvasive diagnostic techniques in vascular surgery (Mosby)
White R.A and Fogarty T.J.: Peripheral endovascular interventions (Mosby)

Three latest years publications of

Journal of Vascular Surgery
European Journal of Vascular and Endovascular Surgery
Phlebology

Working time for vascular trainees: Regular weekly working time is 38 h 15 min. Within the emergency-rota 3–4 times/month, each time 17 h. This makes 51-h weekly working time.

*E-mail address:* mikael.railo@hus.fi (M. Railo).


doi:10.1016/j.ics.2004.04.066

International Congress Series 1272 (2004) 299–303
www.ics-elsevier.com

# Status of vascular surgery in Germany

K. Balzer[a,*], P.C. Maurer[b]

[a] *Vascular Surgical Department, Evangelical Hospital, Wertgasse 30, D-45468 Mülheim/Ruhr, Germany*
[b] *Department of Vascular Surgery, Technical University of Munich, Munich, Germany*

*Keywords:* Vascular surgery

Vascular surgery in Germany has a long tradition, beginning at the turn of the last century with the names of Carrel and Jeger, who carried out fundamental experimental and surgical work for vascular surgical procedures. In the midst of the 1950s, there was a comet-like ascent of vascular surgery, as in other European countries. Yet, it still took another 20 years until it was accepted as an independent branch of surgery in 1978. The scientific society of vascular surgery in Germany was not founded until December 1984—as opposed to the German-speaking neighbor, Austria (1968). Fig. 1 shows the founding document of the German Society for Vascular Surgery. The declaration of the society was made during the traditional Munich vascular meeting under conspiring circumstances against the surgical establishment. Prof. Henner Müller-Wiefel, Duisburg, was elected as the first president. He served for two terms (Fig. 2). The initiator of this Munich meeting was the later president Prof. Peter Maurer (Fig. 3) After 4 years as the second president, Prof. Henning Loeprecht, Augsburg, was elected, followed by Prof. Hans-Martin Becker, Munich (in Fig. 4 together with the first Treasurer, Prof. Hugo Tiemann, right). Unfortunately, these three founding members, who were fighting for an independent Vascular Surgery, died too early. We miss them, not only because of their important work for our society, but mostly because of their humanity.

The president is elected for 2 years, the secretary for 3 years. The Board of the German Society for Vascular Surgery consists of nine members. Several commissions, i.e. for education, scientific research, certification of vascular centers, presentation of the Society on the Internet, quality assurance, etc. are doing an excellent job.

Over the years, there has been a controversy as to whether vascular surgical procedures belong to the methods applied in the independent disciplines of cardiac, thoracic and vascular surgery or should be considered a subspecialty of general surgery. Until today, vascular surgical procedures have been performed in clinics of cardiac surgery. Post-

* Corresponding author. Tel.: +49-208-309443.
*E-mail address:* klaus.balzer@evkmh.de (K. Balzer).


doi:10.1016/j.ics.2004.04.081

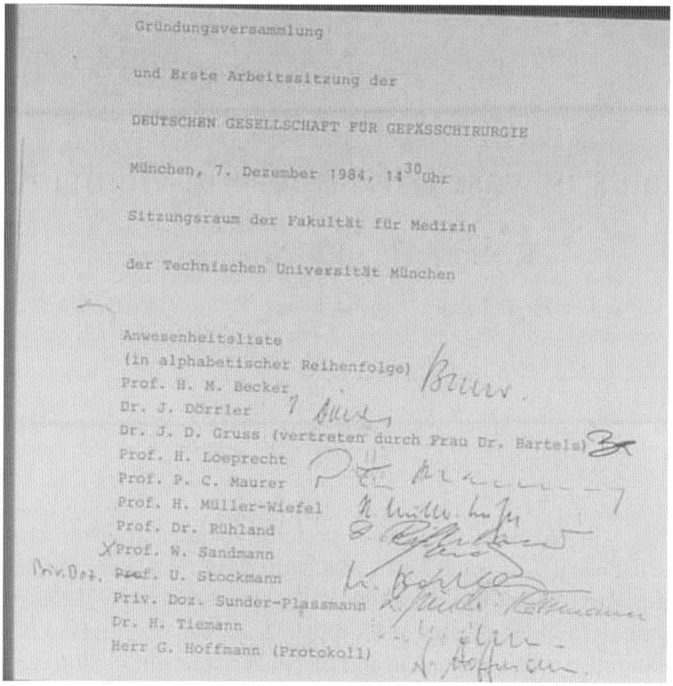

Gründungsversammlung

und Erste Arbeitssitzung der

DEUTSCHEN GESELLSCHAFT FÜR GEFÄSSCHIRURGIE

München, 7. Dezember 1984, 14$^{30}$ Uhr

Sitzungsraum der Fakultät für Medizin

der Technischen Universität München

Anwesenheitsliste
(in alphabetischer Reihenfolge)
Prof. H. M. Becker
Dr. J. Dörrler
Dr. J. D. Gruss (vertreten durch Frau Dr. Bartels)
Prof. H. Loeprecht
Prof. P. C. Maurer
Prof. H. Müller-Wiefel
Prof. Dr. Rühland
Prof. W. Sandmann
Priv.Doz. ~~Prof.~~ U. Stockmann
Priv. Doz. Sunder-Plassmann
Dr. H. Tiemann
Herr G. Hoffmann (Protokoll)

Fig. 1. Founding document of the German Society for Vascular Surgery.

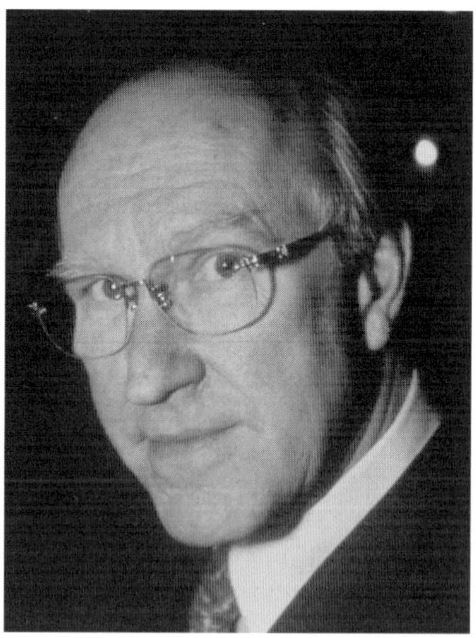

Fig. 2. The first president Professor Henner Müller-Wiefel.

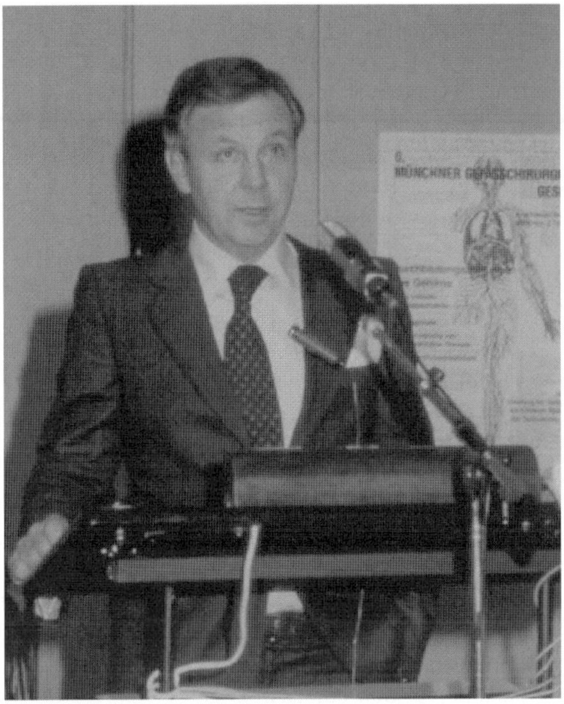

Fig. 3. The initiator of the Munich vascular meeting, which is celebrating its 25th anniversary in December 2003.

graduate education in vascular surgery is possible based only on general surgery. A catalogue of surgical procedures performed within a period of 3 years is required, including not only a number of clearly defined diagnostic means, but surgical procedures, graded according to their anatomic location and performed independently under the

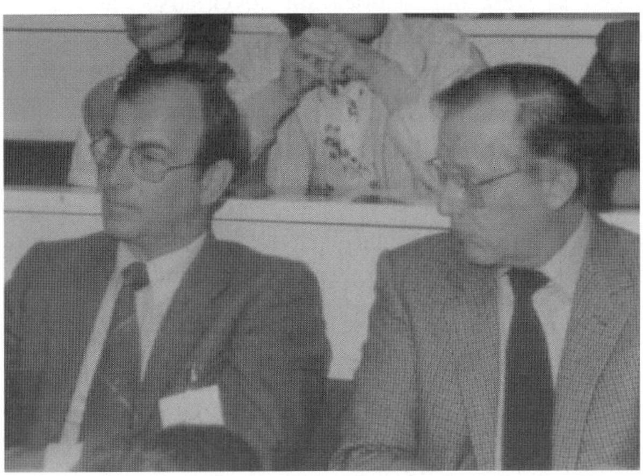

Fig. 4. Professor Hans-Martin Becker, third president (left), and the first treasurer Professor Hugo Tiemann (right).

supervision of a vascular specialist. To be authorized to offer postgraduate training in vascular surgery for a period of 3 years, the vascular specialist must be head of a clinic with a minimum number of surgical procedures performed. After the specialty board has assessed the clinic, the number of operations and the curriculum vitae, the surgeon may receive authorization for a training program in the subspecialty, which can last from half a year up to 3 years. Requirements of certification are conventional surgical procedures, as well as endovascular operations and interventions, which are the standard routine of the vascular surgeon. Irrespective of being part of another clinic, postgraduate training in vascular surgery can only take place in a department of this subspecialty.

Even nowadays, the existence of an independent department of vascular surgery in a clinic is not a rule. Moreover, certified surgeons in cardiac or general surgical clinics perform vascular surgical procedures. It is true for more than half of the clinics, which provide training programs. However, the trend is to establish independent clinics of vascular surgery with qualified leaders.

In the Federal Republic of Germany with a population of ca. 80 million, there are approximately 100 independent vascular surgery clinics, which serve the areas with different population density. It is believed that in about 300 clinics of general or cardiac surgery, vascular operations are actually being performed. Because the exact number of vascular surgical beds is not known, only a rough estimate is possible. In densely populated areas, the number is certainly higher than in rural regions. Altogether, about 2.5 vascular surgery beds per 10,000 citizens exist.

To control the treatment quality of carotid surgeries, we have a national register in Germany with more than 65,000 patients, which proves excellent results. Registers for surgery of abdominal aortic aneurysms, varicose veins and the percutaneous transluminal angioplasties were developed in recent years. Altogether, a high level of surgical quality is available in Germany.

We are experiencing problems with a new reimbursement system, the DRG classification created in Australia. It does not cover costs for expensive vascular and endovascular procedures and for the treatment of multilevel diseases. This may lead to a more restrictive treatment of our patients and a decreasing number of surgeries and interventions.

In cooperation with the Austrian and Swiss Society of Vascular Surgery, the German Society of Vascular Surgery is editing the scientific magazine *Gefaesschirurgie* in German and English.

After vascular surgery has established itself well apart from its “mother disciplines”, there is nowadays a rivalry between it and interventionally treating disciplines such as radiology, angiology and cardiology. Development of endovascular and/or interventional techniques leads to a tremendous change in the spectrum of vascular surgical treatment. Not to give away the competence for these modern techniques, they are part of new postgraduate training program. To withstand the pressure of competition, the three disciplines dealing with the treatment of vascular diseases were combined in Germany in a vascular surgery center: vascular surgery for operative and combined procedures (interventional and surgical), interventional radiology and angiology for conservative therapy of vascular disease. The section of angiology can be represented by specially trained medical consultants, as occasionally a vascular surgeon may be practicing conservative treatment, depending on education and background.

In a center of vascular surgery, not only the above-mentioned specialists should work together productively as a team. Doctors practicing other disciplines like neurology, nephrology, cardiology and general surgery, and physicians treating vascular diseases in a practice, should be assigned to such a center. Therefore, a modern center of vascular surgery is characterized by competent teamwork of qualified colleagues. The German Society of Vascular Surgery has developed a list of requirements to be met by the center. A committee member evaluates those clinics, applying for certification. The board will grant the qualification for 3 years.

Vascular surgery has not only developed into an independent specialty, but completely changed its spectrum in the last years. It is a leader in a general development that can also be expected for other disciplines. Under the term "center of excellence", it ensures competent treatment of different organic systems. In case of vascular surgery, it means comprehensive therapy of all arterial and venous diseases in view of conservative, interventional and surgical therapeutic methods. Because of the demographic factor with increasing aging of the population, we do not have to worry about the future of our specialty.

International Congress Series 1272 (2004) 304–307

www.ics-elsevier.com

# Status of vascular surgery in Greece

C.D. Liapis[a,*], M.K. Lazarides[b]

[a]*Department of Vascular Surgery, UEMS Division and Board of Vascular Surgery, Athens University Medical School, Athens, Greece*
[b]*Department of Vascular Surgery, Democritus University of Alexandroupolis of Thrace, Greece*

## 1. Introduction

Vascular surgery became an independent specialty in Greece in 1989. As is the case with all medical specialties, residency training is under governmental control. Accreditation of training centers is held on an annual basis through the Greek Ministry of Health and Social Welfare following documentation of caseload, teaching records and research activity.

Junior doctors, following graduation from medical school, have to serve for 1 year in a rural area as general practitioners incorporated into the National Health System. Training in vascular surgery requires a 3-year fellowship in general surgery. After completion of the common trunk training, trainees are eligible for higher surgical training in 1 of 14 centers accredited for training in vascular surgery.

The duration of training in vascular surgery is 4 years. The fourth year of training consists of a rotation in cardiac surgery and thoracic surgery, as well. While the whole training period is 7 years, with the inclusion of time lost in waiting lists, the average duration is nearly 10 years. Trainees who have completed the 7-year fellowship are assessed by logbook evaluation and examined viva voce by a three-member committee authorized by the Central Council of Health.

## 2. An update of current status in vascular surgery training

Researchers from vascular units in two university hospitals have conducted a nationwide survey on the current status of training in vascular surgery. Since there is no vascular registry in Greece, data were obtained by direct contact with all 14 vascular units accredited for training during a 1-year period. The survey was performed in the form of a questionnaire addressed to all vascular departments querying the number of trainers, trainees, operations performed in total and per trainee. Data from vascular units dedicated to private practice or those within army hospitals, or units with no accreditation in training, were not included in the query.

* Corresponding author. Tel.: +30-210-7456128; fax: +30-210-6847949.
*E-mail address:* ics1272@hotmail.com (C.D. Liapis).


doi:10.1016/j.ics.2004.04.086

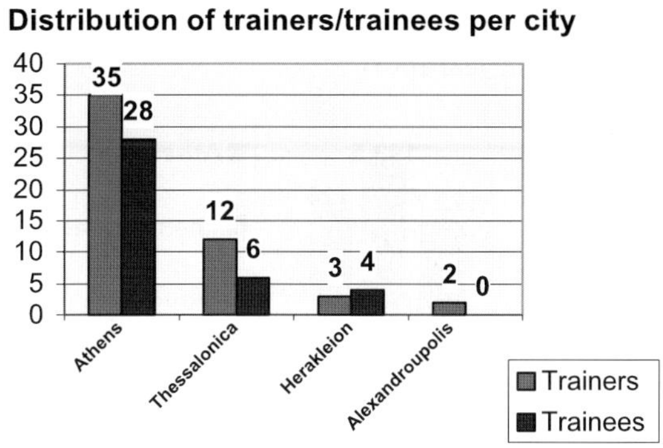


Fig. 1. The geographical distribution of trainers/trainees.

Between January 1st and December 31st 2001, 5315 operations were performed in the aforementioned training centers. Most of these centers are in Athens (nine) and Thessalonica (three). The majority of the units are in academic hospitals as well. A number of 52 trainers and 38 trainees were recorded as serving in the participating vascular centers during the study period. Trainers were either professors, members of the faculty of medical schools in university hospitals, or consultants and non-consultant specialists dedicated to the Greek National Health System. The mean age of trainees was 34.5 years (range 32–39).

The ratio of trainers per trainee was 1.4:1. Fig. 1 depicts the geographical distribution of trainers/trainees. As Greece has a population of approximately 10.5 million, the ratio of vascular trainees/million population was 3.6.

An average of 380 vascular operations (elective and emergency procedures) was performed per center/year. Fig. 2 illustrates the geographical distribution of operations held per city/year. A total of 140 operations were held per trainee/year. Fig. 3 denotes the average number of surgical exposures per trainee/year, while Fig. 4 depicts the relevant caseload performed per trainee/year according to type of vascular unit (academic vs. district).

## 3. Areas of concern

A number of hot topics have been raised following this survey. Since training and certification in vascular surgery are under governmental control, the number of trainees

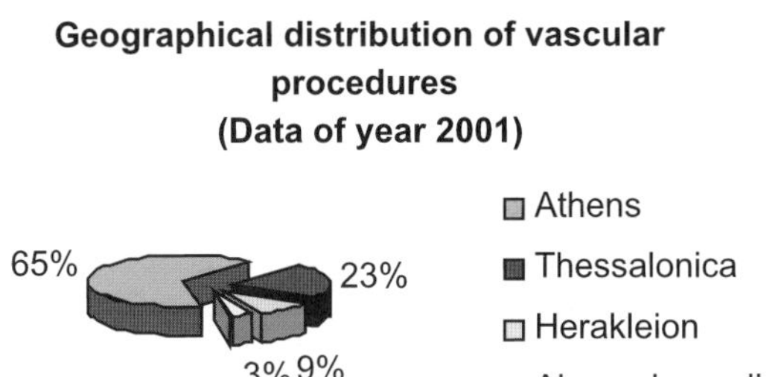


Fig. 2. The geographical distribution of vascular procedures performed in the year 2001.

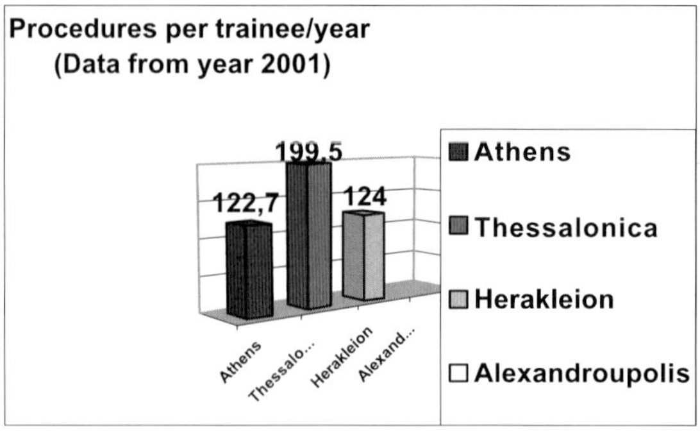


Fig. 3. Surgical exposure per trainee/year.

seems to be greater than the demand for vascular surgeons nationwide. This is in contrast to the need for high-quality training.

An adequate number of vascular procedures are performed in vascular centers each year. However, not all hospital programmes have successfully added an endovascular surgery component to their training protocols, while percutaneous interventional techniques have not been adopted in the majority of training units' disciplines. Moreover, no system of peer-review has been set in order to provide quality standards for higher surgical training.

Trainees, according to law restrictions, are not allowed to act as principal surgeons if not assisted by a scrubbed trainer. This limitation seems inappropriate for a training programme focusing on self-confident surgeons. In addition, young Greek vascular surgeons may have difficulties meeting the eligibility criteria for the European Board of Surgery Qualifications in Vascular Surgery Assessments.

The weaknesses of the training programme in vascular surgery are well recognized by the Greek Society for Vascular Surgery, and currently all professional bodies are pressing for harmonization in vascular training among European countries. We do hope that the

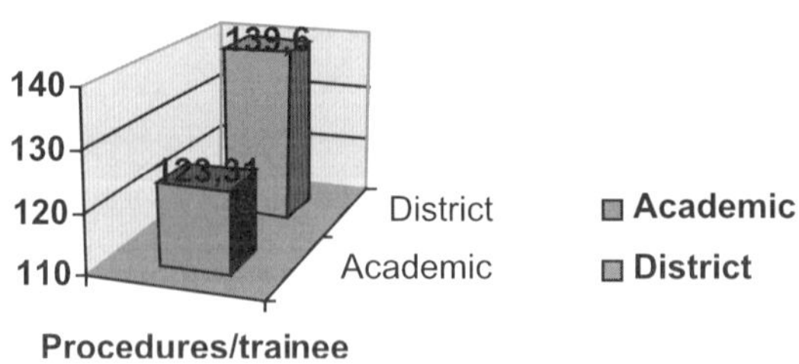


Fig. 4. Vascular procedures performed per trainee/year depending on type of vascular unit.

European Division and Board of Vascular Surgery will undertake a more active role towards high-quality training on our continent.

## Acknowledgements

We thank Dr. E.A. Tzortzis, Research Associate, Athens, Greece, who kindly contributed to the preparation of the manuscript. Data included in this paper were presented at the 2002 ESVS meeting held in Istanbul, Turkey.

International Congress Series 1272 (2004) 308–311

www.ics-elsevier.com

# Status of vascular surgery in Hungary

Attila Nemes[a], Zsolt Antal Varga[b,*]

[a] *National Institute for Vascular Surgery, Budapest, Hungary*
[b] *Tolna County Hospital, Hungary*

**Abstract.** Health Care in Hungary is almost exclusively provided by the National Health Service. The National Health Insurance Bureau finances health care providers retrospectively according to their accomplishment. Health care expenditure in Hungary was only 5.7% of the GDP in 2000, decreasing year by year, while in most European Countries this measure is around 7%. This is unacceptably low keeping in mind that the price of modern diagnostics and treatment is rising and we pay the same price as more developed countries. On top of this financial situation, the Hungarian health status is one of the worst in Europe. Life expectancy is approximately 10 years lower than in Europe (71.7 years) and cardiovascular mortality is higher than in most European countries. © 2004 Published by Elsevier B.V.

*Keywords:* Vascular surgery

Vascular Surgery as an independent sub-speciality has more than 20 years of tradition in Hungary. First Fellowship exam was held in 1980, when approximately 40 Honorary Diploma of Speciality Certificates were also issued. This core of specialists provided the further training and made possible the development of a national network. The National Institute for Vascular Surgery was established in 1982 and by that time a national network of vascular surgery was also built mainly on the basis of the county hospitals. The National Institute for Vascular Surgery keeps a hand on training, on examination and—based on the yearly statistics on vascular surgery's performance nationwide—on the development of the services. Between 1982 and 1996 there was an independent College of Vascular Surgery. Since 1996 Vascular Surgery is only represented in the College of General Surgery and there are only three Vascular Surgeons out of the 23 representatives. This change has had a major negative influence on respect of our speciality and also possibly influence on the decision makers as far as finance, future trends and acknowledgement of this important speciality is concerned.

Currently, there are approximately 180 Vascular Surgeons registered in our country but only 80 specialists take part in everyday practice, performing reconstructive vascular operations regularly. According to the National Health Statistics presently there are 578 hospital beds dedicated to Vascular Surgery and there are 42 Departments or Sections of

* Corresponding author. 42 Domosclo it, Budapest 1037, Hungary. Tel.: +36-1-250-6582.
*E-mail address:* drvzs@vnet.hu (A. Nemes).


doi:10.1016/j.ics.2004.04.068

Vascular Surgery who report any vascular surgical procedures to the National Institute. The major workload however comes only from less than 30 Departments or Sections. These are the six University Departments of the four Medical Faculties, 19 County Hospitals and some Departments from major capital hospital departments.

Vascular Surgery is a second qualification in Hungary based on General Surgical qualification. In the main trunk of General Surgery, there is a 6-month training period of Vascular Surgery. To be eligible for sitting the Fellowship Exam in Vascular Surgery 2 years experience in a recognised Vascular Centre expected after taking the Fellowship Exam in General Surgery. According to the department (quality and quantity of vascular operations, diagnostic facilities) from which the candidate is coming, the National Institute for Vascular Surgery can request the candidate to spend up to 6 months in the National Institute to broaden and deepen experience and knowledge in the whole spectrum of Vascular Surgery. As far as the operative experience is concerned participating in 200 reconstructive vascular operations as an assistant and performing 80 such as first the operator under various degrees of supervision would be requested as eligibility criteria.

As mentioned, an annual report is requested from each and every department where vascular surgery is performed to be sent to the National Institute for Vascular Surgery. On the basis of this information, experts from the National Institute and from centres of excellence take part in legislation with the National Health Insurance Bureau. This ad hoc body quantifies the central expenditure on the individually financed prosthesis (ringed PTFE, bifurcated grafts, stent grafts, homografts) and decides how this assigned to different departments. On the basis of this annual report these are the indicator procedures performed in Hungary:

| Carotid reconstruction | | | |
|---|---|---|---|
| | 2000 | 2001 | 2002 |
| Number | 2006 | 2020 | 2100 |
| Neurologic deficit | 1.5% | 1.3% | 1.2% |
| Mortality | 1.3% | 1.5% | 1.3% |

A rough estimation shows that in 2002 there were 200, and in 2003 there will be 500 carotid endovascular interventions performed in Hungary.

| Open AAA reconstruction ruptured | | | |
|---|---|---|---|
| | 2000 | 2001 | 2002 |
| Number | 81 | 76 | 85 |
| Mortality | 38% | 40% | 32% |

| Open AAA reconstruction elective | | | |
|---|---|---|---|
| | 2000 | 2001 | 2002 |
| Number | 454 | 463 | 480 |
| Mortality | 8% | 6% | 6% |

It should be noted that the first endovascular AAA repair was performed in 1998. Since then, 110 endovascular treatments were performed for thoracic (30) and abdominal aortic aneurysms.

| Femoro-popliteal and infrapopliteal reconstruction | | | |
|---|---|---|---|
| | 2000 | 2001 | 2002 |
| Together | 2102 | 2089 | 2120 |
| Venous | 1260 | 1212 | 1335 |
| Crural | 653 | 687 | 692 |

| Major amputation | | | |
|---|---|---|---|
| | 2000 | 2001 | 2002 |
| All together | 4760 | 4860 | 4820 |
| without angiography | 2760 | 3013 | 3212 |

It should be mentioned that a more detailed national registry is being introduced on carotid, AAA and infrapopliteal reconstruction. This registry is a PC-based system and data entered can be traced on the basis of the national insurance number. On the basis of this, quality and quantity can be more closely monitored on national and departmental level. Participation is voluntary. However, data are going to have an influence on the financing. Therefore, it can be expected that nearly all centres are participating.

Since 1996 there is no independent College of Vascular Surgery in Hungary. The Hungarian Society of Angiology and Vascular Surgery therefore has a crucial role in regulation and professional decision making. The Society itself shows the close cooperation of angiologists, interventional radiologists and vascular surgeons as every speciality is represented in the Society and in the Council as well. According to a survey in 1998 however there are only 14 hospitals where a Vascular Unit (radiology, angiology, surgery) exists and works. Angiology is not an independent, accepted sub-speciality but on the basis of experience and knowledge a specialist in angiology is granted by the College of Internal Medicine.

Vascular Surgeons in Hungary are not as highly academic as in UK for instance. There are two Doctors of Science and 15 PhD degree holders among us.

On the basis of the information provided in this summary of Hungarian Vascular Surgery it can be concluded and summarised that we work within very difficult circumstances as there is a high prevalence of cardiovascular morbidity and mortality; there is a very low level of finance (5.7% of GDP) and there are many financial anomalies (primary amputation has higher reimbursement than crural reconstruction) in spite of the continuous efforts made to change this. Despite difficulties we have our place in Europe. Hungary is one of the first where Vascular Surgery has been accepted as an independent sub-speciality, indicator procedures are performed on a very high level of efficacy and Hungarian Vascular Surgeons have a great reputation in Europe and in the USA. We should not be satisfied as we still have many things to do. We should build up a much closer cooperation with vascular radiologists and angiologists, and follow the international trends of ideally invasive surgery and make these techniques more widely available nationwide. Although there has been a national network of vascular surgery in Hungary for more than 20 years, the quality of service should be more evenly distributed and a nationwide quality control system introduced.

International Congress Series 1272 (2004) 312–313

www.ics-elsevier.com

# Status of vascular surgery in Ireland

Dermot Moore

*Department of Vascular Surgery, St James's Hospital, Dublin 8, Ireland*

*Keywords:* Vascular surgery

Vascular surgery in Ireland remains an integral part of the general surgical discipline. However, new techniques, and especially the use of endovascular devices, are increasing a trend towards the development of an independent speciality. At a recent meeting of the Irish Association of Vascular Surgeons (IAVS), this issue was debated and further attempts are to be made within the Irish medical community to establish Vascular Surgery as a pure specialty. Vascular surgery is considered a subspecialty within General Surgery in the training college, the Royal College of Surgeons in Ireland (RCSI), but the specialty of Vascular Surgery is not recognised by the Irish Medical Council, which is the overall regulatory authority.

Training in Vascular Surgery is very much akin to the UK model. Following a year of internship, the junior doctor proceeds with basic surgical training (BST) on an approved scheme monitored by the RCSI. At the end of 2 years, the junior doctors are examined by the college (AFRCSI).

Once this exam has been passed, the trainee spends a further 1 to 2 years as a junior registrar either in Ireland, the United Kingdom or occasionally in the United States. During this period they are expected to conduct research and publish in surgical journals and will probably start an MD or MCH thesis. After 2 years, they are eligible to apply for the RCSI higher surgical training scheme (HST), which provides 6 years of training in recognised Senior Registrar posts throughout the country. If the candidate shows an inclination or interest in vascular surgery, he or she may apply to rotate through at least two of the approved vascular posts as Senior Registrar. These posts are regularly assessed by the Joint Surgical Accreditation Committee (SAC) to ensure that the experience, teaching and training facilities are up to the standard expected by the training college. There are approximately 12 such approved posts in the country at any one time. Not all of the trainees in post will be designated as vascular surgeons and, on occasion, doctors may hold the posts from countries outside the EU who are not appointed to the approved HST scheme. At the end of 6 years, the trainee sits an exit examination and may declare the speciality interest of Vascular Surgery at that time.

*E-mail address:* prospecthse@hotmail.com (D. Moore).

0531-5131/
doi:10.1016/j.ics.2004.04.071

Consultant posts are advertised by hospitals looking for candidates who are qualified General Surgeons with a specialist interest in vascular surgery. Candidates are expected to have at least 2 years of training in the speciality of vascular surgery. In practice, all trainee appointments to consultant posts have had more than 3 years of training. At this moment, there are fewer than 25 surgeons who profess an interest in vascular surgery and, of these, only seven are pure vascular surgeons in the sense that they do not participate in a general surgical on-call rota.

The Irish Association of Vascular Surgeons (IAVS) is the official professional body, which meets on a number of occasions throughout the year, and is in the process of organising and coordinating the views and aspirations of vascular surgeons. It was responsible for drawing up a document with Comhairle na nOspideal (appointments committee for hospital consultants) making recommendations adapted from the Vascular Surgical Society's document in the United Kingdom. The purpose of the document was to set guidelines for the appointment of Vascular Surgeons and to recommend establishment of regional referral centres with a minimum of three vascular surgeons serving a population of 750,000 people. Many of the document's recommendations have been implemented, but significant deficiencies remain.

Endovascular surgery is still in its infancy in Ireland. Most vascular surgical centres carry out endovascular interventions, which are primarily carried out by interventional radiologists. A small but growing number of vascular surgeons have taken on this skill and are carrying out interventions in an operating room setting. One centre has an established and dedicated surgical, endovascular theatre with state-of-the art imaging equipment and is equipped to be a full operating theatre.

International Congress Series 1272 (2004) 314–317

www.ics-elsevier.com

# Status of vascular surgery in Italy

Fabrizio Benedetti-Valentini*

*Via Cassiodoro 6, 00193 Rome, Italy*

At present in Italy, vascular surgery (VS) is a rapidly evolving specialty spreading over the national territory. Established by law as an autonomous specialty since some 30 years ago, it was not really so for a long period of time, being held subservient to general surgery or cardiac surgery both in the universities and in civic and community hospitals. At that time, development was slow and research restricted to a few centres. Some legacy of that past still remains and burdens VS, sometimes heavily, but things are improving at a good pace.

There are now 28 Chairs of VS in the School of Medicine of universities with a first Class Professor, each with a service or a division of VS, that means between 12 and 25 beds per unit. There are 79 Civic Hospital Centres of VS with beds varying from 6 to 40 depending on the size of the hospital, the size of the affluent territory, the trend of the hospital towards specialties and so forth. Some are excellent, working at the highest international standards, while some are much less so and leave much to be desired. Most are at a good level, measuring it by European criteria. The overall number of beds is definitely sufficient; what is lacking often and particularly in some centres is a reasonably fast turnover. This is not due to the surgeons, but to insufficient service and supporting activities; obtaining investigations, when they are not done in the vascular unit, take a long time; operating time allotted is too short due to shortage of personnel and a variety of unions quarrelling; and intensive care units are small and few, so that in some centres the place must be "booked" in advance for planned operations and may lack for emergencies. Possibly, we should close some centres and improve some others.

We have so many training centres in VS in Italy today where the title of Specialist in Vascular Surgery is obtained. All of them belong to the universities. Fewer and better seems reasonable and we are working in that direction with the Ministry of Health, the Ministry of Education and the National University Council. There are at present 36 Schools of Specialization (or training centres) in VS (Fig. 1, and theoretically they should enroll altogether some 45–50 trainees per year [1]. They are full-time and receive a grant [2]. However, their number sometimes double since it is possible to enroll as trainees, doctors already working, and paid, in some other unit of the National Health System; most of the time, they do not move from their working place and get involved only marginally

* Tel.: +39-6-490255; fax: +39-6-49970230.
*E-mail address:* chvs.rm@flashnet.it (F. Benedetti-Valentini).


doi:10.1016/j.ics.2004.04.088

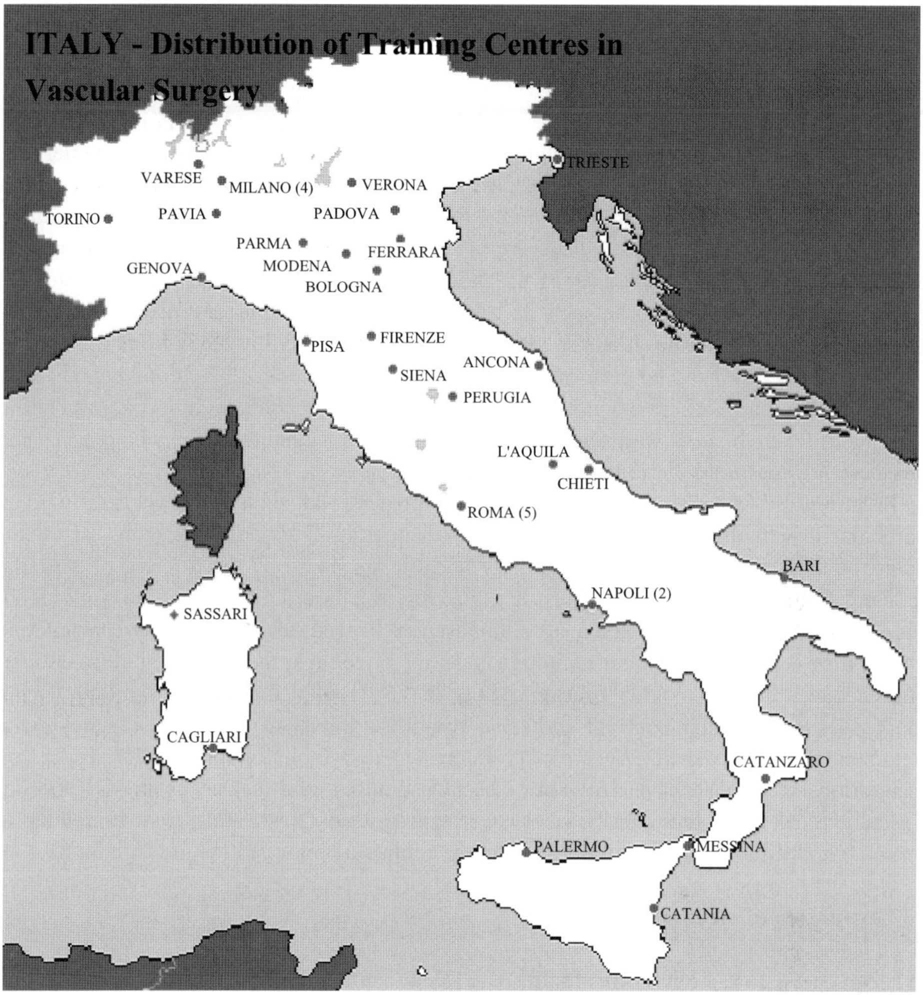


Fig. 1. Distribution of training centres in vascular surgery in Italy. Training centres directed by general surgeons are in Milan (1 out of 4), Verona (1), Ferrara (1), Ancona (1), Chieti (1), Rome (1 out of 5), and Catanzaro (1). In Rome, one training centre is directed by a cardiac surgeon.

in the training programme. This is the easiest way for general surgery units to grow their own homemade vascular surgeons.

Moreover, 28 training centres are directed by Professors of Vascular Surgery, while 8 (22%—1 out of 5) are still directed by General Surgeons (7) or Cardiac Surgeons [1] who are involved only occasionally in VS. They even lack a university unit of VS (6) and in 3 of them there is no vascular surgeon on the teaching faculty. It is difficult to explain this to outsiders, but it is possibly due to some old laws of ours, and it is sad to say that some academic bodies tolerated this to happen. Great effort is being done to correct such misdeeds and I am sure that such a goal will be reached, although with time.

On the other side, the seriously managed training centres run at a high standard and produce excellent professionals.

For many years, there have been laws in Italy setting "European" standards for specialist training in most Specialties and VS is one of them [3,4]. For instance, the number of diagnostic, surgical and endovascular procedures requested per trainee per year is practically the same as that requested for the EBSQ-VASC. It should be explicit that: (1) endovascular procedures are included in the requirements for the specialist training and (2) there is a basic training in general surgery (a kind of common trunk) within the training in vascular surgery. This training is of 12 months duration and can be divided into two periods of 6 months each to be spent in two different departments and distributed during the first 2 years of training. It is also stated by law and precised by regulations the number and type of operations to be performed as first aid or first operator. The good centres meet no difficulties and usually do not accept trainees over a certain number, some centres struggle to reach the goal, and some others possibly do not even try. Others have too many trainees and, presumably, training is mostly on paper.

Relationships with the other scientific and/or professional societies are generally good, particularly with the two major angiological associations. Vascular surgeons sit on the board of the Italian Society of Angiology and on the board of the Society of Vascular Investigations and Diagnosis. They are also on the board of the Italian College of Phlebology. A permanent Forum of Endovascular Procedures is very active promoting cooperation with interventional radiologists. In many centres, there is fairly close cooperation between the angiological units and those of VS. However, there is still a long way to the desirable "vascular centres," where a multidisciplinary approach to diagnosis and treatment can be reached. We are very interested and look forward to the works and suggestions of the Working Group for Vascular Centres, just formed by the Division of Vascular Surgery of the UEMS, because it will give us fresh ideas and guidelines to promote and drive the constitution of vascular centres as pilot centres in our country.

## 1. Our points of strength

(1) An acceptable number of highly qualified centres both in university and civic hospitals, working at high standards in classical vascular surgery, endovascular procedures and mininvasive and/or laparoscopic methods. They are also developing significant scientific research, including national and international trials and clinical investigation programmes.

(2) SICVE (Italian Society of Vascular and Endovascular Surgery), our young but very active scientific–professional society, which is involved in all of the most important problems to date; Continuing Medical Education (CME), a national programme of various activities promoted in cooperation with the governmental agency; registry of all vascular and endovascular procedures carried out in all vascular surgical centres; negotiations with the Ministry of Health and other government authorities on the status of the Surgical Specialist in the incoming restructuring of the National Health System and Profession.

(3) Progressive establishment of Vascular Surgery as an autonomous specialty, separated from general surgery and cardiac surgery, both in universities and in civic hospitals.

This comes from laws and regulations obtained from the Government, Health Agencies and the National University Council, correcting, though slowly, many liabilities of the past.

## 2. Our points of weakness

(1) Significant disparities in the standards of the centres of vascular surgery concerning organization, equipment, number of patients and quality of performances. The causes are mainly historical (centres growing out of general surgery being usually the weakest) or resting with regional or local mismanagement.
(2) Inadequate training of the specialists coming from a certain number of training centres. Possibly some of them are skirting the rules and, quite obviously, they cannot involve regularly the trainees in important basic procedures that they are doing only occasionally or not at all! This emphasizes the need for further and in-depth control both at the national and European level.
(3) Feuding between university and civic hospital vascular surgeons. On one side, this is fanned by a few, old fashioned academics trying to refuse teaching positions to excellent and highly valued hospital vascular surgeons; on the other side, there is a bad trend to exclude from the management of civic hospital units very esteemed professionals coming from the university.

Osmosis is needed, but it is hard to come by and will take some time.

## 3. Final assessment

The quality and trends of development of vascular surgery in Italy are overall good at present. Much work remains to be done, particularly in the fields of training and regulations. Standards of professional performance are rapidly and definitely improving.

## References

[1] D.M. Sanità, 20/4/2001 Gazz. Uff. Rep. Ital. n. 292, 17 dec. 2001.
[2] D. Lgv., 257, 8/8/1991 Gazz. Uff. Rep. Ital. n. 191, 16 aug. 1999.
[3] D. Lgv., 368, 17/8/1999 (Eur. Directive 93/16/CEE) Gazz. Uff. Rep. Ital. n. 187/L, 23 oct. 1999.
[4] D. MURST, 5/5/1997 Art. 44 Tab. B Gazz. Uff. Rep. Ital. n. 139, 17 june 1997.

International Congress Series 1272 (2004) 318

www.ics-elsevier.com

# Status of vascular surgery in Luxembourg

Patrick Berg*

*Centre Hospitalier de Luxembourg 4, rue Barblé L-1210, Luxembourg*

The population of Luxembourg is about 450,000. Hospital treatment is performed in nine hospitals or clinics, five of which are principal hospitals. Most of the physicians are working in private practice, even in hospitals; only in one hospital physicians are employed.

Training of vascular surgeons is made abroad because of the nonexistence of a university hospital in our country. The recognized diploma in Luxembourg corresponds to the diploma of the respective country of the university they attended.

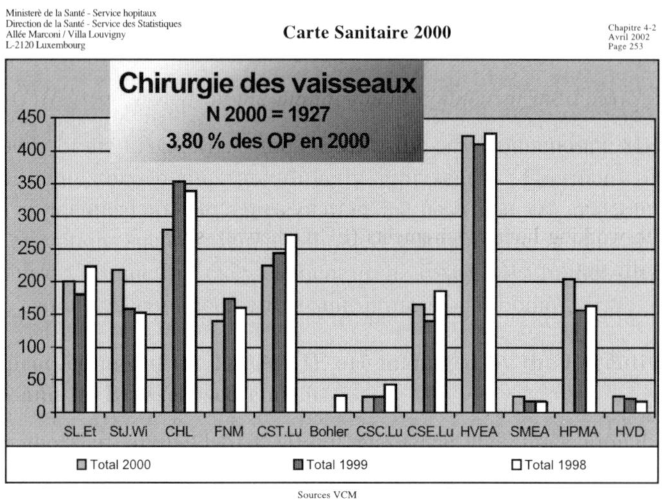


The level of competence is equal to other European centers, performed by well-qualified general surgeons having mostly the subspeciality in vascular surgery.

In the year 2000, 1927 vascular procedures were performed in Luxembourg [1].

The Luxembourg Association for Vascular Surgery contains 17 members.

The Luxembourg vascular surgeons hope that the Division and Board of Vascular Surgery will obtain the formation of a Section of Vascular Surgery within the UEMS. The European Board of Surgery Qualification in Vascular Surgery could help in harmonizing the differences existing in the different European countries and could permit to obtain an equivalent diploma in each country that would be recognized in Luxembourg.

## Reference

[1] Carte Sanitaire 2000. Publ. 15/02/2002. Health Ministry Luxembourg. http://www.etat.lu/MS/.

* Department of Vascular Surgery, Centre Hospitalier de Luxembourg, 4, rue Barblé, L-1210 Luxembourg. Tel.: +35-2-4411-6382; fax: +35-2-4411-6274.


doi:10.1016/j.ics.2004.05.088

International Congress Series 1272 (2004) 319–321

www.ics-elsevier.com

# Status of vascular surgery in The Netherlands

J. Hajo van Bockel[a,*], J.D. Blankensteijn[b]

[a] *Department of Vascular Surgery, Leiden University Medical Centre, P.O. Box 9600, 2300 RC Leiden, The Netherlands*

[b] *Division of Vascular Surgery, University Medical Centre Nijmegen, Nijmegen, The Netherlands*

**Abstract.** In the Netherlands, vascular surgery is not a monospecialty. Vascular interventions are performed by general surgeons with an interest and additional training in vascular surgery. The Dutch Society for Vascular Surgery was founded in 1981, is stimulating and coordinating patient care and research and is also involved in postgraduate training of vascular surgery. An official 2-year training programme has been established in 1986. Currently, there are 12 vascular training programmes certified to certify surgeons as vascular surgeons. The quality of the training programmes is thoroughly evaluated every 5 years. Renewed certification is based on a written report from the director of the programme, supplemented with an 'on-site' visit and established by the Dutch Association of Surgeons of the Netherlands. Currently, (vascular) surgical training is being restructured due to working hour requirements (EC Directive), shortening of the years of training (currently 6+2) and further improvement of the quality of training. 

*Keywords:* Vascular surgery

## 1. Preamble

The Netherlands has a population of 16 million inhabitants. There are approximately 100 hospitals including eight University Medical Centres. There are approximately 900 members of the Dutch association of Surgeons of The Netherlands and, in addition, there are 300 residents in training for general surgery (6-year programme). The number of residents entering the surgical training programme each year is restricted by the Dutch Association of Surgeons of The Netherlands and is determined each year according to a manpower planning schedule (for 2003 there are 72 training positions for starters throughout the country). Most surgeons work together in groups (between 4 and 15 associates). The vascular expertise varies from 0 in very small hospitals to four or five colleagues in large teaching hospitals. The total number of vascular operations in the arterial system is approximately 10,000–15,000 per year in The Netherlands.

* Corresponding author. Tel.: +31-71-52-63-610; fax: +31-71-52-66-750.
*E-mail address:* bockel@lumc.nl (J.H. van Bockel).

0531-5131/ 
doi:10.1016/j.ics.2004.05.080

## 2. Historical situation

In the past, vascular surgery was not organized or structured. It was not incorporated in the general surgical programme. Since the end of the 1970s, individuals who chose to get more experience in vascular surgery contacted a centre and worked there after qualification for surgery for 1 or 2 years.

From the beginning of the 1980s, some vascular surgery was incorporated in the general surgical programme. However, only a minority of the residents obtained full exposure to vascular surgery.

## 3. The Dutch Society for Vascular Surgery

The Dutch Society for Vascular Surgery was founded in 1981. The society has around 350 members. Most of these members combine a vascular surgical practice with a general surgical practice. A minority, mostly associated with university medical centres or large teaching hospitals, practice exclusively vascular surgery.

## 4. Establishment of vascular training programmes

The Dutch Society for Vascular Surgery initiated a pilot study for a vascular surgery training programme in 1986. Two centres were involved and after the pilot study the requirements were put together.

To enter the programme, the candidate had to successfully complete his general surgical training programme of 6 years. Two years of vascular surgical training included: pre- and postoperative care, operation theatre experience, noninvasive diagnostics in the vascular laboratory and research. Recently, endovascular surgery has been added to the training module.

The Dutch Association of Surgeons of The Netherlands, in cooperation with the Dutch Society for Vascular Surgery, set up these guidelines. After successful completion, the candidate receives a certificate from the Dutch Association of Surgeons of The Netherlands. This structure implies that vascular surgery is not a monospecialty in The Netherlands like the general surgery, rather it is closely linked to general surgery.

The quality of vascular training programmes is guaranteed by the system of visitations. For new training programs, there is a visitation at the start and after 2 years thereafter every 5 years. This system is the same for general surgery, as well as for the other postgraduate training programmes in oncology, trauma and gastrointestinal surgical training. A team of three surgeons performs the visitation, one general surgeon and two surgeons appointed by the Dutch Society for Vascular Surgery, after an extensive report by the director of the training programme has been submitted. A decision about qualification of the training programme is made during the monthly meetings of the Concilium Chirurgicum (the training and education committee of the Dutch Association of Surgeons of The Netherlands). This committee may ask for adjustments or additional requirements and checks that these have been implemented within the defined period of time.

Currently, there are 12 vascular training programmes (7 in University Medical Centres and 5 in large teaching hospitals) and there are more to be established in the near future.

## 5. Changes during the years

In the early 1990s, it was felt that the field of general surgery had grown too large to fully train each resident sufficiently in all aspects. It was decided that the last year of the 6-year general surgery training programme should be devoted either to vascular, trauma, oncology or gastrointestinal surgery. Thereafter, the 2-year postgraduate training was additional training. This change in the general surgery programme was not popular and has never been successfully implemented for several reasons.

The 48-h week has been implemented since 1993 (European Directive). This law has had a major impact on training and methods of training. At the same time, it was decided by the government that the duration of training of specialists (6 years of medical school, 1 or 2 years of work, 6 years of general surgery and 2 years postgraduate training) was too long and had to be reduced substantially. Since then, major efforts have been made to design a shorter, still effective (vascular) surgical training programme. Currently, two models are being discussed: either the 2 + 2 + 2 system (2 years of basic training, 2 years of general surgery and 2 years of vascular training) or 2 + 3 + 2 (2 years of basic training, 3 years of general surgery and 2 years of vascular training). In each scenario, vascular training will remain the full 2 years.

International Congress Series 1272 (2004) 322–324

www.ics-elsevier.com

# Status of vascular surgery in Norway

Hans O. Myhre[a,*], Anne Karin Lindahl[b,1]

[a] *Department of Surgery, University Hospital of Trondheim, N-7006 Trondheim, Norway*
[b] *Society for Vacular Surgery, Anne Maries vei 4, N-0373 Oslo, Norway*

**Abstract.** We have some problems getting younger doctors to specialize in vascular surgery. The reasons for this are not completely clear. Some of them feel that the number of open operations is decreasing and that more and more of the treatment is done by endovascular techniques. Although the surgeons are involved in this work in Norway there is an uncertainty about the future. Furthermore, a more systematic training in endovascular surgery seems necessary. This is a very important problem that we should discuss, and we suppose the problem is the same in many other European countries. Economical factors may also pay a role for the younger doctors when they plan their future. GP's are in general earning a lot more than those who are employed at hospitals and there are very little differences in salary between junior doctors and senior colleagues who have been in the hospital for decades putting a lot of effort into clinical work, administration and teaching.


*Keywords:* Vascular surgery

## 1. Background

| | |
|---|---|
| Inhabitants | 4.5 million people live in Norway |
| Number of hospitals performing vascular surgery | 27 |
| Number of hospitals involved in vascular surgical training | 16 |
| Number of university hospitals | 4 |
| Number of registered Vascular Surgeons | approx. 86, about 63 with vascular surgery as their main activity |
| Number of training positions for vascular surgery | 13 |
| Number of new, qualified specialists per year | average of 4 |
| Vascular surgical training | 3 years (with a general surgical speciality qualification as the basis), of which at least 2 years must be at a University Hospital or a Central Hospital with vascular, surgical educational approval |

* Corresponding author. Tel.: +47-73-86-83-63; fax: +47-73-86-74-28.
*E-mail addresses:* hans.myhre@medisin.ntnu.no (H.O. Myhre), a-lindah@online.no (A.K. Lindahl).
[1] Tel.: +47-93011169; Private: +47-22137181.

0531-5131/
doi:10.1016/j.ics.2004.04.075

| | |
|---|---|
| Requirements for procedures | a minimum of 185 vascular procedures, specified (i.e. 10 carotid endarterectomies, 20 aortic aneurysms, of which 5 acute, etc.), in addition to at least 20 interventional procedures |
| Requirements for courses in vascular surgery | 80 h of elective courses in vascular surgery, plus a requirement for an administrative course. During the vascular surgical training, 2 h/week of theoretical, in-house courses are required. Topics of these in-house courses must be specified and approved, and cover all fields of vascular surgery, including medical treatment, primary and secondary prevention, risk modification, preoperative assessment, indications for surgery, outcome measures, etc. |
| Certification | There is no board or qualifying final exam. The certification is awarded on the basis of practice, performed procedures and courses/theoretical education |

## 2. Areas of concern for vascular surgery in Norway

### *2.1. Recruitment of young surgeons to vascular surgery*

We have some problems getting younger doctors to specialize in vascular surgery. The reasons for this are not completely clear. Some of them feel that the number of open operations is decreasing and that more and more of the treatment is done by endovascular techniques. Although the surgeons are involved in this work in Norway, there is an uncertainty about the future. Furthermore, a more systematic training in endovascular surgery seems necessary. This is a very important problem that we should discuss, and we suppose the problem is the same in many other European countries.

Economic factors may also pay a role for the younger doctors when they plan their future. GPs are in general earning a lot more than those who are employed at hospitals, and there is very little difference in salary between junior doctors and senior colleagues who have been in the hospital for decades putting a lot of effort into clinical work, administration and teaching.

### *2.2. Not enough volume and focus on vascular surgery in the training period*

Candidates of vascular surgery also cover general surgery, (vascular, GI surgery, urology, paediatric surgery, trauma, endocrine surgery, etc.) when they are on call. While on call, they are operating cases that do not belong to vascular surgery. The regulation of the working hours and the organisation of the on call duty forces candidates in training to take the day off after they have been on call. These factors lead to too little focus on vascular surgery and too much discontinuity of the training and experience. This scenario gives rise to concern, because the younger doctors are exposed to a lower volume of vascular surgery than used to be the case 10–20 years ago. One has to go through the training programs again to be sure that specialist candidates get sufficient technical skill in one way or another. For some operations, we have seen that the operating time has actually increased over time.

### 2.3. *Need for centralization*

A certain centralization of vascular surgery has taken place in Norway during the last 10 years, yet there are still too many hospitals performing vascular surgery. The population of Norway is 4.5 million. A recent committee from the Norwegian Society for Vascular Surgery recommended that certain centralization should take place to give vascular centers a sufficient caseload. A relationship between volume and quality has been shown for at least some operations. It is also inferior health economy to have a small number of patients operated on at many local district hospitals. We have good communications with helicopters, etc. In our minds, it is unjustified for one single vascular surgeon to perform a small number of operations as the situation in some hospitals today.

### 2.4. *Lack of ICU capacity*

ICU capacity is a problem in most major Norwegian hospitals. The ICUs are most often serving the whole hospital and emergencies from other specialities occupy an increasing amount of resources. In other words, the ICU capacity is unpredictable, which makes it difficult to plan the elective operating program. This problem is affecting most surgical specialities. The solution is probably that one has a certain ICU capacity reserved for the surgical department. Some hospitals establish more intermediate care beds within the regular vascular surgical ward for a more graded intensive care treatment.

### 2.5. *Need for better understanding of the vascular surgical patient population*

The hospital planners are not taking into consideration that there will be an increasing need for diagnosis and treatment of vascular diseases as the elderly part of the population is increasing. A decrease in the number of beds is planned, thinking that more and more of the treatment will take place as day surgery or outpatient treatment. As we are operating on more elderly patients, we will need at least the number of beds we have today. Also, more patients will need follow-up for secondary prevention and lifestyle changes, as well as additional controls and treatments after interventional procedures.

### 2.6. *Venous surgery lacks resources*

The resources within Norwegian public hospitals are constrained. Patients who do not have life-threatening or severe diseases are put on waiting lists for treatment. In vascular surgery, this problem is mainly affecting patients with venous insufficiency. There is little capacity for patients with varicose veins.

### 2.7. *Lack of resources and priority of medical research*

Norwegian authorities are not paying enough attention to resources for research, including medical research. This of course also affects our speciality.

International Congress Series 1272 (2004) 325–326

www.ics-elsevier.com

# Status of vascular surgery in Portugal

José Daniel Menezes*, José Fernandes e Fernandes

*Instituto Cardiovascular de Lisboa, Alges, Portugal*

*Keywords:* Vascular surgery

Vascular surgery has been a recognized monospecialty since 1982 and the certificate of completion of training—title of specialist—is awarded by the Portuguese Medical Association, following completion of training and approval on the final examination.

The training program lasts 6 years: 2 in General Surgery, 6 months of rotations to select between cardiothoracic, orthopaedic, reconstructive surgery, intensive care, and 3 1/2 years on a recognized Vascular Unit.

Evaluation consists of annual assessments incorporating discussion of a report of activities, including logbook of surgical interventions and presentation and discussion of a case history. It is carried out by the Director of the Vascular Service and the candidate's tutor.

After completion of the formal training program, there is a final examination by a court of assessors including the Director of the Unit, tutor and three outside specialists indicated by the College of Vascular Surgery.

Requirements in angiography and endovascular techniques are contemplated as well as experience in non-invasive diagnosis.

Specialist degree—CCST—is recognized by the Ministry of Health and is a qualification required for admission as a vascular surgeon in public hospitals.

At present, Portugal has five medical universities with Vascular Departments (two in Porto, one in Coimbra and two in Lisbon).

There are nine independent Services of Vascular Surgery: three in the Porto area (two academic units), one academic unit in Coimbra, and three in Lisbon (one academic), all with formative capacity recognized by the professional College, plus one at Madeira and one at Azores, and two smaller units within a general surgery department (Guimarães and Santarém).

Vascular surgery is considered a "highly distinguished" specialty under the existing classification, so services and/or units should be located in central or regional hospitals.

* Corresponding author. Tel.: +351-214-104-211; fax: +351-212-727-139.
*E-mail address:* jmvasc@netcabo.pt (J.D. Menezes).

0531-5131/ 
doi:10.1016/j.ics.2004.05.033

The total Portuguese population is 10.5 million people (including Madeira and Azores Islands).

There are no data concerning the number of procedures in private units; there are three major private units in Lisbon, but several private clinics in the country provide specialist services in vascular surgery, although the majority is in venous surgery.

In 2002, there were 220 beds available and 82 specialists, 15 with the position of Chief of Service, 67 as specialists in vascular surgery plus 32 trainees.

The normal working time is 35 h/week (plus extra hours for night shifts).

The accreditation of a service/unit for training is granted by the Medical Association, each year, upon periodic inspections and consideration of the following items:

- Number and qualification of medical staff
- Number of beds
- Number and quality of surgical procedures performed (conventional and endovascular)
- Capability in Vascular Laboratory
- Access to or own angioradiological suite
- Emergency service
- Scientific work (publications, presentations, etc.)
- Library (real and virtual)
- Computerized clinical archive
- Periodic clinical conferences (including morbidity/mortality).

The Scientific Society is the Portuguese Society for Angiology and Vascular Surgery: membership 125 full and associated members with annual meetings.

The professional organization is the College of Angiology and Vascular Surgery, which is part of the structure of the Portuguese Medical Association (ORDEM dos MÉDICOS) and its executive is elected by the registered Vascular Surgeons.

International Congress Series 1272 (2004) 327–330

www.ics-elsevier.com

# State of vascular surgery in Slovak Republic 2003

Vladimir Sefranek[a,*], Peter Mondek[b]

[a] *Slovak Society for Vascular Surgery, Portugal*
[b] *Bratislava, Slovakia*

*Keywords:* Vascular surgery; Slovak Republic; European Union

The Slovak Republic (SR) is one of 10 countries that entered the European Union in May 2004. SR has 5.5 million inhabitants. Because of a marked decreasing population trend the Slovak population has been aging for the last 20 years. There is a relatively higher incidence and mortality rate of cardiovascular diseases in comparison to the European Union countries (54% cardiovascular mortality).

The vascular surgery level may be characterized by the number of vascular surgeries: mean number of 4500 venous operations and 2500 arterial reconstructions yearly (number of venous surgery is satisfactory, but arterial reconstructions are lacking accordingly to ESVS recommendations—5500 operations should be done yearly). The numbers mentioned above are the result of the "Central Registry of Vascular Surgery", which has been realized by the authors of this report since 1996. Since the previous report was written in 2001, no improvement can be recorded despite reformation of the healthcare by the current government.

Vascular surgery in Slovakia, as an extended surgical speciality with a separate certification and board exam, was recognized in 1986 (former Czechoslovakia). We can say that vascular surgery in Slovakia is a monospeciality.

History of vascular surgery in Slovakia is rather different from other countries of middle Europe—the main difference is related to the fact that vascular surgery in Slovakia has been performed mainly in general surgical departments. There are just three departments in the country performing only vascular surgery (2003). We have been trying to reform these unfavorable conditions, however, this reforming effort has been held back due to lack of understanding of the authorities (practically all competence has been centralized in the Ministry of Health of the SR up until now). On the other hand, the top vascular surgery experts in Slovakia have a clear comprehension but not enough competence to bring about this reform.

* Corresponding author. Av. Das Descobertas 30, 1400-092 Lisbon, Portugal. Tel.: +351-21-3011-742; fax: +351-21-3022-348.

*E-mail address:* jffernandes@netcabo.pt (V. Sefranek).

0531-5131/ 
doi:10.1016/j.ics.2004.05.032

The most important center of vascular surgery is the author's department—the Department of Vascular Surgery of the Slovak Institute of Cardiovascular Diseases (a teaching hospital—a base of the postgraduate education specialized in cardiovascular diseases), established 7 years ago after splitting of the Department of Cardiovascular Surgery of the same institution.

The main goal of the reform should be, in our opinion, concentration of vascular surgical service into a smaller number of centers. These centers should have the latest equipment and the highest professional experience. Because there are too many centers, the current system has been lacking order, hierarchy and failing to secure adequate service for the Slovak inhabitants. The quality of health care is unsatisfactory and, however, the effectiveness is low and the costs too high. There are great differences among several regions of the country, as well. In Slovakia, there are actually working approximately 50 vascular surgeons with specialization.

In summary, we can say that in the interest of improving the vascular surgical service in the country, it is necessary:

- to reduce number of centers, to build up and improve the activities of a limited number of them in a mode mentioned above,
- to assure covering of the whole Slovak territory with the qualified vascular surgical service, keeping 100 km distance between centers,
- to reach an improved vascular center network system and better coordination with the general practitioners and out-patient department specialists and in such a way to improve the primary management especially in emergencies, and
- in our opinion, it would be optimal to build up six specialized centers of vascular surgery and another eight vascular surgical units as part of general surgical units.

## 1. Slovak Society for Vascular Surgery (SSVS)

In 1998, the Section for Vascular Surgery as a part of the Slovak Society for Angiology was founded. On 1 January 2002, this section was transformed into the Slovak Society for Vascular Surgery. Nowadays, this society has approximately 100 full members. In our opinion, the number of members will increase in the future.

In Slovakia, there is a system of centralized, institutionalized postgraduate education in all medical specializations. This institution is named "Slovak Healthcare University" (SZU) and it is in Bratislava, the capital of the SR. The Board of Vascular Surgery of the SZU has its residence in the Department of Vascular Surgery of the Slovak Institute of Cardiovascular Diseases (SUSCH) Bratislava and is responsible for the postgraduate education and training in vascular surgery in Slovakia. In the future, there is an idea to involve more accredited departments into the vascular surgical training and postgraduate education.

Until now, there have been two possibilities to achieve specialization in vascular surgery:

1. after having been specialized from general surgery I and II,
2. after having been specialized from surgery (basic surgical training)—this is the new form of postgraduate education that will be applied also in future (this reform has been actually realized).

Postgraduate training in surgery is divided into two grades (I, II—basic and higher surgical training). Duration of the combined training in general and vascular surgery is minimum 7 years (3 years of surgical main trunk plus 4–5 years of higher surgical training, only full-time position is accepted). Duration of the training is dependent on the type of department where the trainee is employed. Basic surgical training is the period in a trainee's career that follows the pre-registration house officer year and precedes appointment to a higher surgical training program as a specialist registrar (SpR). Basic surgical trainees are known as senior house officers (SHOs). SHOs spend a minimum of 24 months (or the equivalent if they choose part-time position) in Department of General Surgery or Traumatology to complete this period. The period is concluded by taking the 1st board examination (this exam is obligatory for each surgeon).

To get a certificate in vascular surgery after successful 1st board exam, the trainee has two options. The first one is to get a position in specialized Vascular Surgery Department (duration of training—minimum 4 years) or to be appointed in the Department of General Surgery that has employed vascular surgeon who may take responsibility for trainees education (duration—minimum 5 years).

During the period of higher surgical training (specialist registrar), the trainee is concerned with the diagnosis, treatment and prevention of diseases affecting blood vessels and lymphatics. It is necessary to obtain detailed specialized knowledge of the anatomy and physiology of arteries, veins and lymphatics. All relevant pathologies treated by vascular surgeon are subjects of interest of the trainee (chronic arterial occlusion, aneurysm, acute arterial occlusion, vascular trauma, inflammatory arteriopathies, arteriovenous malformations, disorders of microcirculation, varicous veins, deep vein thrombosis and post-thrombotic syndrome, extracranial cerebrovascular disease, renal and mesenteric disorders, thoracic outlet syndrome). The training encompasses work in out-patient clinic and ward, in specialized vascular ICU with staff who are engaged full-time, postoperative care and a traineeship is exclusively devoted to vascular problems.

The trainee is concerned with non-invasive vascular laboratory techniques which are necessary for the practising vascular surgeon. Basic knowledge of principles and technique of angiography, endovascular treatment, CT and MRA is mandatory.

After this period of higher surgical training (minimum 4–5 years), the trainee is ready for board examination in vascular surgery (2nd board exam). We have defined minimum requirement of vascular operations for a trainee. It includes 100 arterial procedures performed by trainee of the whole surgical range and anatomic areas.

The exam has two parts: written and oral. The written part includes the test (MCQ) and discussion about trainees written thesis (extent of about 60 pages), which deals with up-to-date vascular topics. The oral part represents viva voce discussion between examining body (three to four members, including national directors of the training program) and the trainee about three vascular surgery topics.

The vascular surgeon plays an important role in the training of undergraduate and postgraduate students and has responsibilities regarding the continuing medical education of primary care to keep them informed about the latest advances in vascular medicine.

Scientific activity and clinical research represent an integral part of vascular surgical practise in our major centers. In the interest of reaching the highest possible standard of practise, all vascular surgeons are encouraged to maintain an accurate audit of their results. During the training period, a trainee at the national meeting should present at least one oral paper, and it is highly recommended to have one article published.

International Congress Series 1272 (2004) 331

www.ics-elsevier.com

# Status of vascular surgery in Sweden, November 2003

Lars Norgren*

*Division and Board of Vascular Surgery, Department of Vascular Diseases, University Hospital MAS, Malmo 20502, Sweden*

*Keywords:* Vascular surgery

Sweden has not had Vascular Surgery as a recognised speciality, but for the last 10 years there has been an informal schedule for training, prepared by the Vascular Society. Training has been accepted in all hospitals with Vascular Surgery, but part of the training is recommended to take place at specific (mostly university-based) hospitals. Examination within the Vascular Society is recommended.

Presently major changes will take place. The Government is close to a decision to accept Vascular Surgery as a subspecialty, which means that new rules have to be prepared. Probably this will start rather soon, and it seems therefore less practical to present details of the informal rules.

* Tel.: +46-40-338074; fax: +46-40-3332-81.
*E-mail address:* Lars.Norgren@kir.lu.se (L. Norgren).


doi:10.1016/j.ics.2004.05.031

International Congress Series 1272 (2004) 332–333
www.ics-elsevier.com

# Status of vascular surgery in Spain

Marc Anton Cairols [a], Jordi Maeso Lebrún [b,*]

[a] *Cap del Servei de Cirurgia Vascular, Hospital Universitari de Bellvitge, Feixa Llarga, s/n, 08907 L'Hospitalet de Llobregat, Barcelona, Spain*
[b] *Hospital General Vall d'Hebron, Servicio de Angiología, Cirugia Vascular y Endovascular, Barcelona, Spain*

**Abstract.** Different countries within the UEMS organisation have different ways of accrediting their postgraduates. In some of them, Vascular Surgery is a monospecialty; in others, it is a branch very close to General Surgery. This undesirable situation represents a drawback for homogenisation of training of Vascular Surgery in Europe. 

*Keywords:* Vascular surgery; Spain; Angiology

## 1. Training in angiology and vascular surgery in Spain

In Spain, Angiology and Vascular Surgery (AVS) is a monospecialty, and is defined as a discipline that includes the medical and surgical aspects of the discipline, which concerns the prophylaxis, diagnosis and treatment of arteries, veins and lymphatic diseases.

As far as training in AVS is concerned, only teaching accredited units can have young doctors in training; we call them medical residents. There are 28 teaching centres in Spain, with a quite homogeneous territorial distribution, with the exception of Barcelona and Madrid where we can find up to five teaching units in each city. As there is just one resident per year in each unit we are forming 28 specialist per year.

A Teaching National Commission, located in Madrid and linked to the Ministry of Health, is the only organism that may give accreditation after auditing the activity of the candidate vascular unit. The National Commission has representation from different entities. Whereas the Spanish Society for Vascular Surgery has one senior member as its elected representative, the residents have two representatives. More than 250 arterial surgical procedures a year, plus an indefinite number of varicose vein operations and other miscellaneous procedures, are the minimum requirement needed for accreditation.

A fully equipped vascular lab under the authority of the Chief of the vascular service is required, as well as ready access to angiographic diagnosis. Recently a C-arm in the operating theatre has been added to the requirements. As far as the number of doctors working, a Teaching Vascular Service must have a minimum of four full time staff.

* Corresponding author. Tel.: +34-93-260-76-65; fax: +34-93-260-75-15.
*E-mail address:* mcairols@csub.scs.es (J.M. Lebrún).

0531-5131/ 
doi:10.1016/j.ics.2004.05.026

The selection for acceding to a resident job is made after a national examination consisting of a full array of multiple-choice questions. According to the qualification obtained each applicant gets an ordinal number, this number gives to the candidate priority for choosing the city, the hospital and the speciality. The higher the number obtained, the easier it is to choose the desired place and job. The number of residents equals the number of teaching centres (one resident for each one of the accredited services).

The Spanish National Commission is in charge not only of maintaining the accreditation, but it can also withdraw it. Periodically the Commission review the 5-year training programme in order to incorporate new technical requirements for achieving the main aim, i.e., to guarantee a proper education in Vascular Surgery of all residents. The program has three parts:

1. *Theoretical program:* There a comprehensive theoretical programme, with different topics for developing not only in their own services but along a Continuous Medical Programme (addressed in particular to Residents in their last year of training) held annually, as well as conferences and round table discussions in national meetings. All residents are required to give more than five oral papers accepted by the Spanish Scientific Committee to be read in the National Congress held annually.
2. *Investigation:* Doctoral thesis is recommended but not compulsory. The Spanish Society has established different Scholarships and Grants to promote investigation within the services performed by the residents.
3. Finally there is a logbook in which the abilities for diagnosing and treating patients are registered. A minimum of diagnostic procedures (invasive and noninvasive) as well as a minimum number of operations per year is mandatory from the third year of residency. During the two first years the resident rotates through different Services, in particular through General Surgery, Cardio-Thoracic Surgery, ICU and Anaesthetics, and Radiology. Even the rotation is required within their own department of outpatients and Vascular Lab.

The National Commission is now readdressing the period of rotations to give more relevance to endovascular techniques and vascular laboratory, reducing the period of time devoted to General Surgery. In Spain, in the vast majority of teaching centres, the Vascular Surgeon carries out endovascular abdominal aortoiliac (aneurysms and occlusive disease) procedures in the operating room. However, carotid stents are performed in collaboration with radiology.

At the end of the 5-year period, there is no examination for a final evaluation of the resident capabilities. Nevertheless, since we are aware we have a good system that has no control, the tendency is to arrange some kind of validation, the equivalent to an examination of excellence in Angiology and Vascular Surgery. Nowadays, there are some discrepancies as the convenience for performing this examination in particular from the residents. They argue that the responsibility for training them is in the hands of the Service as after having approved access through the national examination they are entitled to a proper training. In case the service does not fulfil the requested minimum requirements, the National Commission can open an audit and retire the accreditation.

ELSEVIER

International Congress Series 1272 (2004) 334–337

www.ics-elsevier.com

# Status of vascular surgery in Switzerland July 2003 Information on surgical training and working time in Switzerland based on a questionnaire concerning the 48-h week (Directive initially 93/104/EC then amended by 2000/34/EC)

Jon Largiadèr[a,*], Bernhard Nachbur[b]

[a] Hospital: Klinik Hirslanden Zurich, Bellarastrasse 40, Zurich, CH-8038, Switzerland
[b] Professor Emeritus of Surgery, University of Berne, Zurich, Switzerland

*Keywords:* Vascular surgery; Surgical training; Working time

## 1. Date of introduction of working time directive in Switzerland

Switzerland is a confederacy consisting of 20 cantons and 6 half cantons that all exercise the power of government not delegated to the federal government. Notably, the cantons are in charge of health care and therefore working time directives are—if at all—issued by the cantons. The date and working time differ from one canton to the other. In general, cantonal directives have been introduced nationwide at the beginning of the millennium, but due to the pyramidal structure of surgical services these are not necessarily being enforced.

## 2. Length of training (National ruling of the Swiss Society for Surgery)

1. Surgical training consists of two (2) blocks, one of 2 years, then one following of 4 years. After or during the first 2 years of common trunk and basics in surgery, an examination, the so-called basic exam (120 MC questions in 4 h), must be passed before the continuation of training in general surgery becomes valid. The two blocks add up to *6 years* in 'general surgery' (mainly visceral and endocrine surgery) and may include traumatology of the bones. At the end of this training period, the trainee has to pass a viva voce examination to obtain specialty status in surgery.
2. Following the qualification in surgery, it is possible to begin training in one of four subspecialties which uniformly require *4 years* of training. One of these years may be spent within the second block of 4 years.

* Corresponding author. Tel.: +411-4802-250; fax: +411-480-2252.
*E-mail address:* jonlargiader@swissonline.ch (J. Largiadèr).


doi:10.1016/j.ics.2004.05.025

The subspecialties are: visceral, vascular, thoracic and 'general surgery and traumatology'.
To obtain subspecialty status (Schwerpunkt) a third examination has to be passed. In Switzerland, the EBSQ in Vascular Surgery is considered the equivalent of a subspecialty examination in vascular surgery.
The total minimal number of years is *9 or 10.*

## 3. Leave

(a) Vacations and national or religious: 6–7 weeks/year.
(b) External training or conferences: 60 h/year.
(c) Internal education meetings: 10–15 h/week.
(d) Private study time: 2–6 h/week.

## 4. Assessment

It has to be made quite clear right from the outset that vascular surgery is only just emerging as a specialty in its own right in Switzerland and that structured training such as is commonplace in the UK and the US has not been fully introduced. However, there is no doubt that every trainee is continuously monitored by his peer and closely watched by his or her colleagues. Monitoring is therefore a continuous process which makes sense only if followed by a career assessment. Also to be borne in mind: the number of vascular surgical trainees at any given time is small and somewhere around 2–4 in Switzerland.

## 5. Hours of work

(a) When does the normal working day start and finish? *7:30 a.m. to 7:30 p.m. (19.30)*
(b) What is the length (in hours) of the longest shift allowed? *Not regulated*
(c) Night working.
- How often are surgical trainees on duty at 9 p.m.? *Approximately 1 night in five to seven*
- How often are surgical trainees on duty at 3 am? *Approximately 1 in five to seven*
- Does the trainee work the day after a night on duty? *Yes*

(d) How long are surgical trainees at work for each week? *55–60 h/week*
(e) Does the time include training and private study? *Yes*
(f) What percentage of your country's surgical trainees currently conform to the Working Time Directive, including the 48-hour week? *Approximately 20%*

## 6. Team organization

In UK hospitals, a team of doctors consists of one consultant/specialist, one registrar, one senior house officer and maybe a house officer too. That team cares for 10–30 patients. Each patient is cared for only by doctors of that team.

(a) How are the teams organized in your country? *We have a different nomenclature for our doctors, but functionally and essentially our teams are organized very much like in the UK*

(b) How many consultants/specialists are responsible for each patient? *Two to three: consultant, specialist, senior registrar*
(c) How many consultants/specialists supervise each trainee doctor? *Two to three: consultant, specialist, senior registrar*

## 7. Specialty cover at night

(a) At night, do surgeons cover just their own specialty or more than one surgical specialty or subspecialty?

| | |
|---|---|
| Year 1–5 | *own* |
| Year 6 onwards | *several* |
| Consultant/specialist | *own* |

(b) Do surgical trainees cover any non-surgical specialties? *No*
(c) Are emergency surgical patients admitted straight to the specialty ward or to a general admissions ward? *Admissions ward*
(d) In a hospital receiving emergency patients in *general surgery, vascular surgery, urology* and *orthopaedics*
- How many surgical doctors will be in the hospital to cover these specialties at 3 a.m.? *Four+ 2 to 3 medical students*
- How many surgical doctors will be on duty from home to cover these specialties? *Four*
- Which levels of doctors (including consultants) would be in the hospital at 3 a.m.? *A registrar or a house officer*

(e) Are non-medical staff used to decrease the workload of trainee doctors in any of the following areas?

| | |
|---|---|
| Clerical work: | *no* |
| Admitting patients: | *yes* |
| Venepuncture | *yes* |
| Clinics: | *yes* |
| ECGs: | *yes* |
| Endoscopy: | *no* |
| Prescribing drugs: | *no* |
| Catheters: | *no* |
| First operator: | *no* |
| Assistant operator: | *yes* |

## 8. Further Information

After having had a long talk with a senior registrar at the department of visceral surgery and transplantation of the University of Berne Medical School I can summarize the situation as follows.

The government of the canton of Bern has issued the following directie:

- Trainees are not to work more than 55 h/week. Up to 140 h/year may be added if necessary.

- Senior registrars (surgeons who have completed their training) are "allowed" to work only 50 h/week plus a contingent of 140 h/year where necessary.
- Trainees as well as senior registrars keep a daily account of their working hours and have to submit these records to the hospital management once a month.
- The manner of counting hours is very clearly laid down (for instance: a senior registrar on call duty shall note when leaving home, etc., also whether counsel was given by telephone).

*Comment*: This directive has led to a greater efficiency of the trainees' working hours. Nevertheless the workload cannot be dealt with adequately since the enforcement of the directives and consequently additional posts have had to be attributed (for instance the number of trainess in the department of visceral surgery and transplantation has been upped from 11–14) which has consequently driven the cost and expenses of the canton of Berne upwards as well.With more trainees for the same amount of work (operation) it impissible to train surgeons adequately within 6 years. The 50 hours for registrars (junior and senior) are eaten up by clinical work alone. 10 extra hours would be needed for administrative and clerical work whilst scientific work not be metioned.

*Conclusion*: The disadvantages of the directives far outweigh the advantages and cannot stand in the long run.

International Congress Series 1272 (2004) 338–347

www.ics-elsevier.com

# The status of vascular surgery in the UK: vascular surgical training in the UK

Peter M. Lamont *

*Vascular Surgical Society of Great Britain and Ireland, Bristol Royal Infirmary, Bristol BS2 8HW, UK*

**Abstract.** The past few years have seen a fragmentation of General Surgery into the four main areas of Upper GI, Lower GI, Breast/Endocrine and Vascular Surgery. Within this confederation of specialist interests, Vascular Surgery in Great Britain and Ireland remains a major component of General Surgery and the majority of surgeons continue to work as General Surgeons with a Vascular Interest. Core training in General Surgery during SpR years 1-3 remains the foundation upon which a specialist knowledge of Vascular Surgery is built. Increasing numbers of Consultants are now choosing to become specialist Vascular Surgeons with little or no involvement in General Surgery, particularly as the number of dedicated Vascular Surgery emergency rotas increase. Nevertheless, it remains important at the current time to ensure that Vascular Surgeons have sufficient core training to be able to cope competently with General Surgery emergencies. Likewise any non-Vascular General Surgeon should either be able to cope with the common vascular surgical emergencies, or at least know when to refer on to a specialist Vascular Surgeon. © 2004 Published by Elsevier B.V.

*Keywords:* Vascular surgery

Vascular surgery remains a part of General Surgery in the United Kingdom. Surgical training starts after the pre-registration year with a mandatory 2-year period of Basic Surgical Training. This usually comprises four 6-month attachments in each of Accident and Emergency, General Surgery, Orthopaedic Surgery and one other surgical specialty. During this time the trainee sits the examinations for Membership of a Royal College of Surgeons (MRCS). Trainees may only enter Higher Surgical Training once they have completed this 2-year period and been successful in the exam.

Entry into the Specialist Registrar (SpR) grade for Higher Training is by competitive interview and many trainees undertake a 2-year period of research leading to a Higher Degree (MD or MS or ChM) at this stage to enhance their chance of success in the interviews. This period in research is not compulsory, nor is possession of a Higher Degree.

Higher Surgical Training lasts 6 years and is organized in rotational programmes based on large geographical areas known as Deaneries. There are 17 Deaneries in the UK and training grades in each one are under the supervision of a Postgraduate Dean. Each trainee is given a training number and only a limited number of these numbers are available, according to

* Tel.: +44-117-928-5131; fax: +44-117-928-5132.
*E-mail address:* Peter.Lamont@ubht.swest.nhs.uk (P.M. Lamont).

0531-5131/ © 2004 Published by Elsevier B.V.
doi:10.1016/j.ics.2004.05.023

manpower predictions. Trainees rotate around the hospitals in the Deanery and spend their first 3 years learning core surgical skills in a variety of General Surgical posts covering mainly Upper GI, Lower GI, Breast/Endocrine and Vascular Surgery. The majority of these posts are in busy District General Hospitals with varying degrees of sub-specialization. The fourth year of training is known as the flexible year, and it may be spent undertaking research or visiting a specialist unit abroad. Vascular trainees are encouraged to spend this time in an area relevant to Vascular Surgery. Specialist training in Vascular Surgery takes place during the last 2 years, usually on at least two different specialist vascular units. During this time the SpRs sit the Intercollegiate exam in General Surgery, leading to the FRCS. Success in the exam and successful yearly assessments by a Deanery panel in each of the 6 years of training are required before the CCST is awarded. The CCST is in General Surgery. There is no separate certification in Vascular Surgery, although this may be selected as a specialist topic in one section of the Intercollegiate exam. The trainee may then obtain a Consultant post in either General Surgery or Vascular Surgery or both, according to their interests and ambitions.

There are no official numerical requirements for numbers of vascular training procedures at present, but each training post is regularly inspected and approved for training, which involves some assessment of the volumes of cases available for training. A central Specialist Advisory Committee in General Surgery sets the curriculum and inspects the training posts and takes advice on vascular training from the Vascular Surgical Society of Great Britain and Ireland (see Training in Vascular Surgery document). There is no formal training in vascular radiology, although specialist vascular training units must be capable of offering a voluntary half-day session in Vascular Radiology if the trainee requests it (very few do).

**Peter Lamont**
**05/08/02**
**TRAINING IN VASCULAR SURGERY 2001**
**The Vascular Surgical Society of Great Britain and Ireland at The Royal College of Surgeons, 35–43 Lincoln's Inn Fields, London, WC2A 3PE**
**Approved at the VSSGBI AGM, Brighton, 8th November 2001**
**Valid until 30th November 2004**

## 1. Introduction

The past few years have seen a fragmentation of General Surgery into the four main areas of Upper GI, Lower GI, Breast/Endocrine and Vascular Surgery. Within this confederation of specialist interests, Vascular Surgery in Great Britain and Ireland remains a major component of General Surgery and the majority of surgeons continue to work as General Surgeons with a Vascular Interest. Core training in General Surgery during SpR years 1–3 remains the foundation upon which specialist knowledge of Vascular Surgery is built.

Increasing numbers of Consultants are now choosing to become specialist Vascular Surgeons with little or no involvement in General Surgery, particularly as the number of dedicated Vascular Surgery emergency rotas increase. Nevertheless, it remains important at the current time to ensure that Vascular Surgeons have sufficient core training to be able to cope competently with General Surgery emergencies. Likewise any non-Vascular

General Surgeon should either be able to cope with the common vascular surgical emergencies, or at least know when to refer on to a specialist Vascular Surgeon.

This document does not attempt to address the issues of core training in General Surgery during the early SpR years, but is more concerned with specialist training in Vascular Surgery during years 5 and 6.

Vascular surgery includes areas of low volume; high complexity surgery and it may prove difficult for many trainees to achieve sufficient competence in some vascular surgical procedures in just 2 years. Trainees are therefore encouraged to use their flexible year in a clinical post gaining additional experience in Vascular Surgery. Reductions in working hours with consequent reduction in clinical experience mean that the majority of trainees should now aim to spend six clinical years in SpR training. Only those trainees with a demonstrable commitment to enter Academic Surgery should consider using their flexible year in research.

The VSSGBI continues to encourage SpRs to undertake research training, but taken as an SAC approved period of "out of programme" research rather than as the flexible year. There is immense value of such training to a future Consultant Vascular Surgeon, whether it be a year spent on a formal MSc course or a 2-year period of original research leading to a higher degree. The majority of trainees now undertake such research training before entering higher surgical training. Whilst a period in research is considered to be desirable by the VSSGBI, it is not an essential part of Vascular Surgical training.

## 2. Training and the VSSGBI

The assessment of vascular trainees and vascular training centres has most recently been the responsibility of the Postgraduate Deans and the SAC in General Surgery. These assessments may be handicapped because not every vascular trainee will have a Vascular Surgeon present at their annual RITA assessment. Likewise not every SAC visiting team will have vascular expertise, although the VSSGBI do have representation on the SAC in General Surgery through the auspices of the Association of Surgeons of Great Britain and Ireland.

As defined areas of General Surgery become increasingly specialised, so it becomes more difficult for surgeons to address the needs of training outside their own special interests. There is thus increasing reliance on the Specialist Societies to provide advice and guidance on issues of specialist training to the Colleges and the SAC. Many Regional Training Committees nowadays see the value of having a lead member in each speciality area of General Surgery to give advice. The newly revised SAC Curriculum in General Surgery has purposely omitted any details of specialist training and has instead encouraged the Specialist Societies to produce their own guidelines to which the SAC visitors may refer.

This document aims to provide such advice in the field of Vascular Surgery and should be read in conjunction with the SAC Curriculum in General Surgery.

The VSSGBI has formed a new Training and Education Committee to move these issues forward. In addition, the role of the Vascular Advisor has been expanded to include a more direct responsibility for the supervision of Vascular Surgical Trainees in their geographical area (Appendix A). Direct feedback on these issues to the VSSGBI Council is offered through the Vascular Advisory Committee, which comprises the Vascular Advisors, the Vascular Surgical members of the SAC in General Surgery and members of the VSSGBI Council.

In view of the close relationship between Vascular Surgeons and Vascular Interventional Radiologists, the VSSGBI also has a liaison group with the Royal College of Radiologists. This group has worked, among other things, towards definitions of training in interventional radiology for vascular trainees and their recommendations are included in this document (see Appendix B).

The VSSGBI also has representation on the European Board of Vascular Surgery, which examines training issues in Vascular Surgery across Europe on behalf of the Division of Vascular Surgery of the Union of European Medical Specialities (UEMS). The Board also administers the European Board of Vascular Surgery Qualification (EBSQ-Vasc), which attempts to ensure consistency of vascular training standards across Europe. Successful candidates for this qualification must first obtain the training and examinations pertinent to the award of a CCST from the country where they trained. Further information on applying for this qualification can be obtained from the VSSGBI Office.

## 3. Definition of a vascular surgeon

A surgeon with an interest in Vascular Surgery should have:

A sound training in General Surgery.

The necessary clinical and surgical skills relating to the management of relevant diseases of arteries, veins and lymphatics.

The necessary clinical and surgical skills to maintain an emergency surgical service in General Surgery (where appropriate) and in Vascular Surgery.

A sound knowledge of the role of interventional radiology in the management of vascular disease.

A sound knowledge of the role of angiology in the management of vascular disease.

Knowledge of relevant diagnostic imaging investigations.

Knowledge of the role of a Vascular Laboratory in diagnosis and management of vascular disease.

Knowledge of the relevant aspects of basic sciences and critical care as applied to vascular disease.

## 4. Vascular surgery units

*A Specialist Vascular Unit* must have two or more surgeons who are either dedicated to or take a major interest in the specialty of Vascular Surgery. Vascular Surgery will comprise at least 70% of the unit's combined in-patient elective surgical workload.

A three-surgeon unit might have two SpRs in any year of training, but would be most suited to year 5/6 trainees for a 1-year period or to year 3 trainees for a 6-month period. Two-year 5/6 trainees may be attached to a unit at the same time, provided they rotate to work for all of the surgeons during the course of a year and are exposed to appropriate volumes of operative cases. A two-surgeon unit would have only one SpR. All SpRs training in Vascular Surgery should spend both year 5 and year 6 attached to a Specialist Vascular Unit.

*A General Vascular Unit* must have two or more surgeons who are General Surgeons with a Vascular Interest. Vascular Surgery will comprise at least 50% of the unit's combined in-patient elective workload.

A three-surgeon unit might have two SpRs and a two-surgeon unit would have one SpR. These SpRs would not necessarily be committed to a speciality interest in Vascular Surgery. These posts would only be suitable for year 1–3 SpRs.

Both types of unit will have:

At least two consultants who are members of the VSSGBI and regularly attend its meetings.
A vascular surgical workload sufficient for training. This need not be fully comprehensive in each unit, provided the overall SpR *programme* gives full coverage.
A ward with nursing staff experienced in looking after Vascular Surgery patients.
Appropriate investigative facilities, including access to comprehensive angiology, CT scanning, MR scanning and Duplex ultrasound.
Close collaboration and weekly clinical meetings with Vascular Interventional Radiologists.
A multidisciplinary approach to vascular disease incorporating close links to related specialities, including care of the elderly/rehabilitation, limb fitting, neurology, cardiology, diabetology, nephrology, haematology and dermatology.
An ITU and an HDU facility.
Regular Postgraduate meetings and a climate which encourages health promotion and clinical risk management.
A regular audit programme of vascular surgical caseload and outcomes with submission of data to the National Outcome Audit run by the VSSGBI.
A climate which encourages clinical research.

In addition, a specialist vascular unit will have:

A workload sufficient to provide personal operative experience for each trainee to achieve competence by year 6 in the index procedures of aortic aneurysm repair (elective and emergency), carotid endarterectomy and infra-inguinal bypass.
Non invasive vascular laboratory facilities, including teaching of techniques and familiarity with Duplex ultrasound.
A dedicated Vascular Emergency rota.
Twenty-four hour access to Vascular Radiology.
The opportunity to obtain training in Vascular Interventional Radiology.
A programme of prospective vascular research projects, which are presented regularly at National Societies and which are published in peer-reviewed journals.

## 5. Vascular surgery trainees

All Vascular Surgery trainees will have completed basic surgical training and will have passed the MRCS examination or equivalent.
Training in General Surgery must be sufficient to ensure that trainees are competent to manage the full spectrum of Emergency General Surgery. This will require involvement in the rota for unselected General Surgical emergencies for a minimum of 4 years of Higher Surgical Training.

Training in Vascular Surgery must be sufficient to ensure that trainees are competent to manage all vascular surgery emergencies.
Vascular surgical trainees must pass the Intercollegiate Examination or equivalent and would normally submit Vascular Surgery as a Speciality interest.
Year 6 vascular surgery trainees in possession of the Intercollegiate Examination or equivalent may wish to sit the EBSQ-Vasc.
Training in SpR years 1–3 should be in General Surgery and should include at least one 6-month attachment to a General Vascular Unit.
The flexible year should normally be spent in a clinical post relevant to Vascular Surgery, either in the UK or abroad. Only those trainees with a demonstrable commitment to a career in academic surgery should use their flexible year in research.
SpR years 5 and 6 must be spent on a Specialist Vascular Unit.
All Vascular Surgical trainees must keep a logbook of operative experience, including assisted, personal assisted and personal cases.
By the end of year 6, all vascular trainees should have been involved in at least 200 arterial reconstructions. This experience must include as principal operator a minimum of 20 elective aortic aneurysm repairs, 5 ruptured aortic aneurysm repairs, 20 carotid endarterectomies and 10 infra-popliteal bypass grafts. At least 50% of each of these procedures should be personal assisted cases.
Failure to obtain the operative experience detailed above by the end of year 6 should be addressed by an extra period of focused training on a Specialist Vascular Unit.
The future development of effective competency assessments may allow the above targets to be modified according to individual SpR progress and achievement.
There should be sufficient training in interventional radiology to perform the basic range of intra-operative interventions (arteriography and thrombolysis) as specified at level 2 in Appendix B.
By the end of year 6, vascular surgery trainees should have obtained exposure to the majority of procedures specified in the Vascular Surgery Specialist Curriculum (see page 14).
Trainees in Vascular Surgery are encouraged to become Affiliate Members of the VSSGBI and attend its AGM. They are also encouraged to join the Rouleaux Club and to attend courses and workshops relevant to Vascular Surgery.
Trainees in Vascular Surgery should show evidence of original thinking in the subject, either through the award of a Higher Degree in a vascular topic or through the publication of papers relevant to vascular surgery in peer-reviewed journals.
Trainees in Vascular Surgery will have an annual appraisal by their VSSGBI Vascular Advisor. The advisor will make recommendations to the local Surgical Training Committee regarding future attachments on the SpR programme to ensure an adequate training in Vascular Surgery according to the above parameters.

## 6. Curriculum

### *6.1. Core curriculum*

The core curriculum describes the training compulsory for all General Surgeons by the completion of General Surgical Training and outlines the syllabus for the general surgery part of the Intercollegiate examination. These are the areas to which all trainees should be exposed, both to provide core skills and to assist in the choice of specialisation.

### 6.2. Specialist curriculum

This defines training in areas of specialist interest not required for all General Surgeons, which will be examined in the specialist part of the Intercollegiate examination. Trainees will be expected to have gained exposure to a majority of these procedures by the end of year 6. They will be required to exhibit competence in the procedures of aortic aneurysm repair (elective and emergency), carotid endarterectomy and infra-inguinal bypass.

CORE CURRICULUM VASCULAR SURGERY

| Topics | Procedures |
|---|---|
| Ruptured aortic aneurysm | Vascular suture/anastomosis |
| Acutely ischaemic limb | Approach to/control of infra-renal aortic, iliac and femoral arteries |
| Arterial injuries | Control of venous bleeding |
| Atherosclerosis | Balloon thrombo-embolectomy |
| Aneurysmal disease | Amputations of the lower limb |
| Mesenteric ischaemia | Fasciotomy |
| Ischaemic limb | Primary operation for varicose veins |
| Arteriography | Abdominal aortic aneurysm repair, elective and ruptured |
| Magnetic resonance arteriography | Femoropopliteal bypass |
| Vascular CT scanning | Femoro-femoral bypass |
| Vascular ultrasound | |
| Hyper-/hypo-coagulable states | |
| Venous thrombosis and embolism | |
| Chronic venous insufficiency | |
| Varicose veins | |

SPECIALIST CURRICULUM VASCULAR SURGERY

| Topics | Procedures |
|---|---|
| Angioplasty/stenting | Carotid endarterectomy |
| Thrombolysis | Carotid body tumour |
| Reno-vascular disease | Operations for thoracic outlet syndrome |
| Raynaud's/vasospastic disorders | Upper limb arterial reconstruction |
| Lymphoedema | Thoracoscopic sympathectomy |
| Cerebrovascular disease | Suprarenal aortic aneurysm |
| Vasculitis | Renal/visceral artery reconstruction |
| Graft prosthetics | Abdominal aortic aneurysm repair—elective |
| Graft surveillance | Abdominal aortic aneurysm repair—emergency |
| Graft infection | Aortobifemoral bypass |
| Autonomic dysfunction | Iliofemoral bypass |
| Reperfusion injury | Axillofemoral bypass |
| Diabetic foot | Procedures for peripheral aortic dissection |
| Trophic ulceration | Infra-inguinal bypass (all varieties) |

| Topics | Procedures |
| --- | --- |
| Intimal hyperplasia | Revision surgery |
| Arterial dissection | Surgery for infected grafts |
| Arterio-venous malformations | Procedures for arterial injuries |
| Thoracic outlet syndrome | Interventions for arterio-venous malformations |
| Rehabilitation and limb prosthetics | Angioplasty, thrombolysis and stenting |
| Medical management of vascular disease | Per-operative angiography and thrombolysis |
| | Endoluminal grafting |
| | Reduction surgery for lymphoedema |
| | Recurrent and complex varicose veins |
| | Venous reconstruction |
| | Lumbar sympathectomy |
| | Endoscopic vascular procedures |
| | Vena caval filter placement |
| | Vascular access procedures |

## Acknowledgements

The UEMS Division and Board of Vascular Surgery thank the Vascular Surgical Society of Great Britain and Ireland (VSSGBI) for the inclusion of the above document in this publication, and kindly provided by Peter Lamont, Honorary Secretary VSSGBI.

## Appendix A. The role of vascular advisors

### *A.1. General*

The role of the Vascular Advisor should be to represent the VSSGBI in service, training and education matters relevant to vascular surgery within their Deanery, primarily reporting to the VSSGBI Council via the Vascular Advisory Committee (VAC). The Vascular Advisor should develop close links with the Regional Speciality Advisor in General Surgery.

### *A.2. Education and training*

The Vascular Advisor should:

Have responsibility within their Deanery for implementing the recommendations of the VSSGBI on training and education, and for advising their Regional Training Committee on these matters.

Liaise with the Regional SpR Programme Director on matters related to vascular surgical training and advise on the most appropriate placement for individual vascular surgical trainees according to their specific training needs in Vascular Surgery.

Serve on the Regional Training Committee, wherever this is possible.

Keep an up-to-date record of SpRs in their Deanery with a vascular surgical interest.

Be responsible for mentoring vascular surgical trainees in their Deanery, including the assessment of their log books/competency, and a yearly appraisal of their training in vascular surgery.

### *A.3. Posts with a vascular surgical interest and vascular services*

The Vascular Advisor should:

Provide advice for the Regional Speciality Advisor in General Surgery, and other interested parties, on the content of job descriptions for consultant appointments with a vascular surgical interest. They should liaise with the VSSGBI over any points of concern.
Provide local advice on vascular services, liaising with the VSSGBI as required.
Assist VSSGBI Council, through the VAC, on matters relating to manpower planning.

### *A.4. Liaison with the secretariat*

The VSSGBI secretariat aims to assist the Vascular Advisors as much as possible. Specific and regular assistance might include:

Scanning of the BMJ to inform Vascular Advisors immediately of any advertisement for consultant posts with a vascular interest in their Deanery.
Circulation of minutes of committees (Vascular Advisory Committee and the Education and Training Committee).
Early circulation of briefing notes from the Honorary Secretary following Council meetings.

### *A.5. Distinction awards*

Advisors will be asked if they would inform the secretariat about vascular surgeons in their Deanery who might be suitable candidates for A and B awards, either directly or through the offices of a more senior nominee in their Deanery. They should encourage such surgeons to submit ACDA CVs to the secretariat well before the November deadline each year. They will be supplied with a list of A and B award holders by the secretariat.

### *A.6. Meetings of the vascular advisors at the VAC*

The VAC will comprise Council together with all the Vascular Advisors. It will meet at the time of the AGM.

### *A.7. Term of office and process of election*

Vascular Advisors should serve for a term of 5 years.
Election should be by all Ordinary Members of the VSSGBI in the Deanery.
The secretariat will invite nominations and then assist in conducting a postal ballet.

There will be elections in all Deaneries where Vascular Advisors (formerly VAC Representatives) have served for 5 years or more. Thereafter, elections will be conducted when any Vascular Advisor reaches the end of 5 years of service.

## Appendix B. Training in interventional radiology

### *B.1. Proposal by the VSSGBI/RCR Liaison Group*

There should be four levels of training:

**(i) A basic understanding of endovascular techniques and their applications—essential for all vascular trainees**

This should include attendance at regular joint vascular surgical/radiology meetings where management decisions are discussed. Training should also include attendance at vascular radiology sessions.

**(ii) Sufficient training to perform a basic range of intra-operative interventions, such as arteriography, thrombolysis, and angioplasty of 'simple' arterial lesions**

Skills in simple intraoperative vascular radiology, including angiography and thrombolysis, should be part of normal vascular surgical training.

Surgical trainees may acquire skills in more complex radiological procedures (specifically balloon angioplasty) by regular attendance at vascular radiology sessions in a recognised training unit. In consultant practice these surgeons would use their radiological skills intraoperatively, working in liaison with vascular radiological colleagues in their hospital, in appropriately equipped operating theatres. Although such procedures ideally would be conducted in collaboration, it is accepted that this may not always be possible.

**(iii) Insertion of endovascular stent grafts for aortic aneurysms**

Acquire wire and catheter skills for the insertion and the deployment of stent grafts. Endovascular stent grafting should normally be a collaborative procedure between vascular radiologists and surgeons. Specialists who are accredited both in vascular surgery and vascular radiology {(iv) below} may choose to undertake endovascular aneurysm procedures as the sole operator.

**(iv) Full training in endovascular radiology to practise as a vascular and endovascular specialist**

For vascular surgical trainees this should involve the equivalent of a 1-year full-time fellowship in a recognised vascular radiology training unit. Trainees would be required to perform the core number of procedures specified for 'Sub-Specialty Training in Vascular Interventional Radiology', for practitioners with more than one sub-specialty interest, published in 'Structured Training in Clinical Radiology: Curricula for Subspecialty Training'. *Surgeons undertaking endovascular procedures will have to satisfy the training recommendations outlined in the regulations on ionising radiation.*

# Author index

# Keyword index